HPV Infections: Diagnosis, Prevention, and Treatment

Edited by

Azam Bolhassani

Department of Hepatitis and AIDS, Pasteur Institute of Iran, Tehran, Iran

HPV Infections: Diagnosis, Prevention, and Treatment

Editor: Azam Bolhassani

ISBN (Online): 978-1-68108-617-0

ISBN (Print): 978-1-68108-618-7

Bentham Science Publishers Ltd.
Executive Suite Y - 2
PO Box 7917, Saif Zone
Sharjah, U.A.E.
Email: subscriptions@benthamscience.org

BENTHAM SCIENCE

CONTENTS

PREFACE

Human papillomavirus (HPV) infection is one of the most frequently sexually transmitted diseases in the world. Multiple types of HPVs are divided as low risk, and high risk types. Low risk types cause warts and high risk types can cause cancer. HPV infections are responsible for almost all cases of genital warts and cervical cancer, 90% of anal cancers, 65% of vaginal cancers, 50% of vulva cancers, 35% of penile cancers, and 60% of oropharyngeal cancers. The health guidelines are recommended for HPV testing in patients using different methods. However, there is no way of knowing how long a person has had the virus. The methods of reducing the HPV infections include sexual abstinence, condoms, vaccination and microbicides. Recently, two commercial vaccines such as Gardasil and Cervarix have been used to prevent HPV infections. There are several side effects for preventive vaccines such as swelling, redness and pain at the injection site, headaches, blood problems (bleeding), chills, dizzy, Guillain Barré syndrome, joint pain, lymphadenopathy, muscle pain or tenderness, seizures (fits), tiredness, vomiting, and weakness. In rare cases, it is possible to experience an anaphylactic reaction with related signs. Regarding the poor diagnosis of HPV infections in developing countries, the researchers have focused on therapeutic vaccines. Also, the preventive vaccines are being developed using various methods for reducing side effects and also their use against various HPV types in women and also men. The studies continue on HPV diagnosis and vaccination for eradicating all HPV-related cancers. Already, various approaches have been utilized in clinical trials for the treatment of HPV-related cancers. The aim of this book is to provide up-to-date reviews of the growing field of diagnosis, prevention and treatment in HPV-related infections. Contributions cover a large range of topics including epidemiology, molecular biology, transmission, diagnosis, prevention, and treatment along with preclinical and clinical experiments. Regarding the high prevalence of HPV infections and the absence of correct diagnosis especially in developing countries as well as high cost of preventive vaccines and low information of many people about HPVs, hopefully, this book can further clarify and provide open ways for future studies of scientists on uncertain aspects of HPV.

Dr. Azam Bolhassani
Department of Hepatitis and AIDS,
Pasteur Institute of Iran,
Tehran,
Iran

List of Contributors

Afshin Khavari	Department of Hepatitis and AIDS, Pasteur Institute of Iran, Tehran, Iran
Amitis Ramezani	Clinical Research Department, Pasteur Institute of Iran, Tehran, Iran
Arezoo Aghakhani	Clinical Research Department, Pasteur Institute of Iran, Tehran, Iran
Azam Bolhassani	Department of Hepatitis and AIDS, Pasteur Institute of Iran, Tehran, Iran
Elnaz Agi	Department of Hepatitis and AIDS, Pasteur Institute of Iran, Tehran, Iran
Kimia Kardani	Department of Pharmaceutical Biotechnology, School of Pharmacy, Shahid Beheshti University of Medical Sciences, Tehran, Iran
Niloofar Naderi	Department of Hepatitis and AIDS, Pasteur Institute of Iran, Tehran, Iran

CHAPTER 1

General Description of HPVs

Kimia Kardani and **Azam Bolhassani***

Department of Pharmaceutical Biotechnology, School of Pharmacy, Shahid Beheshti University of Medical Sciences, Tehran, Iran

Department of Hepatitis and AIDS, Pasteur Institute of Iran, Tehran, Iran

Abstract: Viruses are related to 15-20% of human cancers worldwide. Many studies focused on clarifying the molecular mechanisms and genetic alterations caused by oncogenic viruses. Among different oncoviruses, human papillomaviruses (HPVs) are small, non-enveloped, double-stranded DNA viruses, which can infect mucosal or cutaneous epithelia. Many HPVs have been classified as low-risk viruses associated with benign warts in the general population. Other HPVs entitled as the high-risk HPV types cause several important human cancers including cervical cancer, other anogenital cancers and head and neck tumors. A general description of HPV types and their association with different disorders are presented in this chapter.

Keywords: Cancer, Genome, Human papillomavirus.

INTRODUCTION

Major advances in the prevention, diagnosis, and treatment of human cancers are associated with a better understanding of their etiology, pathogenesis, and natural history. Specifically, it is important to determine a correlation between viruses and human tumors [1, 2]. The ratio of cancers caused by infectious agents, including bacteria, parasitic worms and viruses, was recently estimated to be more than 20% [3]. The role of several viruses is especially high in certain cancer types. For instance, human hepatitis B virus (HBV) and human hepatitis C virus (HCV) are associated with 80% of hepatocellular carcinomas (HCCs). In addition, human papillomavirus (HPV) is linked to more than 95% of cervical carcinomas [4]. The protein products of these oncoviruses usually act through disruption of cell processes including apoptosis and cell-cycle checkpoint activation. Although, oncogenic viruses from different virus families use various strategies of cancer development, they have many common pathways, *e.g.*, interactions with cellular targets such as p53 and retinoblastoma (Rb) [4, 5]. HPVs were known as the most

* **Corresponding author Azam Bolhassani:** Department of Hepatitis and AIDS, Pasteur Institute of Iran, Tehran, Iran; Tel: 66953311-20; E-mails: A_bolhasani@pasteur.ac.ir, azam.bolhassani@yahoo.com

Azam Bolhassani (Ed.)

common cause of cancers induced by an infectious agent [6]. HPV is found in a majority of epithelial tissues in both males and females. Its recognition was performed in the 1970s, associated with cervical precursor lesions and cervical intraepithelial neoplasia (CIN) [1]. Cervical cancer represents a major cause of morbidity and mortality in women, with nearly 500,000 new cases and 274,000 deaths occurring worldwide each year [7]. Approximately 80% of the 500,000 new cases occur in developing countries and this percentage will be likely increased to ~ 90% by the year 2020 [8].

HPV and Cancer

In early 1976, various epidemiological, molecular, and biological studies showed that novel HPV types are associated with development of cervical cancers. The main research in this field was done by the German scientist Harald Zur Hausen, who for the first time indicated an etiological association of HPVs with cervical cancer by sequencing the most important high-risk HPV types (*i.e.*, 16 and 18) from cervical tumor specimens [9, 10].

In developing countries, cervical cancer is relatively caused in young poor women, since screening and treatment programs, and health care are relatively inaccessible to these women [11]. On the other hand, HPV was related to several other human cancers including vulvar cancer, vaginal and anal cancer, and head and neck cancers [7, 12]. Moreover, human papillomavirus infection accounts for nearly 5.2% of human tumors, including the anus, genital tract and oropharynx cancers in worldwide [13, 14]. For example, the rates of anal cancer are increasing, especially among HIV positive men who have sex with men (MSM) [15].

HPV Classification

According to the International Committee on Taxonomy of Viruses (ICTV), HPV belongs to the Papillomaviridae family including 120 (or 150) HPVs, 69 non-mammalian papillomaviruses (PVs), 3 PVs in birds and 2 PVs in reptiles [16, 17]. As of 9 March 2015, 200 different HPV types, belonging to 49 species, had been recognized by the International HPV Reference Center. Furthermore, 131 animal PV types were identified from 66 different animal species [18]. HPV is species-specific, epitheliotropic and mucosotropic, and usually infects keratinocytes [19], although recent studies have shown HPV DNA in non-epithelial sites such as blood [20 - 24], spermatozoa [25] and placenta [26]. Several epidemiological studies indicated that persistent infection with HPV is strongly associated with squamous cell carcinoma (SCC) and adenocarcinoma of the cervix [27].

As known, human papillomaviruseses are small, double-stranded DNA viruses containing circular genomes of ~ 8 kilobases (kb) in length and encode about eight major open reading frames (ORFs) [28]. Up till now, forty types of HPV have been known to infect the anogenital tracts of men and women which were classified as "low" or "high" risk by their capacity to induce oncogenic changes [29]. The "high-risk" virus types are defined by unique biological properties where the viruses have inherent ability to interfere with the control of proliferation and the maintenance of genomic stability within the infected cell [30]. High risk HPV types found in cervical cancer include types 16, 18, 31, 33, 35, 39, 45, 51, 52, 56, 58, 59, 68, 73, and 82 [31].

Generally, the existing HPV types belong to five PV genera such as alpha-papillomavirus (α-PV), beta-papillomavirus (β-PV), gamma-papillomavirus (γ-PV), mu-papillomavirus (μ-PV), and nu-papillomavirus (ν-PV). Several additional HPVs have been completely sequenced, mainly using next-generation sequencing (NGS), but have not been officially recognized yet [32, 33]. Humans are known as the main host for the alpha and beta viral genera such as HPV16. Cutaneous HPV types from the alpha (*e.g.*, HPV 2 and 3), gamma (*e.g.*, HPV 4), mu (*e.g.*, HPV 1), and nu (*e.g.*, HPV 41) genera cause common and flat skin warts [34]. Moreover, many HPV types including the beta and gamma genera generate only asymptomatic infections in immunocompetent individuals and could be detected in skin swabs, and for some gamma types, also in mucosal rinses [35 - 38]. According to some reports, HPVs were divided into three main groups: cutaneous, mucocutaneous and a rare autosomal recessive disorder, epidermodysplasia verruciformis (EV). The cutaneous HPVs belong to the beta genus with a few members in the gamma, mu and nu genera, while the alpha genus contains all of the mucosal HPVs and a few cutaneous types [39]. In addition, they were grouped according to the infected regions in the body such as skin, anogenital, and oral regions [40].

Recent advances in molecular techniques have led to identify novel HPV types and their sequences in the last few years. For instance, the γ-PV, α-PV and β-PV genera including HPV types 80, 65 and 51, respectively were recognized and completely sequenced [18].

In general, the α-HPVs infect mucosal tissue, whereas β-, γ-, ν-, and μ-subtypes infect cutaneous sites. The mucosal HPVs are able to cause malignancy. Low-risk HPVs including HPV6, 11, 40, 42, 43, 44, 54, 61, 70, 72, and 81 are found in low-grade lesions (*e.g.,* benign cervical lesions) and rarely in malignancies. In contrast, high-risk HPVs are the primary causative agents of cervical carcinoma [31]. Although, about 75% of sexually active adults become infected with one or more anogenital HPV types, most HPV infections are transient and asymptomatic, and about 90% of HPV infected women become HPV DNA negative within two years. However, a minority of high-risk HPV-infected individuals develop persistent HPV infection that can lead to the development of cervical cancer, other anogenital cancers and a subset of head and neck cancers [41].

HPV Genome

The HPV genome encodes at least six early genes (E1, E2, E4, E5, E6 and E7) and two late genes (L1 and L2) [7]. The early genes regulate viral DNA replication while the late genes encode the viral capsid for packaging newly generated virions. In persistent infection, the expression of the HPV genome is correlated to the maturation of the infected cell. Immature epithelial cells in the basal layer allow expression of the HPV early genes whereas in upper differentiated cells, the late genes are expressed to release the newly assembled virions from the submucosa (*i.e.,* the site of immune surveillance) [7]. The HPV genome is usually found in episomal form, but high-risk HPVs may integrate into the host genome in some persistent infections. This integration causes deletion of some of the early genes (E2, E4 and E5) as well as the late genes L1 and L2. E2 is a main regulator of the viral replication and notably a transcriptional repressor of the E6 and E7 oncogenes. Loss of E2 through integration allows up-regulation of E6 and E7 transcription and subsequently inactivation of tumor suppressor p53 and retinoblastoma (Rb) leading to genomic instability and inhibition of apoptosis. Indeed, HPV uses several mechanisms to escape the immune system resulting in its proliferation freely within cells [7].

CONCLUDING REMARKS

Viral infections are able to generate asymptomatic effects, acute clinical disease, neurological disorders and various cancer types. The interactions between a virus and its host can produce different results, from no clear change in the infected cell to the death of the host cell. Some viruses can persist over time and cause no changes in the infected cell. This latency is a characteristic of some members of the herpes simplex virus which can induce cell proliferation without causing malignancy, or some members of the HPV group which can produce cancer types. In HPV infection, cancer progression is associated with persistent high-risk HPV infection and with deregulated viral gene expression which leads to high cell proliferation, deficient DNA repair, and the accumulation of genetic damage in the infected cell.

CONFLICT OF INTEREST

The author (editor) declares no conflict of interest, financial or otherwise.

ACKNOWLEDGEMENT

Declare none.

REFERENCES

[1] Krueger H, Stuart G, Gallagher R, Williams D. HPV and other infectious agents in cancer. Oxford University Press 2010; pp. 3-129.

[2] Elgui de Oliveira D. DNA viruses in human cancer: an integrated overview on fundamental mechanisms of viral carcinogenesis. Cancer Lett 2007; 247(2): 182-96. [http://dx.doi.org/10.1016/j.canlet.2006.05.010] [PMID: 16814460]

[3] Bouvard V, Baan R, Straif K, *et al.* WHO International Agency for Research on Cancer Monograph Working Group. A review of human carcinogens--Part B: biological agents. Lancet Oncol 2009; 10(4): 321-2. [http://dx.doi.org/10.1016/S1470-2045(09)70096-8] [PMID: 19350698]

[4] McLaughlin-Drubin ME, Munger K. Viruses associated with human cancer. Biochim Biophys Acta 2008; 1782(3): 127-50. [http://dx.doi.org/10.1016/j.bbadis.2007.12.005] [PMID: 18201576]

[5] Javier RT, Butel JS. The history of tumor virology. Cancer Res 2008; 68(19): 7693-706. [http://dx.doi.org/10.1158/0008-5472.CAN-08-3301] [PMID: 18829521]

[6] Whiteside MA, Siegel EM, Unger ER. Human papillomavirus and molecular considerations for cancer risk. Cancer 2008; 113(10) (Suppl.): 2981-94. [http://dx.doi.org/10.1002/cncr.23750] [PMID: 18980282]

[7] Lin K, Doolan K, Hung CF, Wu TC. Perspectives for preventive and therapeutic HPV vaccines. J Formos Med Assoc 2010; 109(1): 4-24. [http://dx.doi.org/10.1016/S0929-6646(10)60017-4] [PMID: 20123582]

[8] D'Andrilli G, Bovicelli A, Giordano A. HPV vaccines: state of the art. J Cell Physiol 2010; 224(3): 601-4. [http://dx.doi.org/10.1002/jcp.22174] [PMID: 20432468]

[9] zur Hausen H. Viruses in human cancers. Science 1991; 254(5035): 1167-73. [http://dx.doi.org/10.1126/science.1659743] [PMID: 1659743]

[10] zur Hausen H. Papillomavirus infections--a major cause of human cancers. Biochim Biophys Acta 1996; 1288(2): F55-78. [PMID: 8876633]

[11] Hakim AA, Dinh TA. Worldwide impact of the human papillomavirus vaccine. Curr Treat Options Oncol 2009; 10(1-2): 44-53. [http://dx.doi.org/10.1007/s11864-009-0094-4] [PMID: 19387841]

[12] Parkin DM, Louie KS, Clifford G. Burden and trends of type-specific human papillomavirus infections and related diseases in the Asia Pacific region. Vaccine 2008; 26 (Suppl. 12): M1-M16. [http://dx.doi.org/10.1016/j.vaccine.2008.05.010] [PMID: 18945410]

[13] Chung CH, Bagheri A, D'Souza G. Epidemiology of oral human papillomavirus infection. Oral Oncol 2014; 50(5): 364-9. [http://dx.doi.org/10.1016/j.oraloncology.2013.09.003] [PMID: 24080455]

[14] Tota JE, Chevarie-Davis M, Richardson LA, Devries M, Franco EL. Epidemiology and burden of HPV infection and related diseases: implications for prevention strategies. Prev Med 2011; 53 (Suppl. 1): S12-21. [http://dx.doi.org/10.1016/j.ypmed.2011.08.017] [PMID: 21962466]

[15] Barroso LF II, Wilkin T. Human papillomavirus vaccination in males: the state of the science. Curr

Infect Dis Rep 2011; 13(2): 175-81.
[http://dx.doi.org/10.1007/s11908-010-0163-7] [PMID: 21365381]

[16] Bernard HU, Burk RD, Chen Z, van Doorslaer K, zur Hausen H, de Villiers EM. Classification of papillomaviruses (PVs) based on 189 PV types and proposal of taxonomic amendments. Virology 2010; 401(1): 70-9.
[http://dx.doi.org/10.1016/j.virol.2010.02.002] [PMID: 20206957]

[17] de Freitas AC, Gurgel AP, Chagas BS, Coimbra EC, do Amaral CM. Susceptibility to cervical cancer: an overview. Gynecol Oncol 2012; 126(2): 304-11.
[http://dx.doi.org/10.1016/j.ygyno.2012.03.047] [PMID: 22484226]

[18] Kocjan BJ, Bzhalava D, Forslund O, Dillner J, Poljak M. Molecular methods for identification and characterization of novel papillomaviruses. Clin Microbiol Infect 2015; 21(9): 808-16.
[http://dx.doi.org/10.1016/j.cmi.2015.05.011] [PMID: 26003284]

[19] Bravo IG, de Sanjosé S, Gottschling M. The clinical importance of understanding the evolution of papillomaviruses. Trends Microbiol 2010; 18(10): 432-8.
[http://dx.doi.org/10.1016/j.tim.2010.07.008] [PMID: 20739182]

[20] Gnanamony M, Peedicayil A, Subhashini J, *et al.* Detection and quantitation of HPV 16 and 18 in plasma of Indian women with cervical cancer. Gynecol Oncol 2010; 116(3): 447-51.
[http://dx.doi.org/10.1016/j.ygyno.2009.10.081] [PMID: 19922992]

[21] Kay P, Allan B, Denny L, Hoffman M, Williamson AL. Detection of HPV 16 and HPV 18 DNA in the blood of patients with cervical cancer. J Med Virol 2005; 75(3): 435-9.
[http://dx.doi.org/10.1002/jmv.20294] [PMID: 15648077]

[22] Sathish N, Abraham P, Peedicayil A, *et al.* HPV DNA in plasma of patients with cervical carcinoma. J Clin Virol 2004; 31(3): 204-9.
[http://dx.doi.org/10.1016/j.jcv.2004.03.013] [PMID: 15465413]

[23] Pornthanakasem W, Shotelersuk K, Termrungruanglert W, Voravud N, Niruthisard S, Mutirangura A. Human papillomavirus DNA in plasma of patients with cervical cancer. BMC Cancer 2001; 1(1): 2.
[http://dx.doi.org/10.1186/1471-2407-1-2] [PMID: 11244579]

[24] Liu VW, Tsang P, Yip A, Ng TY, Wong LC, Ngan HY. Low incidence of HPV DNA in sera of pretreatment cervical cancer patients. Gynecol Oncol 2001; 82(2): 269-72.
[http://dx.doi.org/10.1006/gyno.2001.6289] [PMID: 11531278]

[25] Kaspersen MD, Larsen PB, Ingerslev HJ, *et al.* Identification of multiple HPV types on spermatozoa from human sperm donors. PLoS One 2011; 6(3): e18095.
[http://dx.doi.org/10.1371/journal.pone.0018095] [PMID: 21479232]

[26] Weyn C, Thomas D, Jani J, *et al.* Evidence of human papillomavirus in the placenta. J Infect Dis 2011; 203(3): 341-3.
[http://dx.doi.org/10.1093/infdis/jiq056] [PMID: 21208925]

[27] Bosch FX, Lorincz A, Muñoz N, Meijer CJ, Shah KV. The causal relation between human papillomavirus and cervical cancer. J Clin Pathol 2002; 55(4): 244-65.
[http://dx.doi.org/10.1136/jcp.55.4.244] [PMID: 11919208]

[28] Chang MH, Jeang KT. Viruses and human cancer. Springer Berlin Heidelberg 2014; 193: 136-49.

[29] Lacour DE, Trimble C. Human papillomavirus in infants: transmission, prevalence, and persistence. J Pediatr Adolesc Gynecol 2012; 25(2): 93-7.
[http://dx.doi.org/10.1016/j.jpag.2011.03.001] [PMID: 21600804]

[30] Moody CA, Laimins LA. Human papillomavirus oncoproteins: pathways to transformation. Nat Rev Cancer 2010; 10(8): 550-60.
[http://dx.doi.org/10.1038/nrc2886] [PMID: 20592731]

[31] Haedicke J, Iftner T. Human papillomaviruses and cancer. Radiother Oncol 2013; 108(3): 397-402.

[http://dx.doi.org/10.1016/j.radonc.2013.06.004] [PMID: 23830197]

[32] Kocjan BJ, Bzhalava D, Forslund O, Dillner J, Poljak M. Molecular methods for identification and characterization of novel papillomaviruses. Clin Microbiol Infect 2015; 21(9): 808-16. [http://dx.doi.org/10.1016/j.cmi.2015.05.011] [PMID: 26003284]

[33] Van Doorslaer K, Tan Q, Xirasagar S, *et al.* The Papillomavirus Episteme: a central resource for papillomavirus sequence data and analysis. Nucleic Acids Res 2013; 41(Database issue): D571-8. [PMID: 23093593]

[34] Michael KM, Waterboer T, Pfister H, *et al.* Seroreactivity of 38 human papillomavirus types in epidermodysplasia verruciformis patients, relatives, and controls. J Invest Dermatol 2010; 130(3): 841-8.
[http://dx.doi.org/10.1038/jid.2009.356] [PMID: 19924140]

[35] Nindl I, Gottschling M, Stockfleth E. Human papillomaviruses and non-melanoma skin cancer: basic virology and clinical manifestations. Dis Markers 2007; 23(4): 247-59.
[http://dx.doi.org/10.1155/2007/942650] [PMID: 17627060]

[36] Gottschling M, Göker M, Köhler A, Lehmann MD, Stockfleth E, Nindl I. Cutaneotropic human beta-/gamma-papillomaviruses are rarely shared between family members. J Invest Dermatol 2009; 129(10): 2427-34.
[http://dx.doi.org/10.1038/jid.2009.94] [PMID: 19516265]

[37] Ekström J, Forslund O, Dillner J. Three novel papillomaviruses (HPV109, HPV112 and HPV114) and their presence in cutaneous and mucosal samples. Virology 2010; 397(2): 331-6.
[http://dx.doi.org/10.1016/j.virol.2009.11.027] [PMID: 19969321]

[38] Bottalico D, Chen Z, Dunne A, *et al.* The oral cavity contains abundant known and novel human papillomaviruses from the Betapapillomavirus and Gammapapillomavirus genera. J Infect Dis 2011; 204(5): 787-92.
[http://dx.doi.org/10.1093/infdis/jir383] [PMID: 21844305]

[39] Cubie HA. Diseases associated with human papillomavirus infection. Virology 2013; 445(1-2): 21-34.
[http://dx.doi.org/10.1016/j.virol.2013.06.007] [PMID: 23932731]

[40] Veldhuijzen NJ, Snijders PJ, Reiss P, Meijer CJ, van de Wijgert JH. Factors affecting transmission of mucosal human papillomavirus. Lancet Infect Dis 2010; 10(12): 862-74.
[http://dx.doi.org/10.1016/S1473-3099(10)70190-0] [PMID: 21075056]

[41] Huang HS, Buck CB, Lambert PF. Inhibition of gamma secretase blocks HPV infection. Virology 2010; 407(2): 391-6.
[http://dx.doi.org/10.1016/j.virol.2010.09.002] [PMID: 20875908]

CHAPTER 2

HPV Proteins and Their Functions

Kimia Kardani and **Azam Bolhassani***

Department of Pharmaceutical Biotechnology, School of Pharmacy, Shahid Beheshti University of Medical Sciences, Tehran, Iran

Department of Hepatitis and AIDS, Pasteur Institute of Iran, Tehran, Iran

Abstract: Papillomaviruses (PVs) are small non-enveloped viruses with a circular DNA genome encoding the viral early and late genes. The expression of late gene generates the structural L1 and L2 proteins, whereas early gene expression produces the regulatory proteins (E1-E8). The L1 and L2 proteins have important roles in virion assembly. Among the regulatory proteins, E7 and E6 oncoproteins play an important role in benign and also malignant transformation. For instance, a variant of HPV16 with the minimal differences in E6 sequence (Q14H/H78Y/L83V) found in cervical cancers is more effective for virus replication and maintenance as well as cell immortalization compared to other HPV types. Regarding the role of early proteins in the HPV life cycle, all proteins encoded by the HPV genome and their functions will be described in this chapter.

Keywords: Early and late proteins, Genome, HPV, Infection, Structure.

INTRODUCTION

Papillomaviruses have proved to be the most complex group of human pathogenic viruses [1]. The double-stranded human papillomavirus (HPV) genome includes a non-coding "long control region" (LCR) and two protein-coding regions (E and L). The long control region regulates gene expression and replication. The early (E) or regulatory protein-coding region is required for gene expression, replication and survival, and the late (L) or capsid protein-coding region is needed to assemble virion [2 - 4]. The early proteins can be further organized into E1 and E2 proteins involved in replication and transcription, E5, E6 and E7 oncoproteins and E4 protein required in virion production. The late proteins contain L1 and L2 structural proteins [3, 4]. Expression of L1 and L2 proteins occurs in the terminally differentiated cells of the squamous epithelium [5]. The PV genome sequences differ from one another due to the variation of their L1 genes by 10%

* **Corresponding author Azam Bolhassani:** Department of Hepatitis and AIDS, Pasteur Institute of Iran, Tehran, Iran; Tel: 66953311-20; E-mails: A_bolhasani@pasteur.ac.ir, azam.bolhassani@yahoo.com

or more [2, 3]. Fig. (**1**) shows all major proteins expressed by HPV16 genome.

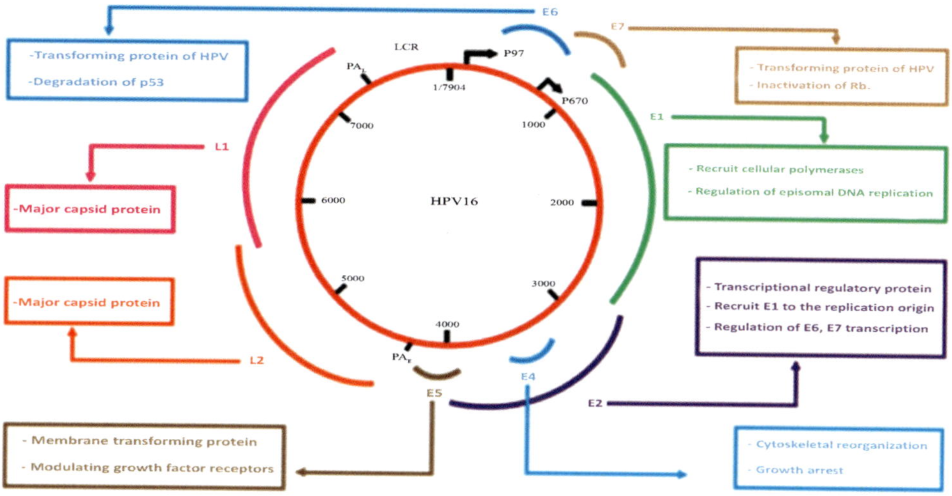

Fig. (1). Schematic presentation of HPV16 genome encoding the early or regulatory (non-structural) genes, the late or capsid (structural) genes, and the long control region (upstream regulatory region or URR).

Late Proteins

The papillomavirus late proteins include the major capsid protein (L1) and the minor capsid protein (L2) as described below. Table **1** indicates all the properties of proteins generated by the high risk HPV genome.

Major Capsid Protein (L1)

The papillomavirus L1 protein (~ 55 kDa) can assemble to form virus-like particles (VLPs) in the lack of any chaperones [6, 7]. Molecular biology analysis showed that messenger RNAs (mRNAs) encoding L1 proteins are generated through splicing events that remove early gene sequences present on the pre-mRNA [8]. The N-terminal region of L1 usually carries a consensus MxxWx$_7$YLPP motif [6]. The N- and C-terminal regions of L1 form the floor between the capsomer knobs. Each of the 72 knobs is composed of a pentameric L1 capsomer. At the outer apex of the knob, an inter-L1 disulfide bond is formed between the adjacent capsomers [6, 9, 10]. The inter-capsomeric disulfide bond involves two conserved homologs of HPV16 L1 cysteines (Cys175 and Cys428) in all papillomaviruses. In the mature virions, L1 molecules form disulfide-linked dimers or ring-shaped L1 trimers [6, 10]. In a few papillomavirus species including bovine papillomavirus type 1 (BPV1), formation of an additional pair of disulfide bonds results in covalent cross-linking of L1 molecules into a unimolecular cage [9]. Further experiments showed that three additional cysteines (homologous to HPV16 L1 residues 161, 185, and 379) are highly conserved among all papillomavirus L1 proteins. These key disulfide bonds are essential for virion stability [6].

Table 1. Properties of proteins generated by the high risk HPV genome [103 - 107].

	Length	Linear	dsDNA	RNA stage	Family	Function	Interactions	Subcellular Location	PTMs	Genebank accession no.
E1	649aa	+	+	No	-Papillomaviridae; Alphapapillomavirus	-ATP-dependent DNA helicase required for initiation of viral DNA replication	- E2 protein -Host DNA polymerase subunit POLA2 -Host single stranded DNA-binding protein RPA1 -Host TOP1	-Host nucleus	-Phosphorylated -Sumoylated	P03114.2
E2	365 aa	+	+	No	-Papillomaviridae; Alphapapillomavirus	-Plays a role in the initiation of viral DNA replication -Regulates viral transcription through binding to the E2RE response element	-Protein E1 -Protein L1 -Protein L2 -Protein E7 -Host TAF1 -Host BRD4 -Host TOPBP1	-Host nucleus	-Phosphorylated -Sumoylated	P03120.1
E4	95 aa	+	+	No	-Papillomaviridae; Alphapapillomavirus	Plays several roles to favor viral DNA replication: -Disruption of host intranuclear speckles organization -Cell cycle arrest at the G2 phase -Inhibition of cellular DNA replication -Regulate host splicing factors -May also act to diminish the integrity of the keratinocyte -Inducing apoptosis	-Host SRPK1 -Host cytokeratin components KRT8 and KRT18	-Host cytoplasm -Host nucleus	-Phosphorylated	P06922.1
E5	83 aa	+	+	No	-Papillomaviridae; Alphapapillomavirus	-Acts to keep host cells in a proliferation-competent state -Epidermal growth factor receptor (EGFR) activation after stimulation by EGF by inhibiting EGFR internalization -Induces a redistribution of host caveolin-1 and glycosphingolipid (ganglioside GM1) components of lipid rafts to the plasma membrane -Alters endosomal pH by interacting with the vacuolar H^+-ATPase -Prevents transport of the major histocompatibility class I to the cell surface and retains the complex in the Golgi apparatus	-Host BCAP31 -Host HLA class I heavy chains A1, A2, A3 and B8	-Host membrane -Host endoplasmic reticulum membrane -Host Golgi apparatus		P06927.2
E6	158 aa	+	+	No	-Papillomaviridae; Alphapapillomavirus	-Plays a major role in the induction and maintenance of cellular transformation -Acts mainly as an oncoprotein -Inhibits immune response by interacting with host IRF3 and TYK2	-Human TP53 -Human NFX1 and MAGI3 -Human IRF3 -Human TYK2	-Host nucleus matrix		P03126.1

(Table 1) contd.....

	Length	Linear	dsDNA	RNA stage	Family	Function	Interactions	Subcellular Location	PTMs	Genebank accession no.
E7	98 aa	+	+	No	-Papillomaviridae; Alphapapillomavirus	-Plays a role in viral genome replication by driving entry of quiescent cells into the cell cycle -Stimulation of progression from G1 to S phase -Has both transforming and trans-activating activities -Induces the disassembly of the E2F1 transcription factor from RB1 -Interferes with host histone deacetylation mediated by HDAC1 and HDAC2 -Plays also a role in the inhibition of both antiviral and antiproliferative functions of host interferon alpha	-Host RB1 -Host EP300 -Protein E2	-Host cytoplasm -Host nucleus	-Highly phosphorylated	P03129.1
L1	505 aa	+	+	No	-Papillomaviridae; Alphapapillomavirus	-Forms an icosahedral capsid -Binds to heparan sulfate proteoglycans on cell surface of basal layer keratinocytes to provide initial virion attachment	-Protein E2 -Host KPNA2 -Host ITGA6 -Host SDC1	-Virion -Host nucleus	-ISGylated by host HERC5	P03101.3
L2	473 aa	+	+	No	-Papillomaviridae; Alphapapillomavirus	-Minor protein of the capsid -Plays a role in capsid stabilization -Escorts the genomic DNA into the nucleus by promoting escape from the endosomal compartments and traffic through the host Golgi network -Localizes viral genomes to host PML bodies -Encapsid the genome	-major capsid protein L1 -Protein E2 -Host GADD45GIP1 -Host HSPA8 -Host importins KPNB2 and KPNB3 -Host DYNLT1	-Virion -Host nucleus	-Highly phosphorylated	P03107.1

Abbreviations: PTMs, Post-translational modifications; SRPK1, SRSF protein kinase 1; H^+-ATPase, Proton-pumping ATPase; BCAP31, B-cell receptor-associated protein 31; MAGI3, Membrane associated guanylate kinase, WW and PDZ domain containing 3; IRF3, The interferon regulatory transcription factor 3; TYK2, Tyrosine kinase 2; KPNA2, Karyopherin subunit alpha 2; ITGA6, Integrin subunit alpha 6; SDC1, Syndecan 1; ISGylation, A similar manner to ubiquitylation; HERC5, E3 ubiquitin-protein ligase; GADD45GIP1, Growth arrest and DNA damage-inducible proteins-interacting protein 1; HSPA8, Heat shock protein family A (Hsp70) member 8; DYNLT1, Dynein light chain tctex-type 1

Conserved Motifs of L1 Protein

All papillomaviruses are able to interact with heparan sulfate (HS) during virus entry through the non-conserved surface-exposed lysine residues (*e.g.,* HPV16 L1 lysines 54, 278, 356, and 361). It has shown that the conserved arginine (Arg) and tyrosine (Tyr) residues (*e.g.,* HPV16 L1 residues 418 and 419) are enriched in high affinity HS-binding peptide motifs. A highly conserved polybasic region at the C-terminus of L1 mediates its import into the cell nucleus in the form of pentameric capsomers for PV virion assembly [6].

Minor Capsid Protein (L2)

The papillomavirus L2 protein (~ 55 kDa) typically exhibits an unreal molecular weight of 64-78 kDa in SDS-PAGE analysis [1, 11]. The reason is unclear as there are no known post-translational modifications of L2 [1, 12]. The PV virion structure is a non-enveloped T=7*d* icosahedral capsid with a diameter of 55-60 nm containing 360 L1 proteins and 72 L2 proteins in a single capsid [1, 13, 14]. There is an L1 binding site at the C-terminal region of L2 protein (residues 396-439) in HPV11 and BPV1 characterized by several proline residues (PxxP) associated with protein-protein interactions [1, 15]. Two highly conserved cysteine residues (C22 and C28) at the N-terminal region of L2 protein form an intra-molecular disulfide hairpin loop in all PV types. The point mutation of these cysteine residues in HPV16 generated non-infectious virions but did not influence virion assembly [1, 16]. It was suggested that the cysteine residues play an important role in capsid stabilization by modulating the accessibility of L2 on the surface of virions [1, 17]. Indeed, L2 is transiently exposed in immature virions. Although L2 is only minimally exposed on the surface of the mature virion, it emerges from the virion during the virus entry process [6].

The Role of L1 in Virus Entry

Capsid interaction with heparan sulfate carbohydrates (HS) leads to a slight conformational change that exposes an N-terminal region of the L2 protein allowing cleavage of L2 by cellular furin protease or related cellular proprotein convertases [18, 19]. Furin cleavage of L2 exhibits a secondary conformational change that may reduce the affinity of the virion for HS. The keratinocyte binding predominantly occurs through interaction of L1-only or furin-cleaved L1/L2 particles *in vivo* [20]. Most studies showed a non-clathrin, non-caveolin pathway for HPV16 entry similar to macropinocytosis. Indeed, L1 and L1/L2 particles have a major role to pass through early endosomes to late endosomes [21]. The studies showed that DNA encapsidated within L1-only HPV16 particles does not escape from late endosomes, whereas in L1/L2 particles, L2 protein and thus the genome are transferred to the trans-Golgi network prior to nuclear delivery [22].

L2 Improves the Encapsidation of HPV Genome

L1 and L2 proteins have the conserved short sequences of positively charged basic residues found at the C-terminal of L1 and at the N- and C-terminal of L2 for effective DNA-binding activity *in vitro* [1, 23 - 25]. Regarding the studies, deletion of DNA binding domain from PV L2 did not affect the encapsidation of genome but made the virions non-infectious [1]. Furthermore, L2 can deliver the virion components to specific locations in the nucleus defined as nuclear domain 10 (ND10), and co-localize L1, E2 and viral genome to facilitate encapsidation of the histone-bound genome and virion assembly [1, 26].

L2 and Cell Host Entry

The studies showed that L2 often buried within the capsid and its exposure requires a conformational change induced by capsid binding to heparan sulfate proteoglycans [18 - 20, 27, 28]. Analysis of the N-terminal of all PV types reveals that the consensus furin cleavage motif site (R-X-K/R-R) is conserved at amino acids of 9-12 required for infection and the exit of the genome from the endosomal compartment [19, 28]. Moreover, furin cleavage exhibits a broadly neutralizing epitope (amino acid 17-36) identified by the RG-1 monoclonal antibody [29]. Two suitable sites were determined on L2 for binding to an effective entry receptor: a) the RG-1 epitope (aa 13-31), and b) the surface exposed region of L2 (aa 108-120) recognized by another neutralizing antibody [30 - 32]. On the other hand, our group also represented that the recombinant L1-L2 fusion DNA is expressed in a high efficiency compared to L1 DNA indicating the role of L2 as an efficient agent for overcoming the cell barriers and poor uptake of DNA *in vitro* and *in vivo* [33].

L2 and Vesicular Trafficking of Papillomavirus

For successful infection, papillomavirus needs to enter the host cell, cross the cytoplasm and transport the viral genome to the nucleus [34, 35]. The studies showed that different host cell proteins were also characterized as interacting partners with L2 to facilitate entry and trafficking by various mechanisms to the nucleus such as the chaperon protein cyclophilins that are peptidyl-prolyl cis/trans isomerases (*e.g.,* CyPB) [36]. It was shown that CyPB binds to L2 amino acid region 90-110, and helps in the uncoating of HPV capsid in the late endosome [37]. The cytosolic adaptor protein Sortin Nexin 17 (SNX17) is another important host protein found in early endosomes for virion trafficking and endosomal recycling. The studies showed that different PV types have a highly conserved NPxY motif at amino acid region 245-257 of L2 that binds to SNX17 [1]. Mutation of the NPxY region decreased viral infectivity suggesting a critical SNX17-L2 interaction [38]. Another possible candidate in PV transport is the tSNARE syntaxin 18 protein which binds to L2 residues 41-45 [39].

L2 and Endosomal Escape

The studies showed that L2 along with HPV viral DNA (vDNA) exit the late endosome in order to escape the viral DNA from the vesicular compartment and transfer into the cell nucleus. Indeed, the deletion or mutation of a 23 amino acid region at the C-terminal of HPV L2 could reduce viral infectivity due to prevention of L2/vDNA endosomal escape [40]. Recently, a transmembrane-like domain at the N-terminal region of L2 (residues 45-67 containing highly conserved GxxxG motifs) was also identified to facilitate the endosomal escape [41]. The L2/vDNA complex may use the cytoskeleton to traverse the cytoplasm, *e.g.*, L2 interaction with β-actin or dynein motors. In fact, L2 linked to the motor protein dynein could interact with the actin microtubule network and transport the

L2/vDNA to the nucleus [26].

Nuclear Entry of HPV Genome by L2

The mechanism of nuclear entry by L2 differs at different stages of the virus life cycle, *i.e.,* initial infection or virion production [42]. It was shown that the L2/vDNA entered the nucleus *via* nuclear pore complexes using the nuclear localization signals (NLS) on both the N- and C-terminal of L2 [43]. Mamoor *et al.* described an arginine-rich nuclear retention signal in HPV16 L2 (296-SRRTGIRYSRIGNKQTLRTRS-316) required for infection, but not virion assembly. Furthermore, a leucine-rich nuclear export signal (NES) was also described at the C-terminal of HPV16 L2 (462-LPYFFSDVSL-471) required for nuclear export in a CRM1 (Exportin)-dependent manner, but not critical for pseudovirion assembly or infection [44]. The nuclear localization signals at N- and C-terminal regions can independently interact with karyopherins (*i.e.,* kapα2β1, kapβ2 and kapβ3) that are specific in various papillomavirus types for entry into the nucleus [45]. A member of heat shock protein 70 (Hsc70) could also assist in transporting newly synthesized L2 into the nucleus *via* forming an active complex with L2 as well as maintaining L2 in a specific state of folding that is optimal for interaction with the L1-capsomers and finally viral assembly [46].

Nuclear Activities of L2

Regarding the studies, L2 protein can recruit other viral components to ND-10 likely to facilitate virion assembly [47, 48]. Day *et al.* showed that PV infection is reduced 10-fold in the lack of PML protein, a critical structural component of ND-10 [49]. In addition, several studies showed the interaction between the N-terminal residues 1-50 of L2 and E2. However, L2 residues 301-400 are also required for the down-regulation of E2-dependent transcriptional activation [1]. Heino *et al* also found that L2 inhibits the transcriptional activation of E2 transactivator (E2TA), but not its ability to support viral DNA replication [50]. The studies represented that overexpression of L2 results in the expulsion from ND-10 followed by degradation of the transcriptional activator, SP100. In addition, overexpression of L2 induces the recruitment of Daxx, a nuclear transcriptional repressor protein to ND-10. Indeed, the accumulation of L2 (especially amino acid 390-420) and Daxx followed by the loss of SP100 could facilitate the assembly of virions [1]. A study showed four nuclear body-associated proteins (PATZ, TIP60, TIN-Ag-RP and PLINP) that could interact with the L2 of different HPV types and co-localize in the ND-10 domains. For example, L2-PATZ interactions might play a role in gene regulation and cell differentiation during papilloma formation [1]. On the other hand, the transcription factors, TBX2 and TBX3, could interact with the C-terminal of HPV

11, 16, 18 L2 proteins, and suppress viral transcription and early viral gene expression (*e.g.,* E6 and E7), and help the transition to viral assembly during infection [1].

Early or Regulatory Proteins

The roles of the major early proteins (E1, E2, E4, E5, E6 and E7) are briefly described in below, respectively. Table **1** indicates all properties of proteins generated by the high risk HPV genome.

E1 Protein

E1 protein binds to the viral origin of replication and represents ATPase and helicase activity, whereas E2 forms a complex with E1, facilitating its binding to the origin of viral replication [51, 52].

E2 Protein

The papillomavirus E2 protein is a DNA binding protein involved in the initiation of DNA replication, control of viral transcription, and separation of viral genomes [53]. E2 protein serves three major functions in the viral life cycle: a) it regulates the expression levels of other viral gene products. This depends on the binding sites occupied by the LCR to act as a transcriptional repressor or activator; b) it recruits E1 to the viral origin and enhances viral DNA replication; c) it has a critical role in the delivery of the viral genome to daughter cells during division of the host cell. The full-length E2 protein is an essential regulatory protein encoded by all papillomaviruses. All E2 proteins bind to 12 bp motifs located at the upstream regulatory region (URR) of the viral genomes. E2 proteins are expressed at early and intermediate stages of the viral life cycle [52, 54]. The full-length E2 protein consists of a conserved N-terminal "transactivation" domain (~ 200 amino acids) linked to a C-terminal DNA binding/dimerization domain (~ 100 amino acids). The domains are connected by a flexible linker sequence (*i.e.*, hinge) which varies in length and sequence composition among different genera of papillomaviruses [54]. On the other hand, all PVs have the potential to encode shorter E2 forms containing the C-terminal domain, the hinge region and a 10-13 residue peptide from an upstream ORF. These E2 fusion proteins are encoded by spliced messages that link sequences from an alternative reading frame in the E1 region of the genome (designated E8) to the C-terminal of E2 (E2C). These proteins have been named E8^E2, E8^E2C, E1^E2, E1M^E2 and E9^E2. The shorter forms of E2 function as repressors of viral transcription and replication [54]. In initiation of viral DNA replication, the regulatory E2 protein helps to recruit the viral helicase E1 to the viral replication origin by protein-protein and protein-DNA interactions [53]. The relative abundance of different E2 isoforms was determined in BPV-1 infected cells. For instance, E2, E2-TR and E8^E2 isoforms were expressed in ratios of 1:10:3, respectively. This means that most full-length E2 proteins are present as heterodimers which can support transcription and replication initiation, but not partitioning of viral genomes [54]. In the alpha-PVs, such as HPV16, the full length E2 protein is encoded from spliced messages expressed from either the early or late promoters. In undifferentiated cells, E2 encoding mRNAs are transcribed from the early promoter and terminated at the early polyadenylation site (pAE). As cells differentiate in the mid-layers of the epithelium, the late promoter is activated and transcribes an intermediate class of messages that still use the early polyadenylation signal. These transcripts encode high levels of E2 that are required for viral DNA replication [54]. The functions of E2 protein are disrupted by mutation or integration of the viral genome. This inactivation leads to improvement of E2-mediated repression and increased expression of the E6 and E7 genes, contributing to malignant progression in "high risk" PV infection [54].

E4 Protein

E4 is a protein translated from spliced mRNA transcripts as an E1^E4 fusion protein and contains the first five residues of E1 fused to the rest of E4 [55]. E4 protein showed various effects on cell behavior, and cellular organization including the suppression of cellular DNA synthesis through inhibition of the G2-to-M transition of the cell cycle, and the promotion of apoptosis by alteration of mitochondrial function [55]. E4 proteins from different HPV types associate with the serine-arginine kinase SRPK1; a kinase that regulates the function of mRNA splicing factors [55]. Proline-rich regions are a general feature of E1^E4 proteins and a threonine dipeptide (residues 22 and 23) within this region of the HPV16 E1^E4 protein is important for the cytoplasmic deletion of cyclins A and B1 [55].

E5 Protein

High-risk HPV E5 could stimulate primary human keratinocytes to proliferate and enhance the efficiency of immortalization of keratinocytes by E6 and E7 proteins [56 - 59]. These activities were enhanced in the presence of epidermal growth factor (EGF) [58].

Indeed, high-risk HPV E5 binds the vacuolar ATPase, decreases the acidity of endosomes and also trafficking through the endocytic pathway, and increases ligand-dependent signaling through the EGF receptor [60, 61]. In addition, the increased signaling may be due to E5-mediated up-regulation of surface gangliosides [62]. Similar to other high-risk HPV oncogenes, E5 was reported to change cellular gene expression by regulating cellular miRNAs. For example, E5 down-regulates miR-203 similar to E7 oncoprotein. Thus, E5 has oncogenic activity *in vitro* and *in vivo* and the β-PVs do not encode this protein [63].

E6 Protein

E6 protein is characterized by four C-X-X-C motifs involved in the formation of two zinc binding sites [64, 65]. These sites are critical in binding to a number of alpha-helix containing cellular proteins that have an LXXLL motif including the ubiquitin ligase named as E6-associated protein (E6-AP). Furthermore, other regions of E6 are important for various E6 functions and for binding to cellular proteins such as p53, E6-AP, p300, and PDZ containing proteins [66]. High-risk HPV E6 was found to be more disordered (unfolded) than low-risk HPV E6 suggesting that oncogenic proteins were more disordered [67, 68]. Several roles of the E6 protein in the virus life-cycle include inhibition of apoptosis induced by the expression of the HPV E7 protein and also facilitation of viral DNA amplification in the upper layers [64]. E6 proteins from high-risk types such as HPV 16 and 18 have transforming potential in various tests [69]. E6 can be localized to nuclear, cytoplasmic, and membrane fractions. E6 localization is different for low- and high-risk viruses that might partially explain differences in regulation of cellular proteins such as p53 by low- and high-risk HPV E6 proteins [70]. The interaction of HPV E6 with p53 leads to the ubiquitin-mediated degradation of p53 by the proteasome. E6 mediates degradation of p53 by associating with E6-AP, a cellular ubiquitin ligase [64]. The data showed that certain E6 mutants are unable to target p53 for degradation but still have transforming properties suggesting that E6 has other functions [71]. On the other hand, certain high-risk HPV types generate one or more truncated E6 transcripts (E6*) modulating apoptotic pathways [72]. The reports showed that E6 proteins from high-risk types do not cause immortalization of human keratinocytes, but significantly increase the efficiency of immortalization of human keratinocytes by high-risk HPV E7. In contrast to these findings, high-risk HPV E6 alone could immortalize human mammary epithelial cells [65]. However, it was demonstrated that loss of expression of p16Ink4a, a cyclin dependent kinase inhibitor, along with E6 expression is necessary for mammary epithelial cell immortalization, indicating a requirement for abrogation of the Rb pathway. In addition, the degradation of p53 is not essential for immortalization of human keratinocytes and mammary epithelial cells and, in fact, immortalization of these cells is further associated with the ability of E6 to activate telomerase [73]. In addition, E6-AP can act to protect the HPV16 and 18 E6 proteins from proteasomal degradation, thus increasing their stability [64]. Recently, a new interaction of both low- and high-risk HPV E6 proteins with the nucleosomal acetyltransferase TIP60 has been demonstrated to influence p53 function. Interaction of E6 proteins with TIP60 destabilizes the TIP60 complex and disrupts TIP60-dependent transcriptional regulation and apoptosis. In addition to the effects of E6 protein in p53 pathway, E6 directly influences apoptotic effector molecules in both low- and high-risk HPV types. For example, HPV E6 proteins degrade the pro-apoptotic protein, Bak that may affect responses to DNA damaging agents (*e.g.*, UV) [74 - 77]. Other studies showed that the E6 PDZ motif is important for binding to several protein phosphatases (*e.g.*, PTPN3 and PTPN13) that are involved in both inhibiting and activating a variety of cell signaling pathways [75]. In fact, these phosphatases are mutated or down-regulated in cancer and E6-mediated degradation of the phosphatases is necessary for tumorigenic transformation by E6 [75, 78]. A recent study indicated that down-regulation of PTPN13 by E6 is associated with activation of MAP kinase signaling [79]. Modulation of keratinocyte differentiation by E6 is a potential mechanism for HPV replication [80]. E6 expression down-regulates a large number of genes that are associated with keratinocyte differentiation. Indeed, E6 inhibits differentiation through down-modulation of the TGF-β pathway. In addition, high-risk HPV E6 proteins bind to cellular proteins including calcium binding protein (ERC-55) and focal adhesion protein (paxillin) which play a role in altering the differentiation capacity of keratinocytes. These findings suggest that E6 is involved in modulating cellular metabolism, and promoting viral replication in differentiated cells [75]. Microarray analysis indicated that E6 activates a large number of NF-κB responsive genes. Indeed, E6 up-regulates the NF-κB responsive gene (c-IAP2) to confer resistance to apoptosis [81]. It has been demonstrated that both low-risk and high-risk HPV E6 can abrogate promyelocytic leukemia (PML)-induced cellular senescence and high-risk HPV E6 can direct the proteolytic degradation of PML in rat kidney primary cells. The interaction of E6 with PMLs is conserved in low- and high-risk viruses, indicating its importance for the viral life cycle [82, 83]. The studies indicated that expression of E6 causes down-regulation of multiple IFN-responsive genes including Stat-1 and 2′-5′ oligoadenylate synthetase, and also IFN-α and IFN-β. High-risk HPV E6 also binds interferon regulatory factor-3 (IRF-3) and inhibits its ability to activate transcription of IFN-β responsive genes. Both E6 and E7 and another viral protein, E1, are thought to play a role in suppressing the IFN response [75, 84]. Moreover, the expression of E6 causes transcriptional up-regulation of TERT, the reverse transcriptase component of telomerase, and acetylation of histones at the TERT promoter. Indeed, E6 protein binds to c-myc and E6-AP leading to activate c-myc at the TERT promoter [75]. Other studies showed that E6 can degrade a cellular protein (NFX1-91) that binds to mSin3a, a histone deacetylase acting as a repressor of TERT transcription in the TERT promoter. Expression of E7 can synergize with E6 to increase telomerase levels. A study showed that E6 protein can directly bind to the TERT protein, stabilize TERT, and change its localization in the cell [85]. Mutational analysis indicated that the telomerase activation by high-risk HPV E6 is essential for immortalization of primary cells. In contrast, low-risk HPV E6 proteins do not activate telomerase [75]. The recent studies indicated that high-risk HPV E6 and E7 proteins affect miRNAs that are involved in growth regulation. For instance, high-risk HPV E6 proteins down-regulate miR-34a, a miRNA that targets various genes involved in control of cell cycle [75]. High-risk HPV E6 proteins also down-regulate the expression of miR-23b, which targets the expression of urokinase plasminogen activator gene, and subsequently may affect cell migration. The ability of high-risk HPV E6 proteins to affect miRNA expression is through its ability to target p53. A recent study indicated that low-risk HPV 11 modulates miRNA expression. Thus, both low and high-risk HPV E6 proteins affect cell function, differentiation, and growth through modulation of miRNAs [75].

E7 Protein

The E7 proteins range in size from 98 to 105 amino acids. The low-risk HPV E7 proteins have a lower degree of disorder as compared to high-risk HPV E7 proteins, indicating a lower number of interactions with other proteins [75]. The N-terminal of E7 has homology with SV40 T antigen and adenovirus E1A, in two regions referred to conserved region 1 (CR1) and conserved region 2 (CR2). This conservation helps that high-risk HPV E7 binds the retinoblastoma tumor suppressor protein (Rb) [75]. Both high and low-risk HPV E7 proteins can change the intracellular location of cellular proteins, and increase their presence in the cytoplasm. The affinity of E7 binding to Rb is lower for low-risk HPVs than for high-risk HPVs [75]. Regarding the reports, the Rb binding motif in CR2 is required for stimulation of DNA synthesis, transactivation and the cooperation with ras in transformation of rodent cells. In addition, the amino acids 6-10 (PTLHE) in CR1 are not required for Rb binding or transactivation, but are needed for cooperation of E7 with ras in transformation. The C-terminal half of E7 contains a zinc binding site, composed of two C-X-X-C motifs that this region is important for protein stability, dimerization, transformation, and immortalization of keratinocytes [75, 86]. Although, high-risk HPV E6, but not E7 targets p53 for degradation, E7 does affect p53 expression and function. High-risk HPV E7 abrogates p53-mediated growth arrest, but low-risk HPV E7 does not [75]. Generally, high-risk HPV E7 disrupts the interaction of mdm2 with p53, abrogates the growth inhibitory effect of p21CIP1 and p27KIP1 and targets Rb family members for degradation, releasing E2F transcription factor. In contrast to high-risk HPV E7, low-risk HPV E7 is much less efficient at binding p21CIP1 and abrogating its ability to inhibit cdk2 activity [75]. High-risk HPV E7 may suppress apoptosis by binding glutathione S-transferase P1 and preventing the phosphorylation of JNK. High-risk HPV E7 was shown to induce autophagy in response to growth factor deprivation. Indeed, the C-terminal of high-risk HPV E7 is able to interact with M2 pyruvate kinase (M2-PK) resulting in a less active form of the enzyme that increases glycolysis [75]. Interestingly, high-risk HPV E7 has been reported to decrease expression of miR-203, a cellular microRNA that is normally increased in differentiating cells and down-regulates a p53 family member (ΔNp63 isoform) and cell proliferation. This E7-mediated down-regulation of miR203 is necessary for strong amplification of viral genomes by creating a replication-competent cellular environment. In contrast, high-risk HPV E7 up-regulates the tumor suppressive miR16-1 in rafts cultures [87]. In human keratinocytes, transfection of the high-risk HPV E6 and E7 genes is necessary and sufficient for immortalization and inhibition of keratinocyte differentiation but not for tumorigenicity. E7, but not E6, alone can immortalize cells; however, the efficiency of immortalization is much greater when E6 and E7 are expressed together. In contrast, low-risk HPV E6 and E7 proteins have little or no immortalizing activity. Two issues are considered: a) the transcription and translation of E6 and E7 are regulated differently between the high-risk and low-risk HPVs. While low-risk HPVs have a promoter upstream of the E6 gene and another upstream of the E7 gene, there is a single promoter upstream of the E6 and E7 genes in high-risk HPVs and thus a polycistronic mRNA is produced; b) in the high-risk HPVs, the relative levels of E6 and E7 translation are determined by whether the splice site within E6 is used, which favors production of E7 [75]. Expression of single genes from the same promoter suggests that the low-risk HPV E6 and E7 genes encode proteins lacking in oncogenic potential. Transgenic mouse models have confirmed the oncogenic potential of high-risk α-HPV E6 and E7 in the skin, cervix, head and neck, and the β-HPV E6 and E7 in the skin. These models have also revealed that the relative impact of E6 and E7 *in vivo* is HPV type and tissue-specific. For example, α-HPV E7 is the more potent oncogene in the cervix, head and neck but α- and β-HPV E6 proteins are more potent in the skin [75]. In addition, the studies showed that the E6 transgene plus estrogen may be more important for tumor progression, while the E7 transgene is more efficient at tumor initiation [88].

Regulation of Cellular miRNA Expression by Human Papillomaviruses

MicroRNAs (miRNAs) show great effects on gene expression at the post-transcriptional level in biological processes. However, miRNA expression is regulated both at the transcriptional and posttranscriptional levels [89 - 91]. Many cellular transcription factors, including c-Myc, p53, and E2F capable of regulating miRNA transcription [92]. Because oncogenic HPV E6 induces degradation of p53 and E7 mediates degradation of pRB to release E2F from the pRB-E2F complex, it is possible that oncogenic HPV infection causes aberrant expression of cellular miRNAs [89].

The studies showed that high-risk E6 interacts with c-Myc to enhance c-Myc binding to the hTERT promoter and induce hTERT mRNA transcription [89, 93]. Viral E7 stimulates the expression of c-Myc by binding pRB protein, thereby releasing E2F to activate c-Myc. High-risk E7 also interacts directly with c-Myc [89, 94, 95]. c-Myc is a potent transcriptional regulator of miRNA expression. Overexpression of c-Myc widely represses miRNA expression that is likely a direct result of c-Myc binding to miRNA promoters, including those of let-7a-1-f-1/d, miR-15a/16-1, miR-22, miR-26a-2, miR-26b, miR-29a/b-1, miR-29b-2/c, miR-30e/30c-1, miR-34a, and miR-146a [96]. The p53 also regulates many cellular miRNAs by increasing the expression of miR-23a, miR-26a, and miR-34a *via* direct transactivation of these miRNA genes [97]. Other studies showed that p53 decreases expression of miRNA clusters, including miR-106b/miR-93/m-R-25, miR-17-5p / 18a / 19a / 20a / 19b-1 / 92-1, and miR-106a / 18b / 20b / 19b-2 / 92-2 [98]. Interestingly, p53 decreases expression of the miRNA clusters by an indirect mechanism through repression of E2F. It has been reported that p53 transactivates expression of the BTG3 gene (B-cell translocation gene 3) which directly binds E2F and inhibits its activity. The p53-induced miR-34a also targets the E2F 3′ UTR and prevents its expression [99]. Moreover, p53 interacts with the Drosha/p68 complex to facilitate Drosha-mediated pri-miRNA processing, thus promoting expression of miR-15a/16-1, miR-103/107, miR-143/145, miR-203, and miR-206 at the post-transcriptional level [100]. E7-mediated degradation of tumor suppressor protein pRB frees E2F from the pRB-E2F complex. The promoter regions of many miRNA genes contain an E2F binding site; therefore the binding of E2F to an E2F binding site in the promoter region transactivates the expression of miRNA genes including miR-17-92, let-7a-d, let-7i, miR-15b/16-2, and miR-106b-25 [101, 102].

CONCLUDING REMARKS

The PV genome encodes the early (E1-E8) and late (L1, L2) proteins. Both L1 and L2 proteins are expressed in the upper layer of the epithelium, form virus capsid, and have immunogenicity. On the other hand, the E6, E7, and E5 oncoproteins play important roles in regulating HPV functions during the viral life cycle and also contribute to the development of cancers. As described, p53 and Rb are two major targets of the E6 and E7 oncoproteins, but other cellular proteins are also involved in cell transformation. Moreover, E5 plays a supplementary role in development of cancers. Generally, improved model systems to study the HPV life cycle as well as the differences between the high-risk and low-risk HPV types will be necessary to progress our understanding from the role of early proteins in the HPV life cycle.

CONFLICT OF INTEREST

The author (editor) declares no conflict of interest, financial or otherwise.

ACKNOWLEDGEMENT

Declare none.

REFERENCES

[1] Krueger H, Stuart G, Gallagher R, Williams D. HPV and other infectious agents in cancer. Oxford University Press 2010; pp. 3-129.

[2] Wang JW, Roden RB. L2, the minor capsid protein of papillomavirus. Virology 2013; 445(1-2): 175-86.
[http://dx.doi.org/10.1016/j.virol.2013.04.017] [PMID: 23689062]

[3] zur Hausen H. Papillomaviruses and cancer: from basic studies to clinical application. Nat Rev Cancer 2002; 2(5): 342-50.
[http://dx.doi.org/10.1038/nrc798] [PMID: 12044010]

[4] Boscolo-Rizzo P, Del Mistro A, Bussu F, *et al.* New insights into human papillomavirus-associated head and neck squamous cell carcinoma. Acta Otorhinolaryngol Ital 2013; 33(2): 77-87.
[PMID: 23853396]

[5] Doorbar J, Quint W, Banks L, *et al.* The biology and life-cycle of human papillomaviruses. Vaccine 2012; 30 (Suppl. 5): F55-70.
[http://dx.doi.org/10.1016/j.vaccine.2012.06.083] [PMID: 23199966]

[6] Klingelhutz AJ, Roman A. Cellular transformation by human papillomaviruses: lessons learned by comparing high- and low-risk viruses. Virology 2012; 424(2): 77-98.
[http://dx.doi.org/10.1016/j.virol.2011.12.018] [PMID: 22284986]

[7] Yee C, Krishnan-Hewlett I, Baker CC, Schlegel R, Howley PM. Presence and expression of human papillomavirus sequences in human cervical carcinoma cell lines. Am J Pathol 1985; 119(3): 361-6.
[PMID: 2990217]

[8] Buck CB, Day PM, Trus BL. The papillomavirus major capsid protein L1. Virology 2013; 445(1-2): 169-74.
[http://dx.doi.org/10.1016/j.virol.2013.05.038] [PMID: 23800545]

[9] Schiller JT, Lowy DR. Understanding and learning from the success of prophylactic human papillomavirus vaccines. Nat Rev Microbiol 2012; 10(10): 681-92.
[http://dx.doi.org/10.1038/nrmicro2872] [PMID: 22961341]

[10] Wang X, Meyers C, Wang HK, Chow LT, Zheng ZM. Construction of a full transcription map of human papillomavirus type 18 during productive viral infection. J Virol 2011; 85(16): 8080-92.
[http://dx.doi.org/10.1128/JVI.00670-11] [PMID: 21680515]

[11] Doorbar J, Gallimore PH. Identification of proteins encoded by the L1 and L2 open reading frames of human papillomavirus 1a. J Virol 1987; 61(9): 2793-9.
[PMID: 3039170]

[12] Marusic MB, Mencin N, Licen M, Banks L, Grm HS. Modification of human papillomavirus minor capsid protein L2 by sumoylation. J Virol 2010; 84(21): 11585-9.
[http://dx.doi.org/10.1128/JVI.01269-10] [PMID: 20739540]

[13] Buck CB, Cheng N, Thompson CD, *et al.* Arrangement of L2 within the papillomavirus capsid. J Virol 2008; 82(11): 5190-7.
[http://dx.doi.org/10.1128/JVI.02726-07] [PMID: 18367526]

[14] Buck CB, Trus BL. The papillomavirus virion: a machine built to hide molecular Achilles' heels. Adv Exp Med Biol 2012; 726: 403-22.
[http://dx.doi.org/10.1007/978-1-4614-0980-9_18] [PMID: 22297524]

[15] Finnen RL, Erickson KD, Chen XS, Garcea RL. Interactions between papillomavirus L1 and L2 capsid proteins. J Virol 2003; 77(8): 4818-26.
[http://dx.doi.org/10.1128/JVI.77.8.4818-4826.2003] [PMID: 12663788]

[16] Campos SK, Ozbun MA. Two highly conserved cysteine residues in HPV16 L2 form an intramolecular disulfide bond and are critical for infectivity in human keratinocytes. PLoS One 2009; 4(2): e4463.
[http://dx.doi.org/10.1371/journal.pone.0004463] [PMID: 19214230]

[17] Conway MJ, Alam S, Christensen ND, Meyers C. Overlapping and independent structural roles for human papillomavirus type 16 L2 conserved cysteines. Virology 2009; 393(2): 295-303.
[http://dx.doi.org/10.1016/j.virol.2009.08.010] [PMID: 19733888]

[18] Johnson KM, Kines RC, Roberts JN, Lowy DR, Schiller JT, Day PM. Role of heparan sulfate in attachment to and infection of the murine female genital tract by human papillomavirus. J Virol 2009; 83(5): 2067-74.
[http://dx.doi.org/10.1128/JVI.02190-08] [PMID: 19073722]

[19] Richards RM, Lowy DR, Schiller JT, Day PM. Cleavage of the papillomavirus minor capsid protein, L2, at a furin consensus site is necessary for infection. Proc Natl Acad Sci USA 2006; 103(5): 1522-7.
[http://dx.doi.org/10.1073/pnas.0508815103] [PMID: 16432208]

[20] Kines RC, Thompson CD, Lowy DR, Schiller JT, Day PM. The initial steps leading to papillomavirus infection occur on the basement membrane prior to cell surface binding. Proc Natl Acad Sci USA 2009; 106(48): 20458-63.
[http://dx.doi.org/10.1073/pnas.0908502106] [PMID: 19920181]

[21] Day PM, Lowy DR, Schiller JT. Papillomaviruses infect cells *via* a clathrin-dependent pathway. Virology 2003; 307(1): 1-11.
[http://dx.doi.org/10.1016/S0042-6822(02)00143-5] [PMID: 12667809]

[22] Day PM, Thompson CD, Schowalter RM, Lowy DR, Schiller JT. Identification of a role for the trans-Golgi network in human papillomavirus 16 pseudovirus infection. J Virol 2013; 87(7): 3862-70.
[http://dx.doi.org/10.1128/JVI.03222-12] [PMID: 23345514]

[23] Schäfer F, Florin L, Sapp M. DNA binding of L1 is required for human papillomavirus morphogenesis *in vivo*. Virology 2002; 295(1): 172-81.
[http://dx.doi.org/10.1006/viro.2002.1361] [PMID: 12033775]

[24] Buck CB, Pastrana DV, Lowy DR, Schiller JT. Efficient intracellular assembly of papillomaviral vectors. J Virol 2004; 78(2): 751-7.
[http://dx.doi.org/10.1128/JVI.78.2.751-757.2004] [PMID: 14694107]

[25] Holmgren SC, Patterson NA, Ozbun MA, Lambert PF. The minor capsid protein L2 contributes to two steps in the human papillomavirus type 31 life cycle. J Virol 2005; 79(7): 3938-48.
[http://dx.doi.org/10.1128/JVI.79.7.3938-3948.2005] [PMID: 15767396]

[26] Florin L, Becker KA, Lambert C, *et al.* Identification of a dynein interacting domain in the papillomavirus minor capsid protein l2. J Virol 2006; 80(13): 6691-6.
[http://dx.doi.org/10.1128/JVI.00057-06] [PMID: 16775357]

[27] Surviladze Z, Dziduszko A, Ozbun MA. Essential roles for soluble virion-associated heparan sulfonated proteoglycans and growth factors in human papillomavirus infections. PLoS Pathog 2012; 8(2): e1002519.
[http://dx.doi.org/10.1371/journal.ppat.1002519] [PMID: 22346752]

[28] Day PM, Schiller JT. The role of furin in papillomavirus infection. Future Microbiol 2009; 4(10): 1255-62.

[http://dx.doi.org/10.2217/fmb.09.86] [PMID: 19995186]

[29] Gambhira R, Karanam B, Jagu S, *et al.* A protective and broadly cross-neutralizing epitope of human papillomavirus L2. J Virol 2007; 81(24): 13927-31.
[http://dx.doi.org/10.1128/JVI.00936-07] [PMID: 17928339]

[30] Yang R, Day PM, Yutzy WH IV, Lin KY, Hung CF, Roden RB. Cell surface-binding motifs of L2 that facilitate papillomavirus infection. J Virol 2003; 77(6): 3531-41.
[http://dx.doi.org/10.1128/JVI.77.6.3531-3541.2003] [PMID: 12610128]

[31] Kurg R, Uusen P, Võsa L, Ustav M. Human papillomavirus E2 protein with single activation domain initiates HPV18 genome replication, but is not sufficient for long-term maintenance of virus genome. Virology 2010; 408(2): 159-66.
[http://dx.doi.org/10.1016/j.virol.2010.09.010] [PMID: 20940072]

[32] Woodham AW, Da Silva DM, Skeate JG, *et al.* The S100A10 subunit of the annexin A2 heterotetramer facilitates L2-mediated human papillomavirus infection. PLoS One 2012; 7(8): e43519.
[http://dx.doi.org/10.1371/journal.pone.0043519] [PMID: 22927980]

[33] Namvar A, Bolhassani A, Hashemi M. HPV16 L2 improves HPV16 L1 gene delivery as an important approach for vaccine design against cervical cancer. Bratisl Lek Listy (Tlacene Vyd) 2016; 117(3): 179-84.
[PMID: 26925750]

[34] Horvath CA, Boulet GA, Renoux VM, Delvenne PO, Bogers JP. Mechanisms of cell entry by human papillomaviruses: an overview. Virol J 2010; 7: 11.
[http://dx.doi.org/10.1186/1743-422X-7-11] [PMID: 20089191]

[35] Fahey LM, Raff AB, Da Silva DM, Kast WM. A major role for the minor capsid protein of human papillomavirus type 16 in immune escape. J Immunol 2009; 183(10): 6151-6.
[http://dx.doi.org/10.4049/jimmunol.0902145] [PMID: 19864613]

[36] Bienkowska-Haba M, Patel HD, Sapp M. Target cell cyclophilins facilitate human papillomavirus type 16 infection. PLoS Pathog 2009; 5(7): e1000524.
[http://dx.doi.org/10.1371/journal.ppat.1000524] [PMID: 19629175]

[37] Bienkowska-Haba M, Williams C, Kim SM, Garcea RL, Sapp M. Cyclophilins facilitate dissociation of the human papillomavirus type 16 capsid protein L1 from the L2/DNA complex following virus entry. J Virol 2012; 86(18): 9875-87.
[http://dx.doi.org/10.1128/JVI.00980-12] [PMID: 22761365]

[38] Bergant M, Banks L. SNX17 facilitates infection with diverse papillomavirus types. J Virol 2013; 87(2): 1270-3.
[http://dx.doi.org/10.1128/JVI.01991-12] [PMID: 23115288]

[39] Bossis I, Roden RB, Gambhira R, *et al.* Interaction of tSNARE syntaxin 18 with the papillomavirus minor capsid protein mediates infection. J Virol 2005; 79(11): 6723-31.
[http://dx.doi.org/10.1128/JVI.79.11.6723-6731.2005] [PMID: 15890910]

[40] Kämper N, Day PM, Nowak T, *et al.* A membrane-destabilizing peptide in capsid protein L2 is required for egress of papillomavirus genomes from endosomes. J Virol 2006; 80(2): 759-68.
[http://dx.doi.org/10.1128/JVI.80.2.759-768.2006] [PMID: 16378978]

[41] Bronnimann MP, Chapman JA, Park CK, Campos SK. A transmembrane domain and GxxxG motifs within L2 are essential for papillomavirus infection. J Virol 2013; 87(1): 464-73.
[http://dx.doi.org/10.1128/JVI.01539-12] [PMID: 23097431]

[42] Day PM, Roden RB, Lowy DR, Schiller JT. The papillomavirus minor capsid protein, L2, induces localization of the major capsid protein, L1, and the viral transcription/replication protein, E2, to PML oncogenic domains. J Virol 1998; 72(1): 142-50.
[PMID: 9420209]

[43] Pyeon D, Pearce SM, Lank SM, Ahlquist P, Lambert PF. Establishment of human papillomavirus

infection requires cell cycle progression. PLoS Pathog 2009; 5(2): e1000318. [http://dx.doi.org/10.1371/journal.ppat.1000318] [PMID: 19247434]

[44] Mamoor S, Onder Z, Karanam B, *et al.* The high risk HPV16 L2 minor capsid protein has multiple transport signals that mediate its nucleocytoplasmic traffic. Virology 2012; 422(2): 413-24. [http://dx.doi.org/10.1016/j.virol.2011.11.007] [PMID: 22154072]

[45] Bordeaux J, Forte S, Harding E, Darshan MS, Klucevsek K, Moroianu J. The l2 minor capsid protein of low-risk human papillomavirus type 11 interacts with host nuclear import receptors and viral DNA. J Virol 2006; 80(16): 8259-62. [http://dx.doi.org/10.1128/JVI.00776-06] [PMID: 16873281]

[46] Florin L, Becker KA, Sapp C, *et al.* Nuclear translocation of papillomavirus minor capsid protein L2 requires Hsc70. J Virol 2004; 78(11): 5546-53. [http://dx.doi.org/10.1128/JVI.78.11.5546-5553.2004] [PMID: 15140951]

[47] Schäfer F, Florin L, Sapp M. DNA binding of L1 is required for human papillomavirus morphogenesis *in vivo.* Virology 2002; 295(1): 172-81. [http://dx.doi.org/10.1006/viro.2002.1361] [PMID: 12033775]

[48] Buck CB, Pastrana DV, Lowy DR, Schiller JT. Efficient intracellular assembly of papillomaviral vectors. J Virol 2004; 78(2): 751-7. [http://dx.doi.org/10.1128/JVI.78.2.751-757.2004] [PMID: 14694107]

[49] Day PM, Baker CC, Lowy DR, Schiller JT. Establishment of papillomavirus infection is enhanced by promyelocytic leukemia protein (PML) expression. Proc Natl Acad Sci USA 2004; 101(39): 14252-7. [http://dx.doi.org/10.1073/pnas.0404229101] [PMID: 15383670]

[50] Heino P, Zhou J, Lambert PF. Interaction of the papillomavirus transcription/replication factor, E2, and the viral capsid protein, L2. Virology 2000; 276(2): 304-14. [http://dx.doi.org/10.1006/viro.2000.0342] [PMID: 11040122]

[51] Xue B, Williams RW, Oldfield CJ, Goh GK, Dunker AK, Uversky VN. Viral disorder or disordered viruses: do viral proteins possess unique features? Protein Pept Lett 2010; 17(8): 932-51. [http://dx.doi.org/10.2174/092986610791498984] [PMID: 20450483]

[52] Amarakoon GU, Fathima F. An overview of human papillomavirus. World Scientific News 2016; 53(3): 275-308.

[53] Kurg R, Uusen P, Võsa L, Ustav M. Human papillomavirus E2 protein with single activation domain initiates HPV18 genome replication, but is not sufficient for long-term maintenance of virus genome. Virology 2010; 408(2): 159-66. [http://dx.doi.org/10.1016/j.virol.2010.09.010] [PMID: 20940072]

[54] McBride AA. The papillomavirus E2 proteins. Virology 2013; 445(1-2): 57-79. [http://dx.doi.org/10.1016/j.virol.2013.06.006] [PMID: 23849793]

[55] Knight GL, Pugh AG, Yates E, *et al.* A cyclin-binding motif in human papillomavirus type 18 (HPV18) E1^E4 is necessary for association with CDK-cyclin complexes and G2/M cell cycle arrest of keratinocytes, but is not required for differentiation-dependent viral genome amplification or L1 capsid protein expression. Virology 2011; 412(1): 196-210. [http://dx.doi.org/10.1016/j.virol.2011.01.007] [PMID: 21276999]

[56] Maufort JP, Williams SM, Pitot HC, Lambert PF. Human papillomavirus 16 E5 oncogene contributes to two stages of skin carcinogenesis. Cancer Res 2007; 67(13): 6106-12. [http://dx.doi.org/10.1158/0008-5472.CAN-07-0921] [PMID: 17616666]

[57] Maufort JP, Shai A, Pitot HC, Lambert PF. A role for HPV16 E5 in cervical carcinogenesis. Cancer Res 2010; 70(7): 2924-31. [http://dx.doi.org/10.1158/0008-5472.CAN-09-3436] [PMID: 20332225]

[58] Bouvard V, Matlashewski G, Gu ZM, Storey A, Banks L. The human papillomavirus type 16 E5 gene cooperates with the E7 gene to stimulate proliferation of primary cells and increases viral gene

expression. Virology 1994; 203(1): 73-80.
[http://dx.doi.org/10.1006/viro.1994.1456] [PMID: 8030286]

[59] Straight SW, Hinkle PM, Jewers RJ, McCance DJ. The E5 oncoprotein of human papillomavirus type 16 transforms fibroblasts and effects the downregulation of the epidermal growth factor receptor in keratinocytes. J Virol 1993; 67(8): 4521-32.
[PMID: 8392596]

[60] Conrad M, Bubb VJ, Schlegel R. The human papillomavirus type 6 and 16 E5 proteins are membrane-associated proteins which associate with the 16-kilodalton pore-forming protein. J Virol 1993; 67(10): 6170-8.
[PMID: 7690419]

[61] Straight SW, Herman B, McCance DJ. The E5 oncoprotein of human papillomavirus type 16 inhibits the acidification of endosomes in human keratinocytes. J Virol 1995; 69(5): 3185-92.
[PMID: 7707548]

[62] Suprynowicz FA, Krawczyk E, Hebert JD, *et al.* The human papillomavirus type 16 E5 oncoprotein inhibits epidermal growth factor trafficking independently of endosome acidification. J Virol 2010; 84(20): 10619-29.
[http://dx.doi.org/10.1128/JVI.00831-10] [PMID: 20686024]

[63] Greco D, Kivi N, Qian K, Leivonen SK, Auvinen P, Auvinen E. Human papillomavirus 16 E5 modulates the expression of host microRNAs. PLoS One 2011; 6(7): e21646.
[http://dx.doi.org/10.1371/journal.pone.0021646] [PMID: 21747943]

[64] Nicolaides L, Davy C, Raj K, Kranjec C, Banks L, Doorbar J. Stabilization of HPV16 E6 protein by PDZ proteins, and potential implications for genome maintenance. Virology 2011; 414(2): 137-45.
[http://dx.doi.org/10.1016/j.virol.2011.03.017] [PMID: 21489588]

[65] Howley PM, Lowy DR. Papillomaviruses. Fields Virology ppincott. Philadelphia: Williams & Wilkins 2007; pp. 2299-354.

[66] Chen JJ, Hong Y, Rustamzadeh E, Baleja JD, Androphy EJ. Identification of an alpha helical motif sufficient for association with papillomavirus E6. J Biol Chem 1998; 273(22): 13537-44.
[http://dx.doi.org/10.1074/jbc.273.22.13537] [PMID: 9593689]

[67] Nominé Y, Masson M, Charbonnier S, *et al.* Structural and functional analysis of E6 oncoprotein: insights in the molecular pathways of human papillomavirus-mediated pathogenesis. Mol Cell 2006; 21(5): 665-78.
[http://dx.doi.org/10.1016/j.molcel.2006.01.024] [PMID: 16507364]

[68] Uversky VN, Roman A, Oldfield CJ, Dunker AK. Protein intrinsic disorder and human papillomaviruses: increased amount of disorder in E6 and E7 oncoproteins from high risk HPVs. J Proteome Res 2006; 5(8): 1829-42.
[http://dx.doi.org/10.1021/pr0602388] [PMID: 16889404]

[69] Bedell MA, Jones KH, Grossman SR, Laimins LA. Identification of human papillomavirus type 18 transforming genes in immortalized and primary cells. J Virol 1989; 63(3): 1247-55.
[PMID: 2536832]

[70] Guccione E, Massimi P, Bernat A, Banks L. Comparative analysis of the intracellular location of the high- and low-risk human papillomavirus oncoproteins. Virology 2002; 293(1): 20-5.
[http://dx.doi.org/10.1006/viro.2001.1290] [PMID: 11853395]

[71] Storey A, Banks L. Human papillomavirus type 16 E6 gene cooperates with EJ-ras to immortalize primary mouse cells. Oncogene 1993; 8(4): 919-24.
[PMID: 8384359]

[72] Pim D, Banks L. HPV-18 E6*I protein modulates the E6-directed degradation of p53 by binding to full-length HPV-18 E6. Oncogene 1999; 18(52): 7403-8.
[http://dx.doi.org/10.1038/sj.onc.1203134] [PMID: 10602499]

[73] Kiyono T, Foster SA, Koop JI, McDougall JK, Galloway DA, Klingelhutz AJ. Both Rb/p16INK4a inactivation and telomerase activity are required to immortalize human epithelial cells. Nature 1998; 396(6706): 84-8.
[http://dx.doi.org/10.1038/23962] [PMID: 9817205]

[74] Crook T, Tidy JA, Vousden KH. Degradation of p53 can be targeted by HPV E6 sequences distinct from those required for p53 binding and trans-activation. Cell 1991; 67(3): 547-56.
[http://dx.doi.org/10.1016/0092-8674(91)90529-8] [PMID: 1657399]

[75] Klingelhutz AJ, Roman A. Cellular transformation by human papillomaviruses: lessons learned by comparing high- and low-risk viruses. Virology 2012; 424(2): 77-98.
[http://dx.doi.org/10.1016/j.virol.2011.12.018] [PMID: 22284986]

[76] Sun Y, Jiang X, Price BD. Tip60: connecting chromatin to DNA damage signaling. Cell Cycle 2010; 9(5): 930-6.
[http://dx.doi.org/10.4161/cc.9.5.10931] [PMID: 20160506]

[77] Thomas M, Banks L. Human papillomavirus (HPV) E6 interactions with Bak are conserved amongst E6 proteins from high and low risk HPV types. J Gen Virol 1999; 80(Pt 6): 1513-7.
[http://dx.doi.org/10.1099/0022-1317-80-6-1513] [PMID: 10374970]

[78] Spanos WC, Hoover A, Harris GF, *et al.* The PDZ binding motif of human papillomavirus type 16 E6 induces PTPN13 loss, which allows anchorage-independent growth and synergizes with ras for invasive growth. J Virol 2008; 82(5): 2493-500.
[http://dx.doi.org/10.1128/JVI.02188-07] [PMID: 18160445]

[79] Hoover AC, Strand GL, Nowicki PN, *et al.* Impaired PTPN13 phosphatase activity in spontaneous or HPV-induced squamous cell carcinomas potentiates oncogene signaling through the MAP kinase pathway. Oncogene 2009; 28(45): 3960-70.
[http://dx.doi.org/10.1038/onc.2009.251] [PMID: 19734941]

[80] Alfandari J, Shnitman Magal S, Jackman A, Schlegel R, Gonen P, Sherman L. HPV16 E6 oncoprotein inhibits apoptosis induced during serum-calcium differentiation of foreskin human keratinocytes. Virology 1999; 257(2): 383-96.
[http://dx.doi.org/10.1006/viro.1999.9675] [PMID: 10329549]

[81] James MA, Lee JH, Klingelhutz AJ. Human papillomavirus type 16 E6 activates NF-kappaB, induces cIAP-2 expression, and protects against apoptosis in a PDZ binding motif-dependent manner. J Virol 2006; 80(11): 5301-7.
[http://dx.doi.org/10.1128/JVI.01942-05] [PMID: 16699010]

[82] Guccione E, Lethbridge KJ, Killick N, Leppard KN, Banks L. HPV E6 proteins interact with specific PML isoforms and allow distinctions to be made between different POD structures. Oncogene 2004; 23(27): 4662-72.
[http://dx.doi.org/10.1038/sj.onc.1207631] [PMID: 15107834]

[83] Nakahara T, Lambert PF. Induction of promyelocytic leukemia (PML) oncogenic domains (PODs) by papillomavirus. Virology 2007; 366(2): 316-29.
[http://dx.doi.org/10.1016/j.virol.2007.04.032] [PMID: 17543368]

[84] Nees M, Geoghegan JM, Hyman T, Frank S, Miller L, Woodworth CD. Papillomavirus type 16 oncogenes downregulate expression of interferon-responsive genes and upregulate proliferation-associated and NF-kappaB-responsive genes in cervical keratinocytes. J Virol 2001; 75(9): 4283-96.
[http://dx.doi.org/10.1128/JVI.75.9.4283-4296.2001] [PMID: 11287578]

[85] Xu M, Luo W, Elzi DJ, Grandori C, Galloway DA. NFX1 interacts with mSin3A/histone deacetylase to repress hTERT transcription in keratinocytes. Mol Cell Biol 2008; 28(15): 4819-28.
[http://dx.doi.org/10.1128/MCB.01969-07] [PMID: 18505829]

[86] Firzlaff JM, Lüscher B, Eisenman RN. Negative charge at the casein kinase II phosphorylation site is important for transformation but not for Rb protein binding by the E7 protein of human papillomavirus

type 16. Proc Natl Acad Sci USA 1991; 88(12): 5187-91.
[http://dx.doi.org/10.1073/pnas.88.12.5187] [PMID: 2052600]

[87] Zheng ZM, Wang X. Regulation of cellular miRNA expression by human papillomaviruses. Biochim Biophys Acta 2011; 1809(11-12): 668-77.
[http://dx.doi.org/10.1016/j.bbagrm.2011.05.005] [PMID: 21616186]

[88] Riley RR, Duensing S, Brake T, Münger K, Lambert PF, Arbeit JM. Dissection of human papillomavirus E6 and E7 function in transgenic mouse models of cervical carcinogenesis. Cancer Res 2003; 63(16): 4862-71.
[PMID: 12941807]

[89] Zheng ZM. Regulation of cellular miRNA expression by human papillomaviruses. Biochimica et Biophysica Acta 2011; 1809: 668-77.

[90] Lewis BP, Burge CB, Bartel DP. Conserved seed pairing, often flanked by adenosines, indicates that thousands of human genes are microRNA targets. Cell 2005; 120(1): 15-20.
[http://dx.doi.org/10.1016/j.cell.2004.12.035] [PMID: 15652477]

[91] Selbach M, Schwanhäusser B, Thierfelder N, Fang Z, Khanin R, Rajewsky N. Widespread changes in protein synthesis induced by microRNAs. Nature 2008; 455(7209): 58-63.
[http://dx.doi.org/10.1038/nature07228] [PMID: 18668040]

[92] Cullen BR. Viruses and microRNAs. Nat Genet 2006; 38 (Suppl.): S25-30.
[http://dx.doi.org/10.1038/ng1793] [PMID: 16736021]

[93] McMurray HR, McCance DJ. Human papillomavirus type 16 E6 activates TERT gene transcription through induction of c-Myc and release of USF-mediated repression. J Virol 2003; 77(18): 9852-61.
[http://dx.doi.org/10.1128/JVI.77.18.9852-9861.2003] [PMID: 12941894]

[94] Gewin L, Galloway DA. E box-dependent activation of telomerase by human papillomavirus type 16 E6 does not require induction of c-myc. J Virol 2001; 75(15): 7198-201.
[http://dx.doi.org/10.1128/JVI.75.15.7198-7201.2001] [PMID: 11435602]

[95] Blackwood EM, Eisenman RN. Max: a helix-loop-helix zipper protein that forms a sequence-specific DNA-binding complex with Myc. Science 1991; 251(4998): 1211-7.
[http://dx.doi.org/10.1126/science.2006410] [PMID: 2006410]

[96] Chang TC, Yu D, Lee YS, *et al.* Widespread microRNA repression by Myc contributes to tumorigenesis. Nat Genet 2008; 40(1): 43-50.
[http://dx.doi.org/10.1038/ng.2007.30] [PMID: 18066065]

[97] Beno I, Rosenthal K, Levitine M, Shaulov L, Haran TE. Sequence-dependent cooperative binding of p53 to DNA targets and its relationship to the structural properties of the DNA targets. Nucleic Acids Res 2011; 39(5): 1919-32.
[http://dx.doi.org/10.1093/nar/gkq1044] [PMID: 21071400]

[98] Brosh R, Shalgi R, Liran A, *et al.* p53-Repressed miRNAs are involved with E2F in a feed-forward loop promoting proliferation. Mol Syst Biol 2008; 4: 229.
[http://dx.doi.org/10.1038/msb.2008.65] [PMID: 19034270]

[99] Ou YH, Chung PH, Hsu FF, Sun TP, Chang WY, Shieh SY. The candidate tumor suppressor BTG3 is a transcriptional target of p53 that inhibits E2F1. EMBO J 2007; 26(17): 3968-80.
[http://dx.doi.org/10.1038/sj.emboj.7601825] [PMID: 17690688]

[100] Suzuki HI, Yamagata K, Sugimoto K, Iwamoto T, Kato S, Miyazono K. Modulation of microRNA processing by p53. Nature 2009; 460(7254): 529-33.
[http://dx.doi.org/10.1038/nature08199] [PMID: 19626115]

[101] O'Donnell KA, Wentzel EA, Zeller KI, Dang CV, Mendell JT. c-Myc-regulated microRNAs modulate E2F1 expression. Nature 2005; 435(7043): 839-43.
[http://dx.doi.org/10.1038/nature03677] [PMID: 15944709]

[102] Petrocca F, Visone R, Onelli MR, *et al.* E2F1-regulated microRNAs impair TGFbeta-dependent cell-cycle arrest and apoptosis in gastric cancer. Cancer Cell 2008; 13(3): 272-86. [http://dx.doi.org/10.1016/j.ccr.2008.02.013] [PMID: 18328430]

[103] Munoz N, Castellsague X, de Gonzalez AB, Gissmann L. Chapter 1: HPV in the etiology of human cancer. Vaccine 2006; 24: S3/1–3/10.

[104] No JH, Kim MK, Jeon YT, Kim YB, Song YS. Human papillomavirus vaccine: widening the scope for cancer prevention. Mol Carcinog 2011; 50(4): 244-53. [http://dx.doi.org/10.1002/mc.20657] [PMID: 21465574]

[105] Lin K, Doolan K, Hung CF, Wu TC. Perspectives for preventive and therapeutic HPV vaccines. J Formos Med Assoc 2010; 109(1): 4-24. [http://dx.doi.org/10.1016/S0929-6646(10)60017-4] [PMID: 20123582]

[106] de Sanjosé S, Alemany L. HPV and cancer: Epidemiology and mechanism of carcinogenesis of the virus HPV.Tropical Hemato-Oncology. Springer International Publishing 2015; pp. 143-56. [http://dx.doi.org/10.1007/978-3-319-18257-5_16]

[107] Stanley M. Pathology and epidemiology of HPV infection in females. Gynecol Oncol 2010; 117(2) (Suppl.): S5-S10. [http://dx.doi.org/10.1016/j.ygyno.2010.01.024] [PMID: 20304221]

CHAPTER 3

Types of Benign or Malignant Diseases Associated with HPV Infections

Kimia Kardani and **Azam Bolhassani***

Department of Pharmaceutical Biotechnology, School of Pharmacy, Shahid Beheshti University of Medical Sciences, Tehran, Iran

Department of Hepatitis and AIDS, Pasteur Institute of Iran, Tehran, Iran

Abstract: During the last years, several researchers have properly focused on classifying variants of human papillomaviruses (HPVs). HPV variants are different in their biological, molecular and chemical properties. Thus, this genomic diversity can represent differences in the natural history and pathogenicity of HPVs. For instance, high-risk HPV variants such as HPVs 16 and 18 can confer various risks of viral persistence in the human cervix and cause cervical cancer. Moreover, low-risk HPV variants including HPVs 6 and 11 can play an important role in the development of anogenital and cutaneous warts, and recurrent respiratory papillomatosis (RRP). Herein, we will discuss main and novel types of HPVs and their correlation with intensity of diseases.

Keywords: Benign disease, Genomic diversity, High-risk HPV, Low-risk HPV, Malignant disease.

INTRODUCTION

HPVs are small double-stranded DNA viruses that infect cutaneous and mucosal epithelial tissues [1, 2]. In general, HPVs generate a wide range of diseases from benign lesions (or papillomas) to invasive tumors in the anogenital tract, oropharynx, and skin [3 - 7]. Persistent infection with HPV can cause a variety of tumors in vagina, vulva, penis, anus, head and neck [8]. HPVs are classified into three major groups: cutaneous (skin), mucocutaneous and epidermodysplasia verruciformis (EV) [9].

The cutaneous HPV types are commonly found in several skin lesions such as benign skin warts, actinic keratosis (AKs), non-melanoma skin cancers (NMSCs) and keratoacanthomas (KAs) [3, 10 - 12]. The mucocutaneous HPV types can be

* **Corresponding author Azam Bolhassani:** Department of Hepatitis and AIDS, Pasteur Institute of Iran, Tehran, Iran; Tel: 66953311-20; E-mails: A_bolhasani@pasteur.ac.ir, azam.bolhassani@yahoo.com

divided into low-risk (LR-HPV) mainly associated with benign warts (*i.e.,* HPV 6, 11) and high-risk (HR-HPV) accompanied by their risk of progression to malignancy (*i.e.,* HPV 16, 18, 31, 33, 45) [7, 9]. Among different types of HPVs, HPV16 and HPV18 showed the highest oncogenic risk [1, 2]. Primary experiments indicated that HR-HPVs can cooperate with activated ras to transform primary rodent cells, but low-risk HPVs cannot. In addition, other authors reported that LR-HPVs can cooperate with ras to transform primary rodent cells requiring more time in culture [7]. The IARC Working Group has classified HPV types 16, 18, 31, 33, 35, 39, 45, 51, 52, 56, 58, 59 as carcinogenic and type 68 as likely carcinogenic to humans in different genital and mucosal regions of body [13]. Table **1** shows some major HPV types in two categories including high-risk and low-risk HPV types.

Table 1. Major high-risk and low-risk HPV types [5, 37 - 39].

HPV type	HPV species	IARC classification	HPV broad risk categories	International Agency for Research on Cancer (Vol 100B)	Disease	Tropism	Relative contribution in cervical cancer (%)
HPV16	Alpha-9	1	High risk	Carcinogenic to humans	-Anogenital cancers and precancers -Oral papillomas -Oropharyngeal carcinoma	Mucosal	96.9
HPV18	Alpha-7	1	High risk	Carcinogenic to humans	-Anogenital cancers and precancers -Oral papillomas -Oropharyngeal carcinoma	Mucosal	96.9
HPV45	Alpha-7	1	High risk	Carcinogenic to humans	-Anogenital cancers and precancers	Mucosal	96.9
HPV33	Alpha-9	1	High risk	Carcinogenic to humans	-Anogenital cancers and precancers	Mucosal	96.9
HPV31	Alpha-9	1	High risk	Carcinogenic to humans	-Anogenital cancers and precancers	Mucosal	96.9
HPV39	Alpha-7	1	High risk	Carcinogenic to humans	-Epidermodysplasia verruciformis	Mucosal	96.9
HPV51	Alpha-5	1	High risk	Carcinogenic to humans	-Anogenital cancers and precancers	Mucosal	96.9
HPV52	Alpha-9	1	High risk	Carcinogenic to humans	-Anogenital cancers and precancers	Mucosal	96.9
HPV68	Alpha-7	2A	High risk	Probably carcinogenic to humans	-Anogenital cancers and precancers	Mucosal	0.7
HPV26	Alpha-5	2B	High risk	Possibly carcinogenic to humans	-Anogenital cancers and precancers	Mucosal	1.3

(Table 1) contd.....

HPV type	HPV species	IARC classification	HPV broad risk categories	International Agency for Research on Cancer (Vol 100B)	Disease	Tropism	Relative contribution in cervical cancer (%)
HPV69	Alpha-5	2B	High risk	Possibly carcinogenic to humans	-Anogenital cancers and precancers	Mucosal	0,5
HPV5	Beta-1	2B	High risk	Possibly carcinogenic to humans	-Epidermodysplasia verruciformis		0
HPV8	Beta-1	2B	High risk	Possibly carcinogenic to humans	-Epidermodysplasia verruciformis		0
HPV6	Alpha-10	3	Low risk		-Anogenital warts -Laryngeal papillomas -Oral papillomas	Mucosal	0.1
HPV11	Alpha-10	3	Low risk		-Anogenital warts -Laryngeal papillomas -Oral papillomas	Mucosal	0.1

Five Genera of HPVs

Cutaneous HPVs indicate more than 75% of the HPV types and are divided into five different genera such as alpha-papillomavirus (α-PV), beta-papillomavirus (β-PV), gamma-papillomavirus (γ-PV), mu-papillomavirus (μ-PV) and nu-papillomavirus (ν-PV). This classification is based on DNA sequence analysis and different life-cycle properties [14 - 16]. Up to now, 200 different HPV types belonging to 49 species have been recognized by the International HPV Reference Center.

At present, there is no reference centre for animal papillomavirus types. According to the papillomavirus episteme (PaVE) database, 131 animal PV types exist, identified from 66 different animal species. Among the characterized HPV types, about 60 types were predominantly detected in mucosal epithelia and classified in the genus alpha-papillomavirus [17, 18]. The studies showed that the beta and gamma genera cause asymptomatic infections in immunocompetent individuals as detected in skin swabs, and sometimes in mucosal rinses for gamma types [19, 20]. The alpha-PVs are divided into cutaneous and mucosal/genital types, and the mucosal types are further subdivided into high-risk and low-risk groups [14, 16]. The cutaneous alpha types are low-risk, *e.g.,* HPV 2 and 57, which cause common warts, and HPV 3 and 10, which generate flat warts [14]. Human alpha-PV infections are involved in the development of both benign (*e.g.,* condylomata acuminatum/respiratory papillomatosis) and malignant (*e.g.,* cervical/anal/head and neck cancers) diseases [17, 21]. The beta types, notably HPV5 and HPV8, are typically asymptomatic in healthy individuals, but have been associated with non-melanoma squamous cell carcinoma (SCC) in patients with epidermodysplasia verruciformis [22 - 24]. The most well studied HPV types are the mucosal alpha types that cause cervical cancer [4, 15].

Low-Risk HPV Types

Some HPV types have a low prevalence in cervical cancers. They are classified as carcinogenic (HPV 26, 30, 34, 53, 66, 67, 69, 70, 73, 82, 85) or non-carcinogenic (low-risk) viruses [13]. Some of the other 'low-risk' HPVs from genus alpha cause genital warts and are infrequently associated with cancer. In contrast, the HPVs from genus beta infect the cutaneous epithelium [18]. The low-risk mucosal types, which despite their name can also cause cutaneous genital lesions, do not typically generate neoplasia [25]. Low-risk types 6 and 11 are not thought to cause cancer, but cause more than 90% of genital warts as well as respiratory papillomatosis (RRP) [8, 26, 27]. Furthermore, low-risk HPVs including HPV 6, 11, 40, 42, 43, 44 54, 61, 70, 72 and 81 can cause low-grade lesions such as benign cervical lesions and are rarely found in malignancies [6, 28].

High-Risk HPV Types

Most of the alpha-HPV types infect mucosal tissues, and a subset of the alpha HPVs are the 'high-risk' types that cause cervical cancer and other anogenital cancers [17, 18]. Twelve HPVs (16, 18, 31, 33, 35, 39, 45, 51, 52, 56, 58, and 59) were defined by the World Health Organization (WHO) as being high-risk cancer causing types, with additional types (68, 73) being recognized as 'possibly' cancer-causing [4]. HPV types 16 and 18 account for 50% and 20% of cervical carcinomas, respectively [22]. There is convincing data that HPV16 variants influence persistence, progression to pre-cancer, development of cancer and histologic type of cervix cancer. Most studies implicated the non-European (NE) lineages as being more pathogenic in comparison with isolates from the European (E) lineage [17]. In general, the most common high-risk HPV types such as HPV16, HPV18, HPV31, HPV33 and HPV35 are estimated to cause about 99% of cervical cancers, 25%-60% of head and neck cancers, 70% of vaginal cancers, 88% of anal cancers, 43% vulvar and 50% of penile cancers [29 - 32]. Recent studies suggest that variant lineages may differ in the risk of persistence and association with high-grade disease [16].

Novel Papillomaviruses

HPV125

HPV125 was initially identified in 2004 as isolate SIBX9 in a hand common wart obtained from a 19-year-old immunocompetent patient, and completely characterized in 2011. HPV125 is phylogenetically classified in the α-PV genus, species α-2, etiologically causing skin warts [17].

HPV150 and HPV151

These novel HPV types were initially identified in 2005 as isolates SIBX1 and SIBX2, respectively, in the eyebrows of patients with anogenital warts and completely characterized as novel β-PV types in 2011. Phylogenetically, HPV150 clusters to species β-5 and is most closely related to HPV96, whereas HPV151 clusters to species β-2 and is most closely related to HPV22. Both novel types were further detected in hair follicles and benign and malignant skin neoplasms as single or multiple infections, usually with low viral loads [17].

HPV120

HPV120 was initially identified in 2005 as isolate SIBX3 in the eyebrows of a patient with anogenital warts. The complete viral genome, phylogenetically placed in the β-PV genus, species β-2 (its closest relative is HPV23), was characterized simultaneously in 2012 from an anal canal sample of patient with anogenital warts in Slovenia and from oral cavity samples of patients with prostate cancer in the USA. HPV120 has further been detected in heterogeneous human biological niches, including the oral cavity, eyebrow hairs, anal canal and penile, vulvar and perianal warts, indicating a broader spectrum of epithelial tropism than previously reported for β-PVs [17].

HPV159

HPV159 was initially identified in 2006 as isolate SIBX8 in anogenital hair follicles, and completely characterized 7 years later from the anal canal sample of a patient suffering from anogenital warts. HPV159, which exhibits both cutaneous and mucosal tropism, is phylogenetically placed in the β-PV genus, species β-2, and is most closely related to HPV9 [17].

HPV174

HPV174 was completely characterized in 2013 from a cutaneous squamous cell carcinoma sample containing HPV9 and HPV150. HPV174 belongs to the β-PV genus, species β-2, and is most closely related to HPV145 [17].

HPV179 and HPV184

These HPVs were initially identified in 2013 as isolates SIBX16 and SIBX17 from two distinct facial common warts of a 64-year-old renal-transplant recipient and completely characterized in 2014. HPV179 and HPV184 are taxonomically placed within the γ-PV genus. HPV179 is a novel member of species γ-15 (additionally containing HPV135 and HPV146), whereas HPV184 is a single member of a novel species γ-25. HPV179 and HPV184 are relatively rare HPV types etiologically linked to common warts [17].

HPV199

HPV199 was initially identified in 2013 as isolate KC82 (GenBank Accession No. KC752084) from a skin swab sample of healthy individual in China and completely characterized in 2014 from a nasopharyngeal swab sample of a 25-year-old immunocompetent Slovenian patient. HPV199 belongs to the γ-PV genus, species γ-12, and is most closely related to HPV127 [17]. Its potential clinical importance and tissue tropism are underway.

HPV204

HPV204 was initially identified in 2009 as isolate GC03 (GenBank Accession No. FJ947082) from a skin swab sample of healthy individual in Argentina, and was completely characterized in 2014 from anogenital warts of a 42-year-old immunocompetent Slovenian patient. HPV204 is phylogenetically positioned in the μ-PV genus as a new type. Its potential clinical importance and tissue tropism is in progress [17].

PsuPV1

Recently, the first PV-Phodopus sungorus papillomavirus type 1, PsuPV1, whose natural host is the Siberian hamster (Phodopus sungorus) has been identified. PsuPV1 is taxonomically placed in the πi-PV genus, currently consisting of PV types isolated from various rodent species, including Syrian hamster, various mouse species and Brown rat (Rattus norvegicus). PsuPV1 is most closely related to MaPV1 isolated from the oral cavity of a Syrian hamster (Mesocricetus auratus) [17].

HPV153

HPV153 species γ-13 was originally identified by FAP-PCR from a genital wart swab sample [17].

HPV154

HPV154 species γ-11 was first identified by FAP-PCR from a swab of a wart at the intergluteal cleft of a three-year-old boy. HPV154 has been detected in 3% (2/62) of forehead skin swabs from healthy children [17].

HPV180

HPV180 species γ-10, initially designated FA69, was identified in 2003 by FAP-PCR from healthy skin and several years later by whole genomic amplification of DNA isolated from a genital wart swab sample [17].

HPV155

HPV155 species γ-7, initially designated isolate SE42, was identified by metagenomic analysis of an actinic keratosis swab sample. Further studies revealed that HPV155 is present in 1.1% (4/341) and 2.1% (7/341) of swab samples obtained from various skin lesions and healthy skin, respectively [17].

HPV175

HPV175 species γ-23, initially designated isolate SE87, was identified by the next generation sequencing (NGS) from a genital wart swab sample [17].

HPV178

HPV178 species γ-24 was obtained from a swab sample of healthy skin, adjacent to an actinic keratosis, after an attempt to amplify the closely related SE46 isolate [17].

HPV197

HPV197 species γ-24, initially designated isolate SE46, was identified as a complete genome by NGS from a tissue sample of cutaneous squamous cell carcinoma [17].

HPV198 and HPV203

HPV198 species β-2 and HPV203, initially designated SE22 and SE3, respectively, were identified by NGS of FAP amplicons from frozen biopsies of actinic keratosis and squamous cell carcinoma, respectively [17].

HPV200, HPV201 and HPV202

HPV200 species γ-2, HPV201 species γ-27 and HPV202 species γ-11 identified by NGS in swab samples of genital warts were initially 'HPV-negative' by PCR [17].

Diseases Associated with HPV Infection

Various types of epithelial diseases caused by HPVs (*i.e.*, chronic asymptomatic infection or transient visible papillomas) are associated with their transmission and propagation within the epithelium and their interactions with the immune system [33, 34]. Several diseases related to HPV infections will be described in following:

HPV in External Skin

Cutaneous warts are spread either by direct contact from person to person or indirectly by contact with contaminated surfaces or objects [9]. Histologically, warts are benign lesions, with hypertrophy of all layers of the dermis. Vacuolation of cells occurs in the upper layers and inclusion bodies are sometimes observed. Warts usually disappear spontaneously but occasionally may be resistant to treatment [9].

Anogenital Warts

Anogenital warts reveal as multiple flesh-colored, exophytic papillomatous lesions. In men, anogenital warts commonly involve the coronal sulcus, the glans of the penis, penile shaft and perianal region, and in women involve the external genitalia. They influence about 1% of the sexually active population in the world [21].

Laryngeal Papillomatosis

Laryngeal papillomatosis, also known as recurrent respiratory papillomatosis, is a relatively rare but debilitating disease characterized by repeated growth of benign squamous cell papillomas in the upper respiratory tract, with a tendency to the larynx [21]. The overall mortality rate with laryngeal papillomatosis ranges from 4% to 14%. Laryngeal papillomas can occur before the age of five without gender preference (juvenile-onset laryngeal papillomatosis), and also between the ages of 20 and 40 with a slight male predominance (adult-onset laryngeal papillomatosis) [21].

Common Warts of Hands and Face

Common warts are usually exophytic, multiple, irregular, rough nodules which show a variety of clinical patterns on skin surfaces at different sites of body including fingers, hands, elbows and knees. Common warts are most frequently caused by HPV-2 and HPV-4 and sometimes by HPV- 3, -10, -28 and -7 [9]. Histologically, common warts showed major papillomatosis, acanthosis, hypergranulosis and hyperkeratosis. HPV-2 warts are persistent, especially when present as more superficial 'mosaic' warts. Plane warts caused by HPVs 3, 10 and 28 are small and flat-topped papules [9]. Plane warts exhibited an unusual phenomenon including spontaneous regression of lesions, likely due to T-cell infiltration and activated Langerhans cells. In adults, plane warts are more frequent in women but are rarely observed in men except those who are immunosuppressed by HIV infection. Topical salicylic acid solutions are effective for most cutaneous warts as the first line therapy, followed by cryotherapy with dry ice or liquid nitrogen for disruptive warts [9].

Plantar Warts

Plantar warts rarely occur before the age of 5 years and have a peak distribution at 10-14 years. Activities which cause maceration of the skin such as swimming provide an additional risk of transmission [9]. Deep plantar warts caused by HPV-1 or HPV-63 occur frequently on weight-bearing areas or pressure points of the feet. Deep plantar warts are painful, but their response to treatment is generally good. In contrast, warts caused by HPV-2 and HPV-4, which have a superficial mosaic pattern tend to be less painful, but are more persistent and respond poorly to treatment. The rare HPV types 57 and 60 are also associated with plantar lesions such as epidermoid cysts. The HPV-60 sometimes pigmented due to melanin granules in the keratinocytes [9].

Epidermodysplasia Verruciformis

Epidermodysplasia verruciformis (EV) is a rare autosomal recessive condition linked to mutation in one of two genes (EVER1 and EVER2) on the long arm of chromosome 17, in which selective depletion of specific T cell clones is associated with extensive infection restricted to a subset of about 20 β-HPV types. The EVER genes encode transmembrane proteins which are important regulators of zinc homoeostasis and enhance expression of viral E6 and E7 genes. There are two presenting conditions in EV: a) scattered benign plane warts caused by HPV-3 and -10 which develop in early childhood and persist throughout life. The main characteristics are enlarged keratinocytes with granular and often vacuolated cytoplasm [9]; b) Verrucous lesions caused by with HPV-5 and -8 which occur on light-exposed areas and have greater malignant potential. EV-like conditions develop in HIV-infected individuals and other immunodeficiencies. EV-HPV types have also been found in a high proportion of lesions associated with epithelial hyperproliferation such as psoriasis [9]. Several β-HPVs were found in hyperproliferative lesions in patients with EV [18, 35]. Infection by the β-HPVs is relatively frequent but typically asymptomatic, either because of efficient clearance of infected cells or due to persistent infections that are undetected by the immune system and do not cause abnormal pathology [18].

Persistence and Malignant Conversion of Cutaneous Warts

HPV infections are normally controlled by intact cell-mediated and humoral immune systems. Regression was shown to be largely driven by cytotoxic T cells and NK cells many years ago, while protection from subsequent infection with the same HPV type results from stimulation of the adaptive response and production of antibodies [9]. Persistence of HPV lesions is a major issue for effective clinical trials of immunosuppressed patients and can significantly affect their quality of life. While β-HPV is universal, a few types of HPV are associated with squamous cell carcinomas (SCC) in EV patients. Cutaneous HPV types are only poorly transforming *in vitro* and their linkage to skin carcinogenesis is restricted by the frequency of infection with β-HPV types and by common risk factors for activation (UV exposure, immunosuppression and hyperproliferation). Sometimes, persistent plantar lesions are associated with the development of verrucous carcinoma [9].

HPV in Mucosal and Anogenital Skin

Mucosal infections associated with α-HPV types are more common than cutaneous HPV and the majority is asymptomatic. External genital warts are the most common sexually transmitted infection with a main increase in incidence and an estimated transmission rate of 60% between partners. External genital warts may occur as discrete, small, papular or large cauliflower-like lesions on moist surfaces, or as keratotic lesions similar to skin warts on dry surfaces. Additional lesions associated with anogenital HPV infection include: a) Urethral warts which are rare complications leading to the reduced urinary flow and infertility due to obstruction of urethral and ejaculatory ducts; b) Bowenoid papulosis occurs in sexually active people of both sexes as reddish-brown verrucous papules on the penis. It is usually referred to as a low grade carcinoma *in situ* and treated by locally destructive methods. Although, Bowenoid papulosis is usually benign, but it can be associated with HR-HPV types inducing malignancy in 2-3% of individuals; c) Giant condyloma acuminatum (Bushcke-Löwenstein tumours) which is a large exophytic lesions frequently found on the penis or in the perianal area and usually associated with HPV 6 and 11. Chemoradiotherapy treatment showed good results in this lesion [9].

Systemic Lupus Erythematosus

Systemic lupus erythematosus (SLE), the prototype of the autoimmune disease is a chronic inflammatory, multi-systemic disease with unknown cause. SLE, as well as other immunological conditions, alone or in combination with immunosuppressive therapy, may influence the development of proliferative diseases. A possible association between SLE and increased frequency of HPV infection, squamous intraepithelial lesions, and cervical cancer has not well defined [36].

HPV Associated Anogenital Pre-Cancers and Cancers

HPV-associated pre-cancers present intraepithelial neoplasia and are named based on the site including cervical intraepithelial neoplasia (CIN), VIN and VAIN (vulval and vaginal intraepithelial neoplasia respectively), PIN (penile intraepithelial neoplasia) and AIN (anal intraepithelial neoplasia). Appropriate intervention can usually prevent progression to invasive cancer, but there is considerable morbidity associated with treatment of the precancerous stages. For example, pre-term births, low birth weight and increased deaths were observed in HPV-related CIN [9].

CONCLUDING REMARKS

As of 9 March 2015, approximately 200 different HPV types have been established. The γ-PV, α-PV and β-PV genera have been growing with 80, 65 and 51 recognized and completely sequenced HPV types, respectively. It is surprising that only one new μ-PV type (HPV204) has been found in recent years. However, novel HPV types of the μ-PV genus were rarely detected due to low viral load in the skin and/or rapid clearance of infection by the immune system. Regarding that variant lineages of HPVs have different pathologic potentials; their comprehensive classification is required to determine their effects in virus persistence and invasive cancers.

CONFLICT OF INTEREST

The author (editor) declares no conflict of interest, financial or otherwise.

ACKNOWLEDGEMENT

Declare none.

REFERENCES

[1] Mammas IN, Spandidos DA, Sourvinos G. Genomic diversity of human papillomaviruses (HPV) and clinical implications: an overview in adulthood and childhood. Infect Genet Evol 2014; 21: 220-6. [http://dx.doi.org/10.1016/j.meegid.2013.11.002] [PMID: 24291228]

[2] Knight GL, Pugh AG, Yates E, *et al.* A cyclin-binding motif in human papillomavirus type 18 (HPV18) E1^E4 is necessary for association with CDK-cyclin complexes and G2/M cell cycle arrest of keratinocytes, but is not required for differentiation-dependent viral genome amplification or L1 capsid protein expression. Virology 2011; 412(1): 196-210. [http://dx.doi.org/10.1016/j.virol.2011.01.007] [PMID: 21276999]

[3] Bouvard V, Baan R, Straif K, *et al.* A review of human carcinogens--Part B: biological agents. Lancet Oncol 2009; 10(4): 321-2.

[http://dx.doi.org/10.1016/S1470-2045(09)70096-8] [PMID: 19350698]

[4] Bzhalava D, Guan P, Franceschi S, Dillner J, Clifford G. A systematic review of the prevalence of mucosal and cutaneous human papillomavirus types. Virology 2013; 445(1-2): 224-31. [http://dx.doi.org/10.1016/j.virol.2013.07.015] [PMID: 23928291]

[5] Doorbar J, Quint W, Banks L, *et al.* The biology and life-cycle of human papillomaviruses. Vaccine 2012; 30(5) (Suppl. 5): F55-70. [http://dx.doi.org/10.1016/j.vaccine.2012.06.083] [PMID: 23199966]

[6] Lacey CJ, Lowndes CM, Shah KV. Chapter 4: Burden and management of noncancerous HPV-related conditions: HPV-6/11 disease. Vaccine 2006; 24(3): S3/35-41.

[7] Haedicke J, Iftner T. Human papillomaviruses and cancer. Radiother Oncol 2013; 108(3): 397-402. [http://dx.doi.org/10.1016/j.radonc.2013.06.004] [PMID: 23830197]

[8] Klingelhutz AJ, Roman A. Cellular transformation by human papillomaviruses: lessons learned by comparing high- and low-risk viruses. Virology 2012; 424(2): 77-98. [http://dx.doi.org/10.1016/j.virol.2011.12.018] [PMID: 22284986]

[9] Sundaram ME, Mason SM, Basta NE. HPV vaccine uptake among overweight and obese US adolescents: An analysis of the National Health and Nutrition Examination Survey (NHANES) 2009-2014. Vaccine 2016; 34(22): 2501-6. [http://dx.doi.org/10.1016/j.vaccine.2016.03.064] [PMID: 27020709]

[10] Cubie HA. Diseases associated with human papillomavirus infection. Virology 2013; 445(1-2): 21-34. [http://dx.doi.org/10.1016/j.virol.2013.06.007] [PMID: 23932731]

[11] Asgari MM, Kiviat NB, Critchlow CW, *et al.* Detection of human papillomavirus DNA in cutaneous squamous cell carcinoma among immunocompetent individuals. J Invest Dermatol 2008; 128(6): 1409-17. [http://dx.doi.org/10.1038/sj.jid.5701227] [PMID: 18185530]

[12] Forslund O, Lindelöf B, Hradil E, *et al.* High prevalence of cutaneous human papillomavirus DNA on the top of skin tumors but not in "Stripped" biopsies from the same tumors. J Invest Dermatol 2004; 123(2): 388-94. [http://dx.doi.org/10.1111/j.0022-202X.2004.23205.x] [PMID: 15245440]

[13] Luevano M, Bernard HU, Barrera-Saldaña HA, *et al.* High-throughput profiling of the humoral immune responses against thirteen human papillomavirus types by proteome microarrays. Virology 2010; 405(1): 31-40. [http://dx.doi.org/10.1016/j.virol.2010.05.011] [PMID: 20554302]

[14] Boscolo-Rizzo P, Del Mistro A, Bussu F, *et al.* New insights into human papillomavirus-associated head and neck squamous cell carcinoma. Acta Otorhinolaryngol Ital 2013; 33(2): 77-87. [PMID: 23853396]

[15] Bernard HU, Burk RD, Chen Z, van Doorslaer K, zur Hausen H, de Villiers EM. Classification of papillomaviruses (PVs) based on 189 PV types and proposal of taxonomic amendments. Virology 2010; 401(1): 70-9. [http://dx.doi.org/10.1016/j.virol.2010.02.002] [PMID: 20206957]

[16] Ekström J, Bzhalava D, Svenback D, Forslund O, Dillner J. High throughput sequencing reveals diversity of Human Papillomaviruses in cutaneous lesions. Int J Cancer 2011; 129(11): 2643-50. [http://dx.doi.org/10.1002/ijc.26204] [PMID: 21630257]

[17] Kocjan BJ, Bzhalava D, Forslund O, Dillner J, Poljak M. Molecular methods for identification and characterization of novel papillomaviruses. Clin Microbiol Infect 2015; 21(9): 808-16. [http://dx.doi.org/10.1016/j.cmi.2015.05.011] [PMID: 26003284]

[18] Burk RD, Harari A, Chen Z. Human papillomavirus genome variants. Virology 2013; 445(1-2): 232-43. [http://dx.doi.org/10.1016/j.virol.2013.07.018] [PMID: 23998342]

[19] White EA, Howley PM. Proteomic approaches to the study of papillomavirus-host interactions. Virology 2013; 435(1): 57-69.
[http://dx.doi.org/10.1016/j.virol.2012.09.046] [PMID: 23217616]

[20] Nindl I, Gottschling M, Stockfleth E. Human papillomaviruses and non-melanoma skin cancer: basic virology and clinical manifestations. Dis Markers 2007; 23(4): 247-59.
[http://dx.doi.org/10.1155/2007/942650] [PMID: 17627060]

[21] Ekström J, Forslund O, Dillner J. Three novel papillomaviruses (HPV109, HPV112 and HPV114) and their presence in cutaneous and mucosal samples. Virology 2010; 397(2): 331-6.
[http://dx.doi.org/10.1016/j.virol.2009.11.027] [PMID: 19969321]

[22] Komloš KF, Kocjan BJ, Košorok P, *et al.* Tumor-specific and gender-specific pre-vaccination distribution of human papillomavirus types 6 and 11 in anogenital warts and laryngeal papillomas: a study on 574 tissue specimens. J Med Virol 2012; 84(8): 1233-41.
[http://dx.doi.org/10.1002/jmv.23318] [PMID: 22711351]

[23] Wang JW, Roden RB. L2, the minor capsid protein of papillomavirus. Virology 2013; 445(1-2): 175-86.
[http://dx.doi.org/10.1016/j.virol.2013.04.017] [PMID: 23689062]

[24] Gottschling M, Stamatakis A, Nindl I, Stockfleth E, Alonso A, Bravo IG. Multiple evolutionary mechanisms drive papillomavirus diversification. Mol Biol Evol 2007; 24(5): 1242-58.
[http://dx.doi.org/10.1093/molbev/msm039] [PMID: 17344207]

[25] Chen Z, Schiffman M, Herrero R, *et al.* Evolution and taxonomic classification of human papillomavirus 16 (HPV16)-related variant genomes: HPV31, HPV33, HPV35, HPV52, HPV58 and HPV67. PLoS One 2011; 6(5): e20183.
[http://dx.doi.org/10.1371/journal.pone.0020183] [PMID: 21673791]

[26] Middleton K, Peh W, Southern S, *et al.* Organization of human papillomavirus productive cycle during neoplastic progression provides a basis for selection of diagnostic markers. J Virol 2003; 77(19): 10186-201.
[http://dx.doi.org/10.1128/JVI.77.19.10186-10201.2003] [PMID: 12970404]

[27] Major T, Szarka K, Sziklai I, Gergely L, Czeglédy J. The characteristics of human papillomavirus DNA in head and neck cancers and papillomas. J Clin Pathol 2005; 58(1): 51-5.
[http://dx.doi.org/10.1136/jcp.2004.016634] [PMID: 15623482]

[28] Hsueh PR. Human papillomavirus, genital warts, and vaccines. J Microbiol Immunol Infect 2009; 42(2): 101-6.
[PMID: 19597640]

[29] Syrjänen S, Lodi G, von Bültzingslöwen I, *et al.* Human papillomaviruses in oral carcinoma and oral potentially malignant disorders: a systematic review. Oral Dis 2011; 17(1) (Suppl. 1): 58-72.
[http://dx.doi.org/10.1111/j.1601-0825.2011.01792.x] [PMID: 21382139]

[30] Dok R, Nuyts S. HPV positive head and neck cancers: Molecular pathogenesis and evolving treatment strategies. Cancers (Basal) 2016; 8(4)

[31] Glynne-Jones R, Nilsson PJ, Aschele C, *et al.* Anal cancer: ESMO-ESSO-ESTRO clinical practice guidelines for diagnosis, treatment and follow-up. Eur J Surg Oncol 2014; 40(10): 1165-76.
[http://dx.doi.org/10.1016/j.ejso.2014.07.030] [PMID: 25239441]

[32] zur Hausen H. Papillomaviruses in the causation of human cancers - a brief historical account. Virology 2009; 384(2): 260-5.
[http://dx.doi.org/10.1016/j.virol.2008.11.046] [PMID: 19135222]

[33] Chouhy D, Gorosito M, Sánchez A, *et al.* New generic primer system targeting mucosal/genital and cutaneous human papillomaviruses leads to the characterization of HPV 115, a novel Beta-papillomavirus species 3. Virology 2010; 397(1): 205-16.
[http://dx.doi.org/10.1016/j.virol.2009.11.020] [PMID: 19948351]

[34] Bosch FX, Burchell AN, Schiffman M, *et al.* Epidemiology and natural history of human papillomavirus infections and type-specific implications in cervical neoplasia. Vaccine 2008; 26(10) (Suppl. 10): K1-K16.
[http://dx.doi.org/10.1016/j.vaccine.2008.05.064] [PMID: 18847553]

[35] Doorbar J. The papillomavirus life cycle. J Clin Virol 2005; 32(1) (Suppl. 1): S7-S15.
[http://dx.doi.org/10.1016/j.jcv.2004.12.006] [PMID: 15753007]

[36] Oberyszyn TM. Non-melanoma skin cancer: importance of gender, immunosuppressive status and vitamin D. Cancer Lett 2008; 261(2): 127-36.
[http://dx.doi.org/10.1016/j.canlet.2008.01.009] [PMID: 18267352]

[37] Muñoz N, Bosch FX, de Sanjosé S, *et al.* Epidemiologic classification of human papillomavirus types associated with cervical cancer. N Engl J Med 2003; 348(6): 518-27.
[http://dx.doi.org/10.1056/NEJMoa021641] [PMID: 12571259]

[38] Muñoz N, Bosch FX, Castellsagué X, *et al.* Against which human papillomavirus types shall we vaccinate and screen? The international perspective. Int J Cancer 2004; 111(2): 278-85.
[http://dx.doi.org/10.1002/ijc.20244] [PMID: 15197783]

[39] Geraets D, Alemany L, Guimera N, *et al.* Detection of rare and possibly carcinogenic human papillomavirus genotypes as single infections in invasive cervical cancer. J Pathol 2012; 228(4): 534-43.
[http://dx.doi.org/10.1002/path.4065] [PMID: 22711526]

CHAPTER 4

The Life Cycle and Transmission of HPV Types

Kimia Kardani, Niloofar Naderi and **Azam Bolhassani***

Department of Pharmaceutical Biotechnology, School of Pharmacy, Shahid Beheshti University of Medical Sciences, Tehran, Iran

Department of Hepatitis and AIDS, Pasteur Institute of Iran, Tehran, Iran

Abstract: Genital HPV infections are the most common of all sexually transmissible agents. The HPV life cycle is dependent on host cell differentiation with late viral events such as structural gene expression and viral genome amplification in the upper layers of the stratified epithelium. Indeed, the virus destabilizes host chromatin-remodeling factors to facilitate viral replication and transcription. Generally, the life cycle of the virus is divided into major steps including entry, establishment of the non-productive infectious state, maintenance of the non-productive infectious state, and productive stage. In this chapter, we briefly explain transmission and the life cycle of HPVs in host cells.

Keywords: HPV infection, Life cycle, Transmission.

INTRODUCTION

HPV is specifically epitheliotropic and its life cycle takes place within squamous epithelia. Thus, the HPV life cycle is strongly related to the differentiation of the host cell keratinocyte. Due to the small coding capacity of the virus, HPV is dependent on cellular factors for viral replication. The life cycle of the virus is divided into four main steps which are entry, establishment of the non-productive infectious state, maintenance of the non-productive infectious state and productive stage [1, 2]. Fig. (**1**) shows differentiation-dependent HPV life cycle. Genital HPV infections are the most common of all sexually transmissible agents [2, 3]. Mucosal HPV spreads through direct skin-to-skin contact in oral, vaginal or anal regions. Vertical transmission between mother and infant are less common methods of transmission [3 - 5]. On the other hand, condoms offer protection about 60% against the development of cervical intraepithelial neoplasia (CIN2/3) and invasive cervical cancer (ICC) and promote the regression of intraepithelial lesions in concordant couples [2, 4]. The rate of HPV transmission probability is

* **Corresponding author Azam Bolhassani:** Department of Hepatitis and AIDS, Pasteur Institute of Iran, Tehran, Iran; Tel: 66953311-20; E-mails: A_bolhasani@pasteur.ac.ir, azam.bolhassani@yahoo.com

Azam Bolhassani (Ed.)

higher than that of human immunodeficiency virus (HIV) or herpes simplex virus, type 2 (HSV-2) [2, 6]. HPV seroprevalence data showed a per-partner male to female transmission probability of 60% to 80% for HPV type 16 [2, 7, 8]. The factors enhancing transmission are related predominantly to sexual behaviors [4]. It is not clear whether HPVs can infect and transform non-stem cells of the columnar epithelium or the basal and parabasal layers of the stratified epithelium [2]. The reports indicated a higher rate of female-to-male (0.19-0.81) versus male-to-female (0.05-0.28) transmission [9 - 11]. Indeed, transmission depends on the viral load and/or duration of infection in the partner [3, 10 - 13].

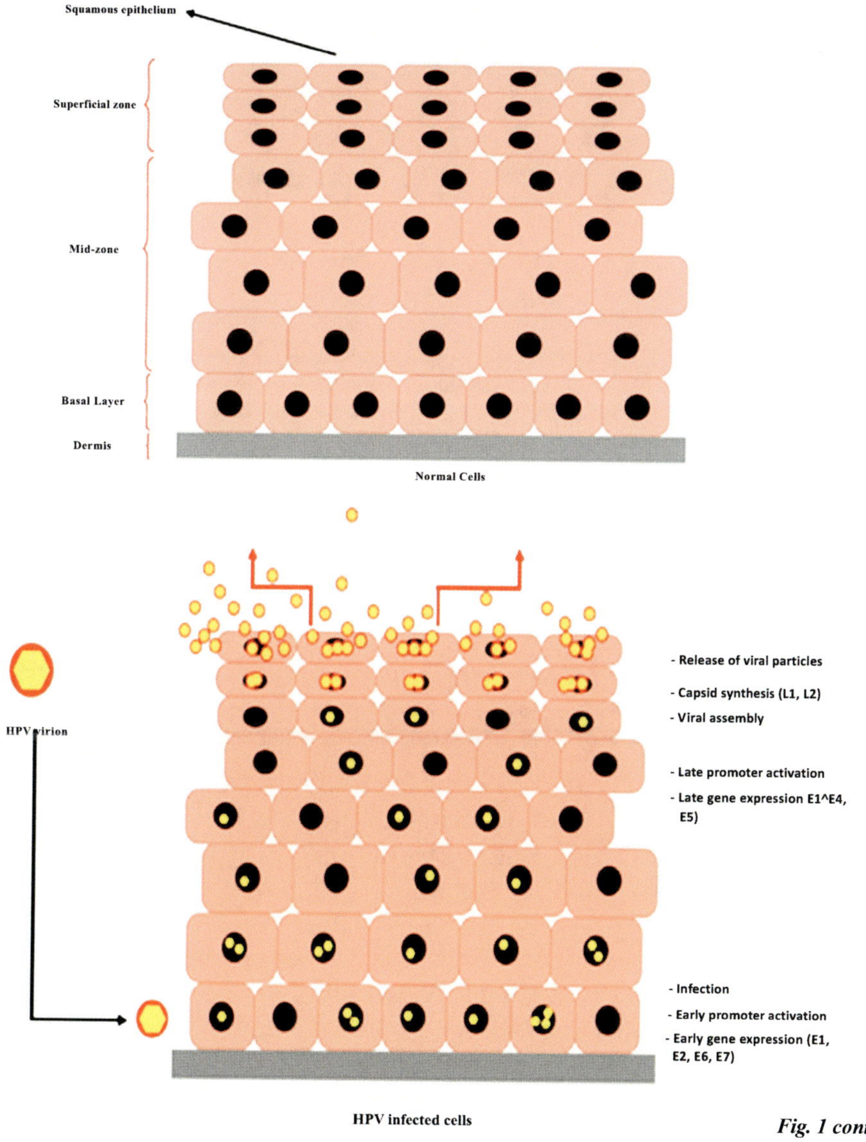

Fig. 1 contd.....

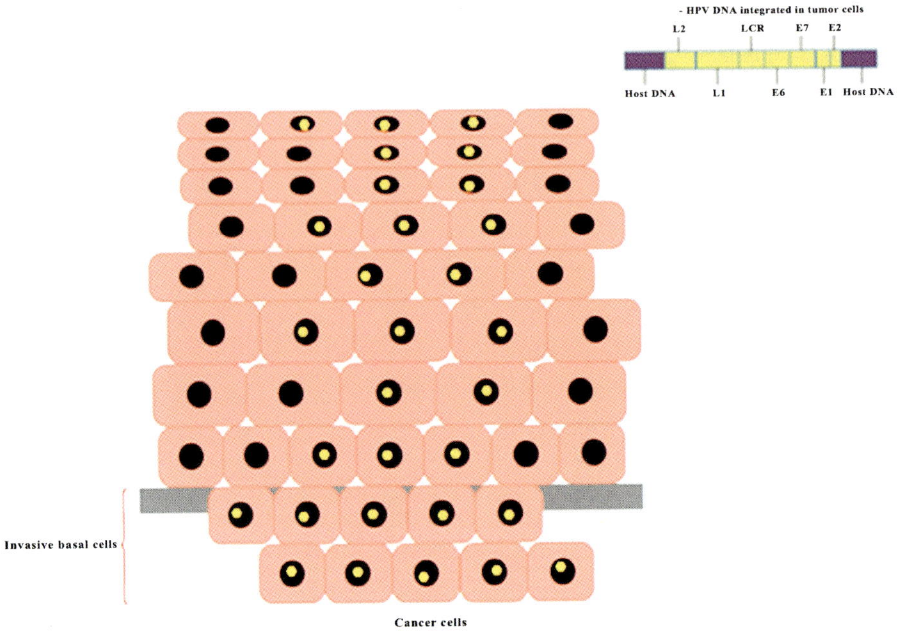

Fig. (1). HPV Life Cycle: The HPV life cycle is related to the differentiation of epithelial cells. At first, HPV infects dividing cells in basal layer of the epithelium. Then, the viral genes are expressed and HPV genome is episomally maintained in the infected cells (~ 50-100 copies / cell). Once the infected cells begin to differentiate, the late promoter is activated leading to the amplification of viral DNA, and the increased expression of viral proteins. Next, synthesis of viral capsids and assembly occurs in the highest differentiated layer of the epithelium, and finally the progeny virions are released to infect other cells [121, 122].

Life Cycle of HPV

The HPV life cycle is completely related to the differentiation of the epithelium after infecting the basal layer cells by virus [12, 13] and thus depends on the presence of external factors including hormones and cytokines [14, 15]. After infection of basal cells, the viral genomes begin to replicate along with host DNA as episomes [12]. In the basal epithelium, the early promoter of HPV genome is activated to express the viral E1, E2, E6 and E7 genes (*i.e.,* early proteins). Then, once HPV-positive cells start to differentiate, the late promoter is activated to express the viral late genes leading to the onset of the virus productive phase. Finally, in the differentiated epithelial cells (or suprabasal layer), HPV genomes are assembled into the progeny virions which are released from the cells (Fig. **1**) [12]. Finally, the virions infect the basal lamina again through the interaction with heparin sulphate proteoglycans and likely laminin [16 - 21]. Structural changes in the viral capsid including the L2 protein-DNA complex and furin cleavage of L2 are necessary for virus internalization, endosomal escape, and subsequently nuclear entry of the viral genome [22 - 28]. It should be noted that active cell division is essential for nuclear entry of HPV genome [29]. The researchers showed that lesion formation by the low-risk HPV types begins with the infection of a basal stem cell that its durability is a key factor for the stability of a lesion [14]. Table **1** shows the steps of HPV life cycle.

Table 1. Steps of HPV life cycle.

HPV Life cycle steps		Ref.
Entry	-HPV initiate infection by penetrating through microtraumas in the epithelial -To reach the basal cells which are believed to be the target cells for HPV infection	11
Establishment	-The non-productive infectious state is once HPV particle enters the host cell -The virus relies primarily on the host's cellular machinery to replicate the virus DNA -The HPV genome becomes established as a low copy number nuclear plasmid inside in the infected basal cells -Within these cells only early viral gene products are expressed and consequently referred to as the non-productive stage of infection	11
Maintenance	-The non-productive infectious state is a hallmark of HPV infection -It requires the viral genome to be maintained over multiple cell divisions, but the mechanism is still unclear	11
	-Establishment and maintenance of the viral genome in proliferating basal keratinocytes is followed by vegetative viral DNA amplification in cells that have moved up from the basal layer and differentiated. -In normal epithelia, cells exit the cell cycle upon differentiation, but as the virus is dependent on the cellular replication machinery for the synthesis of its own DNA the virus induces these cells to re-enter the cell cycle in order to gain access to host replication factors	9, 119
Production	-It begins when the daughter cells derived from the infected basal cells. -Virus starts to differentiate and delays the terminal differentiation programme of the cell. -It redirects the cell's DNA replicative capacity. -It allows amplification of the viral genome and expression of the late viral genes which are necessary for the production of progeny virus and subsequent viral release	11

Maintenance of the Viral Genome and Cell Proliferation in the Lower Epithelial Layers

Irrespective of the nature of the infected basal cell, viral infection is caused by a primary phase of genome amplification, and then by maintenance of the viral episome at low copy number [29 - 31]. In persistent infection caused by high-risk HPV types, the integration of viral DNA into the host cell genome may occur which is associated with a deletion in the regulatory genes responsible for the viral replication (*i.e.,* E1 and E2) [26, 32]. In the onset of viral replication, the regulatory E2 protein helps to recruit the viral helicase E1 to the viral replication origin by protein-protein and protein-DNA interactions [33 - 35]. The use of a helicase E1 which is distinct from the cellular replication helicases (*i.e.,* MCM proteins) allows viral DNA replication to be independent on cellular DNA replication [14, 36, 37]. The studies showed that E2 cooperatively binds to four

E2-binding sites in the long control region (LCR) of the HPV genome leading to the activation (at low levels of E2) or the repression (at high levels of E2) of E6 and E7 expression from the early promoter [12, 38 - 40]. During the malignant progression, the high-risk HPV DNA often integrates into the host genome, leading to the disruption of the E2 gene, high expression of the viral oncogene E6 and E7, and subsequently stimulation of cellular proliferation [12]. The studies showed that repressor proteins such as a small conserved fragment of HPV 11, 16, 31 E8 gene or of HPV11 E1 gene fused to the C-terminus of E2 gene (*i.e.*, E8^E2 or E1^E2) act as negative regulators of E2-dependent transcriptional activation by competing with E2 binding at E2BSs [33, 35, 41]. On the other hand, there are many functional differences between promoter activity and expression of the high and low-risk HPV E6 and E7 proteins that play an important role in various HPV-associated pathologies. Recent studies have shown that the deregulation of E6/E7 expression is a critical event in determining neoplastic grade, even in the lack of genome integration [14, 42 - 44].

Genome Maintenance and Proliferation in the Upper Epithelial Layers

As observed, E7 is required to maintain virus in the basal cells infected by some HPV types, as well as it is needed to proliferate other virus types in the differentiated cells [45]. Functional differences between the high- and low-risk HPV E7 proteins depend on their different affinities to bind the Retinoblastoma (Rb) protein family. The high-risk E7 proteins interact with the Rb-family tumor suppressor proteins, p105, p107 and p130 and disrupt their interaction with E2F transcription factors leading to the activation of E2F-dependent gene expression and cell cycle progression [45, 46]. The low-risk E7 proteins generally have a lower affinity for p105 and p107 than the high-risk types, but can degrade p130 in the mid-epithelial layers for viral replication [47 - 50]. The studies showed that p16, a protein up-regulated upon pRb degradation, accumulates in HPV-positive cancers [20, 51].

The high-risk E6 proteins also have potency to up-regulate telomerase activity and to degrade p53 in a proteosome-dependent pathway during cell division [52 - 56]. Another study showed that the high-risk HPV E6 proteins up-regulate the E2F-responsive genes such as MCM-7 and Cyclin E and push the cells into S phase independent on the p53 pathway [45, 57]. Finally, the conserved C-terminal region of high-risk HPVs E6 protein mediates its interaction with PDZ domain-containing proteins involved in cell signaling and proliferation [58 - 61]. Indeed, the expression of the E6 and E7 proteins in the upper epithelial layers leads to push the infected cells into S phase, and to increase the copy-number of viral genome [62]. It is possible that E7 protein maintains the viral genome by decreasing the amount of available TATA binding protein (TBP) [45]. It appears that the E4 and E5 proteins indirectly influence the amplification of viral genome by enhancing the stability of the epidermal growth factor receptor (EGFR), EGF signaling and the activity of MAP kinase, as well as by supporting virus synthesis, release or transmission and indirect optimization of genome amplification [63 - 72]. Fig. (**2**) summarizes the main interference of high-risk HPV E6 and E7 proteins with the host cell cycle.

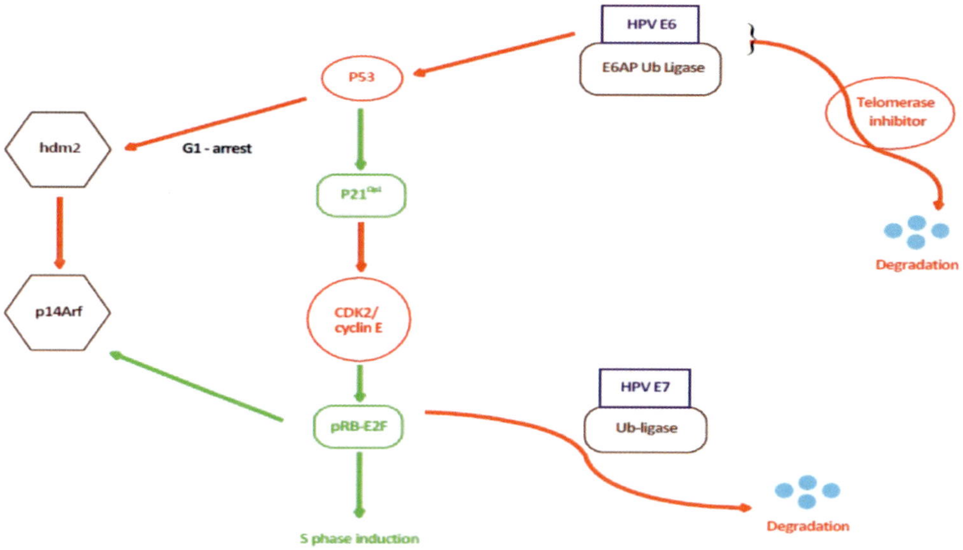

Fig. (2). Interference of E6 and E7 proteins from high-risk HPVs with the host cell cycle: The HPV E6 proteins interact with the p53 tumor suppressor and induce its proteolytic degradation as well as stimulate telomerase activity. Moreover, E6-induced transcriptional changes in HPV-positive cells depend on the ubiquitin ligase E6-associated protein (E6AP) [26]; On the other hand, the high-risk HPV E7 oncoproteins bind the pRB tumor suppressor and inactivate p21Cip1, resulting in a spontaneous transition from G1 to S phase in the cell cycle. The E7 proteins also activate the histone demethylases (KDM6A and KDM6B) which stimulate the expression of p16INK4a, an inhibitor of CDK4/6 in HPV- transformed cells [120].

Generally, both low and high-risk HPV E7 proteins have the ability to target the Rb family member p130 suggesting that its degradation may be critical for the viral life cycle [73 - 76]. Moreover, both high- and low-risk HPV E7 proteins can prolong the G2 phase of cell cycle in the differentiated cells [77, 78], and inhibit the division of daughter cells into one basal and one suprabasal cell through binding to nuclear mitotic apparatus protein 1 (NuMA) and delocalizing dynein from mitotic spindles [79]. Finally, the high-risk HPV E7 up-regulates nucleophosmin, a positive regulator of proliferation and negative regulator of differentiation through AKT activation [80, 81].

The HPV E6 proteins interact with the p53 tumor suppressor and induce its proteolytic degradation as well as stimulate telomerase activity. Moreover, E6-induced transcriptional changes in HPV-positive cells depend on the ubiquitin ligase E6-associated protein (E6AP) [26]; On the other hand, the high-risk HPV E7 oncoproteins bind the pRB tumor suppressor and inactivate p21Cip1, resulting in a spontaneous transition from G1 to S phase in the cell cycle. The E7 proteins also activate the histone demethylases (KDM6A and KDM6B) which stimulate the expression of p16INK4a, an inhibitor of CDK4/6 in HPV- transformed cells [120].

Virus Packaging and Release

Genome encapsidation involves the recruitment of the minor coat protein (L2) to regions of replication *via* E2, prior to the expression of the major coat protein (L1) and the assembly of the icosohedral capsid in the nucleus [82 - 84]. Virus maturation occurs in the most superficial keratinocytes which convert from a reducing to an oxidizing environment due to the lack of mitochondrial oxidative phosphorylation. This modification results in the progressive accumulation of disulphide bonds between the L1 proteins and subsequently the generation of stable infectious virions before virus release [85]. Moreover, the E4 protein is thought to contribute to virion release and infectivity in the upper epithelial layers *via* disruption of keratin structure [14].

Cancer Progression

The controlled expression of viral gene products is disrupted in HPV-associated neoplasia. In cervical disease, the expression of E6 and E7 proteins enhances from cervical intraepithelial neoplasia grade 1 to 3 (CIN1 to CIN3) inducing the neoplastic phenotype. The CIN1 lesions similar to flat warts possess a lower level of cell proliferation in the basal and parabasal layers and retain the ability to complete the HPV life cycle and generate virus particles [86]. The increased expression of E6 and E7 proteins in the high-risk HPV infection leading to the CIN2+ phenotype influences the accumulation of genetic changes in the cells, which increasingly contribute to cancer progression. The viral deregulation in CIN2/3+ is also thought to facilitate integration of the viral DNA into the host cell genome resulting in further deregulation of the expression of E6 and E7 proteins [14]. The HPV16 LCR contains hormone response elements that can be stimulated by estrogen indicating the cooperation between estrogen and HPV in the development of cervical cancer [73, 87 - 92]. In CIN, the LCR is differentially methylated according to disease severity suggesting that epigenetic changes may also regulate gene expression [14, 44]. Several reports suggested that duplications within the HPV genome or special integration may be important in cancer progression [93]. Also, the genetic susceptibility of the host can play an important role in some cancers associated with low-risk HPV types [94]. The current studies indicated that the HPV16, 18 E6 and E7 proteins interact with a variety of host cell proteins in order to manipulate cell proliferation, senescence, and apoptosis [26, 94-96].

Lesion Regression and Clearance

Most HPV infections are cleared by a cell-mediated immune response, and do not persist for deregulated gene expression and the secondary genetic errors [14, 58, 97]. Regression of anogenital warts is accompanied by a $CD4^+$ Th1 immune response [38, 39]. The failure to develop an effective cell-mediated immunity results in persistent infection as observed for oncogenic HPVs [14]. Generally, HPV down-regulates the innate immune signaling pathways in the infected keratinocyte, prevents the release of pro-inflammatory cytokines, especially the type I interferons, and reduces the activation and migration of Langerhans cell and the recruitment of stromal DCs and macrophages. Furthermore, the infected cells that express effectively viral proteins are shed from the epithelial surface, away from circulating immune cells [14, 37, 98]. Indeed, the low-level presentation of viral antigens in the lack of inflammation likely favors immune tolerance rather than an effector T cell response [84 - 86]. On the other hand, dermal DCs and macrophages recruited to HPV-infected epithelium may represent an important role in the recognition of HPV antigens, the induction of effector responses and the regression of lesions [14]. The lesion is cleared by the replacement of actively infected cells with 'apparently normal cells' as the basal cells continue to divide. The apparently normal cells may contain viral genomes without concurrent viral gene expression suggesting that the virus life cycle may be subsequently reactivated following immune suppression or changes in hormone levels [14, 99].

Papillomavirus Interaction with Cellular Chromatin

Papillomavirus genomes are organized in the form of nucleosomes packaged into chromatin [12], suggesting their regulatory roles in the transcription of viral oncogene [100]. In undifferentiated cells, hypersensitive regions were detected in the upstream regulatory region (URR) involved in the early gene transcription. Upon differentiation, the late transcript initiation region becomes accessible to DNase I, indicating a differentiation-induced chromatin remodeling around the late promoter [101, 102]. In undifferentiated cells, the chromatin surrounding both early and late viral promoter regions reveals an open, transcriptionally active state with dimethylated forms of histone H3K4 as well as acetylated histone H3 and H4. Upon differentiation, the levels of dimethylated H3K4 and acetylated H3 are increased around both the early and late promoter regions, while the acetylated H4 is enhanced at the early promoter [102, 103]. On the other hand, Brd4 is a member of the BET family proteins that harbor double bromodomains for association with mitotic chromosomes. In general, the bromodomains of Brd4 act as a molecular adapter targeting acetylated chromatin, while its C-terminal domain recruits the N-terminal region of viral E2 protein. Thus, the multiple functions of E2 protein may rely on its ability to interact with Brd4 and associate with cellular chromatin. Indeed, the interaction of HPV16 E2 protein with the C-terminal region of Brd4 has offered a molecular platform for developing antiviral compounds and blocking HPV latent infection [104 - 115].

Episome Maintenance in Proliferating Basal Epithelial Cells

The functions of the high-risk HPV E6 and E7 oncoproteins are essential for the viral genome maintenance through abrogating the cellular checkpoints that block the long-term retention of viral episomes in the infected cells [116 - 118]. In addition, to establish persistence in host cells, PVs have developed a strategy for hitching on cellular mitotic chromosomes. This mechanism ensures that the replicated viral episomes are retained inside the nuclei of dividing host cells and accurately partition to the daughter cells during mitosis. For many papillomaviruses, this non-covalent association of viral DNA with chromosomes is mediated by the viral E2 protein [12].

CONCLUDING REMARKS

The virus-chromatin interaction provides an excellent model to study the HPV life cycle and develop novel compounds directed to abrogate the virus-host interaction. On the other hand, the viral oncogenes E6 and E7 are the major mediators of HPV-induced oncogenesis. Determination of mechanisms that repress the viral oncogenes will offer new strategies to prevent HPV-induced cancer.

CONFLICT OF INTEREST

The author (editor) declares no conflict of interest, financial or otherwise.

ACKNOWLEDGEMENT

Declare none.

REFERENCES

[1] Anacker DC, Moody CA. Modulation of the DNA damage response during the life cycle of human papillomaviruses. Virus Res 2017; 231: 41-9. [http://dx.doi.org/10.1016/j.virusres.2016.11.006] [PMID: 27836727]

[2] Wheeler CM. The natural history of cervical human papillomavirus infections and cervical cancer: gaps in knowledge and future horizons. Obstet Gynecol Clin North Am 2013; 40(2): 165-76.

[http://dx.doi.org/10.1016/j.ogc.2013.02.004] [PMID: 23732023]

[3] Moscicki AB, Schiffman M, Burchell A, *et al.* Updating the natural history of human papillomavirus and anogenital cancers. Vaccine 2012; 30(5) (Suppl. 5): F24-33. [http://dx.doi.org/10.1016/j.vaccine.2012.05.089] [PMID: 23199964]

[4] Stanley M. Pathology and epidemiology of HPV infection in females. Gynecol Oncol 2010; 117(2) (Suppl.): S5-S10. [http://dx.doi.org/10.1016/j.ygyno.2010.01.024] [PMID: 20304221]

[5] Cleveland JL, Junger ML, Saraiya M, Markowitz LE, Dunne EF, Epstein JB. The connection between human papillomavirus and oropharyngeal squamous cell carcinomas in the United States: implications for dentistry. J Am Dent Assoc 2011; 142(8): 915-24. [http://dx.doi.org/10.14219/jada.archive.2011.0298] [PMID: 21804058]

[6] Burchell AN, Richardson H, Mahmud SM, *et al.* Modeling the sexual transmissibility of human papillomavirus infection using stochastic computer simulation and empirical data from a cohort study of young women in Montreal, Canada. Am J Epidemiol 2006; 163(6): 534-43. [http://dx.doi.org/10.1093/aje/kwj077] [PMID: 16421235]

[7] Barnabas RV, Laukkanen P, Koskela P, Kontula O, Lehtinen M, Garnett GP. Epidemiology of HPV 16 and cervical cancer in Finland and the potential impact of vaccination: mathematical modelling analyses. PLoS Med 2006; 3(5): e138. [http://dx.doi.org/10.1371/journal.pmed.0030138] [PMID: 16573364]

[8] Hughes JP, Garnett GP, Koutsky L. The theoretical population-level impact of a prophylactic human papilloma virus vaccine. Epidemiology 2002; 13(6): 631-9. [http://dx.doi.org/10.1097/00001648-200211000-00006] [PMID: 12410003]

[9] Hernandez BY, Wilkens LR, Zhu X, *et al.* Transmission of human papillomavirus in heterosexual couples. Emerg Infect Dis 2008; 14(6): 888-94. [http://dx.doi.org/10.3201/eid1406.0706162] [PMID: 18507898]

[10] Heck JE, Berthiller J, Vaccarella S, *et al.* Sexual behaviours and the risk of head and neck cancers: a pooled analysis in the International Head and Neck Cancer Epidemiology (INHANCE) consortium. Int J Epidemiol 2010; 39(1): 166-81. [http://dx.doi.org/10.1093/ije/dyp350] [PMID: 20022926]

[11] Burchell AN, Coutlée F, Tellier PP, Hanley J, Franco EL. Genital transmission of human papillomavirus in recently formed heterosexual couples. J Infect Dis 2011; 204(11): 1723-9. [http://dx.doi.org/10.1093/infdis/jir644] [PMID: 21984739]

[12] You J. Papillomavirus interaction with cellular chromatin. Biochim Biophys Acta 2010; 1799(3-4): 192-9. [http://dx.doi.org/10.1016/j.bbagrm.2009.09.009] [PMID: 19786128]

[13] Knight GL, Pugh AG, Yates E, *et al.* A cyclin-binding motif in human papillomavirus type 18 (HPV18) E1^E4 is necessary for association with CDK-cyclin complexes and G2/M cell cycle arrest of keratinocytes, but is not required for differentiation-dependent viral genome amplification or L1 capsid protein expression. Virology 2011; 412(1): 196-210. [http://dx.doi.org/10.1016/j.virol.2011.01.007] [PMID: 21276999]

[14] Doorbar J, Quint W, Banks L, *et al.* The biology and life-cycle of human papillomaviruses. Vaccine 2012; 30 (Suppl. 5): F55-70. [http://dx.doi.org/10.1016/j.vaccine.2012.06.083] [PMID: 23199966]

[15] de Jong A, van Poelgeest MI, van der Hulst JM, *et al.* Human papillomavirus type 16-positive cervical cancer is associated with impaired CD4+ T-cell immunity against early antigens E2 and E6. Cancer Res 2004; 64(15): 5449-55. [http://dx.doi.org/10.1158/0008-5472.CAN-04-0831] [PMID: 15289354]

[16] Buck CB, Cheng N, Thompson CD, *et al.* Arrangement of L2 within the papillomavirus capsid. J Virol

2008; 82(11): 5190-7.
[http://dx.doi.org/10.1128/JVI.02726-07] [PMID: 18367526]

[17] Finnen RL, Erickson KD, Chen XS, Garcea RL. Interactions between papillomavirus L1 and L2 capsid proteins. J Virol 2003; 77(8): 4818-26.
[http://dx.doi.org/10.1128/JVI.77.8.4818-4826.2003] [PMID: 12663788]

[18] Johnson KM, Kines RC, Roberts JN, Lowy DR, Schiller JT, Day PM. Role of heparan sulfate in attachment to and infection of the murine female genital tract by human papillomavirus. J Virol 2009; 83(5): 2067-74.
[http://dx.doi.org/10.1128/JVI.02190-08] [PMID: 19073722]

[19] Combita AL, Touzé A, Bousarghin L, Sizaret PY, Muñoz N, Coursaget P. Gene transfer using human papillomavirus pseudovirions varies according to virus genotype and requires cell surface heparan sulfate. FEMS Microbiol Lett 2001; 204(1): 183-8.
[http://dx.doi.org/10.1111/j.1574-6968.2001.tb10883.x] [PMID: 11682199]

[20] Giroglou T, Florin L, Schäfer F, Streeck RE, Sapp M. Human papillomavirus infection requires cell surface heparan sulfate. J Virol 2001; 75(3): 1565-70.
[http://dx.doi.org/10.1128/JVI.75.3.1565-1570.2001] [PMID: 11152531]

[21] Culp TD, Budgeon LR, Marinkovich MP, Meneguzzi G, Christensen ND. Keratinocyte-secreted laminin 5 can function as a transient receptor for human papillomaviruses by binding virions and transferring them to adjacent cells. J Virol 2006; 80(18): 8940-50.
[http://dx.doi.org/10.1128/JVI.00724-06] [PMID: 16940506]

[22] Doorbar J. The papillomavirus life cycle. J Clin Virol 2005; 32 (Suppl. 1): S7-S15.
[http://dx.doi.org/10.1016/j.jcv.2004.12.006] [PMID: 15753007]

[23] Schiller JT, Day PM, Kines RC. Current understanding of the mechanism of HPV infection. Gynecol Oncol 2010; 118(1) (Suppl.): S12-7.
[http://dx.doi.org/10.1016/j.ygyno.2010.04.004] [PMID: 20494219]

[24] Bienkowska-Haba M, Patel HD, Sapp M. Target cell cyclophilins facilitate human papillomavirus type 16 infection. PLoS Pathog 2009; 5(7): e1000524.
[http://dx.doi.org/10.1371/journal.ppat.1000524] [PMID: 19629175]

[25] Richards RM, Lowy DR, Schiller JT, Day PM. Cleavage of the papillomavirus minor capsid protein, L2, at a furin consensus site is necessary for infection. Proc Natl Acad Sci USA 2006; 103(5): 1522-7.
[http://dx.doi.org/10.1073/pnas.0508815103] [PMID: 16432208]

[26] Haedicke J, Iftner T. Human papillomaviruses and cancer. Radiother Oncol 2013; 108(3): 397-402.
[http://dx.doi.org/10.1016/j.radonc.2013.06.004] [PMID: 23830197]

[27] Bergant Marušič M, Ozbun MA, Campos SK, Myers MP, Banks L. Human papillomavirus L2 facilitates viral escape from late endosomes *via* sorting nexin 17. Traffic 2012; 13(3): 455-67.
[http://dx.doi.org/10.1111/j.1600-0854.2011.01320.x] [PMID: 22151726]

[28] Schelhaas M, Shah B, Holzer M, *et al.* Entry of human papillomavirus type 16 by actin-dependent, clathrin- and lipid raft-independent endocytosis. PLoS Pathog 2012; 8(4): e1002657.
[http://dx.doi.org/10.1371/journal.ppat.1002657] [PMID: 22536154]

[29] Pyeon D, Pearce SM, Lank SM, Ahlquist P, Lambert PF. Establishment of human papillomavirus infection requires cell cycle progression. PLoS Pathog 2009; 5(2): e1000318.
[http://dx.doi.org/10.1371/journal.ppat.1000318] [PMID: 19247434]

[30] McBride AA. Replication and partitioning of papillomavirus genomes. Adv Virus Res 2008; 72: 155-205.
[http://dx.doi.org/10.1016/S0065-3527(08)00404-1] [PMID: 19081491]

[31] Maglennon GA, McIntosh P, Doorbar J. Persistence of viral DNA in the epithelial basal layer suggests a model for papillomavirus latency following immune regression. Virology 2011; 414(2): 153-63.
[http://dx.doi.org/10.1016/j.virol.2011.03.019] [PMID: 21492895]

[32] Fertey J, Hurst J, Straub E, Schenker A, Iftner T, Stubenrauch F. Growth inhibition of HeLa cells is a conserved feature of high-risk human papillomavirus E8^E2C proteins and can also be achieved by an artificial repressor protein. J Virol 2011; 85(6): 2918-26. [http://dx.doi.org/10.1128/JVI.01647-10] [PMID: 21191025]

[33] Kurg R, Uusen P, Võsa L, Ustav M. Human papillomavirus E2 protein with single activation domain initiates HPV18 genome replication, but is not sufficient for long-term maintenance of virus genome. Virology 2010; 408(2): 159-66. [http://dx.doi.org/10.1016/j.virol.2010.09.010] [PMID: 20940072]

[34] Egawa N, Nakahara T, Ohno S, *et al.* The E1 protein of human papillomavirus type 16 is dispensable for maintenance replication of the viral genome. J Virol 2012; 86(6): 3276-83. [http://dx.doi.org/10.1128/JVI.06450-11] [PMID: 22238312]

[35] Lace MJ, Anson JR, Thomas GS, Turek LP, Haugen TH. The E8--E2 gene product of human papillomavirus type 16 represses early transcription and replication but is dispensable for viral plasmid persistence in keratinocytes. J Virol 2008; 82(21): 10841-53. [http://dx.doi.org/10.1128/JVI.01481-08] [PMID: 18753207]

[36] Blakaj DM, Fernandez-Fuentes N, Chen Z, *et al.* Evolutionary and biophysical relationships among the papillomavirus E2 proteins. Front Biosci (Landmark Ed) 2009; 14: 900-17. [http://dx.doi.org/10.2741/3285] [PMID: 19273107]

[37] Doorbar J. Molecular biology of human papillomavirus infection and cervical cancer. Clin Sci 2006; 110(5): 525-41. [http://dx.doi.org/10.1042/CS20050369] [PMID: 16597322]

[38] Kurg R, Tekkel H, Abroi A, Ustav M. Characterization of the functional activities of the bovine papillomavirus type 1 E2 protein single-chain heterodimers. J Virol 2006; 80(22): 11218-25. [http://dx.doi.org/10.1128/JVI.01127-06] [PMID: 16943289]

[39] Spalholz BA, Yang YC, Howley PM. Transactivation of a bovine papilloma virus transcriptional regulatory element by the E2 gene product. Cell 1985; 42(1): 183-91. [http://dx.doi.org/10.1016/S0092-8674(85)80114-8] [PMID: 2990724]

[40] Thierry F, Yaniv M. The BPV1-E2 trans-acting protein can be either an activator or a repressor of the HPV18 regulatory region. EMBO J 1987; 6(11): 3391-7. [PMID: 2828029]

[41] Ammermann I, Bruckner M, Matthes F, Iftner T, Stubenrauch F. Inhibition of transcription and DNA replication by the papillomavirus E8-E2C protein is mediated by interaction with corepressor molecules. J Virol 2008; 82(11): 5127-36. [http://dx.doi.org/10.1128/JVI.02647-07] [PMID: 18353941]

[42] Valencia C, Bonilla-Delgado J, Oktaba K, Ocádiz-Delgado R, Gariglio P, Covarrubias L. Human papillomavirus E6/E7 oncogenes promote mouse ear regeneration by increasing the rate of wound re-epithelization and epidermal growth. J Invest Dermatol 2008; 128(12): 2894-903. [http://dx.doi.org/10.1038/jid.2008.156] [PMID: 18548112]

[43] Rosenberger S, De-Castro Arce J, Langbein L, Steenbergen RD, Rösl F. Alternative splicing of human papillomavirus type-16 E6/E6* early mRNA is coupled to EGF signaling *via* Erk1/2 activation. Proc Natl Acad Sci USA 2010; 107(15): 7006-11. [http://dx.doi.org/10.1073/pnas.1002620107] [PMID: 20351270]

[44] Isaacson Wechsler E, Wang Q, Roberts I, *et al.* Reconstruction of human papillomavirus type 16-mediated early-stage neoplasia implicates E6/E7 deregulation and the loss of contact inhibition in neoplastic progression. J Virol 2012; 86(11): 6358-64. [http://dx.doi.org/10.1128/JVI.07069-11] [PMID: 22457518]

[45] Klingelhutz AJ, Roman A. Cellular transformation by human papillomaviruses: lessons learned by comparing high- and low-risk viruses. Virology 2012; 424(2): 77-98.

[http://dx.doi.org/10.1016/j.virol.2011.12.018] [PMID: 22284986]

[46] Bodily JM, Mehta KP, Cruz L, Meyers C, Laimins LA. The E7 open reading frame acts in cis and in trans to mediate differentiation-dependent activities in the human papillomavirus type 16 life cycle. J Virol 2011; 85(17): 8852-62.
[http://dx.doi.org/10.1128/JVI.00664-11] [PMID: 21697473]

[47] Klingelhutz AJ, Roman A. Cellular transformation by human papillomaviruses: lessons learned by comparing high- and low-risk viruses. Virology 2012; 424(2): 77-98.
[http://dx.doi.org/10.1016/j.virol.2011.12.018] [PMID: 22284986]

[48] Felsani A, Mileo AM, Paggi MG. Retinoblastoma family proteins as key targets of the small DNA virus oncoproteins. Oncogene 2006; 25(38): 5277-85.
[http://dx.doi.org/10.1038/sj.onc.1209621] [PMID: 16936748]

[49] Zhang B, Chen W, Roman A. The E7 proteins of low- and high-risk human papillomaviruses share the ability to target the pRB family member p130 for degradation. Proc Natl Acad Sci USA 2006; 103(2): 437-42.
[http://dx.doi.org/10.1073/pnas.0510012103] [PMID: 16381817]

[50] Korzeniewski N, Spardy N, Duensing A, Duensing S. Genomic instability and cancer: lessons learned from human papillomaviruses. Cancer Lett 2011; 305(2): 113-22.
[http://dx.doi.org/10.1016/j.canlet.2010.10.013] [PMID: 21075512]

[51] Klussmann JP, Gültekin E, Weissenborn SJ, *et al.* Expression of p16 protein identifies a distinct entity of tonsillar carcinomas associated with human papillomavirus. Am J Pathol 2003; 162(3): 747-53.
[http://dx.doi.org/10.1016/S0002-9440(10)63871-0] [PMID: 12598309]

[52] Galloway DA, Gewin LC, Myers H, *et al.* Regulation of telomerase by human papillomaviruses. Cold Spring Harb Symp Quant Biol 2005; 70: 209-15.
[http://dx.doi.org/10.1101/sqb.2005.70.041] [PMID: 16869756]

[53] Fu L, Van Doorslaer K, Chen Z, *et al.* Degradation of p53 by human Alphapapillomavirus E6 proteins shows a stronger correlation with phylogeny than oncogenicity. PLoS One 2010; 5(9): e12816.
[http://dx.doi.org/10.1371/journal.pone.0012816] [PMID: 20862247]

[54] Zanier K, ould M'hamed ould Sidi A, Boulade-Ladame C, *et al.* Solution structure analysis of the HPV16 E6 oncoprotein reveals a self-association mechanism required for E6-mediated degradation of p53. Structure 2012; 20(4): 604-17.
[http://dx.doi.org/10.1016/j.str.2012.02.001] [PMID: 22483108]

[55] Pim D, Banks L. Interaction of viral oncoproteins with cellular target molecules: infection with high-risk *vs* low-risk human papillomaviruses. APMIS 2010; 118(6-7): 471-93.
[http://dx.doi.org/10.1111/j.1600-0463.2010.02618.x] [PMID: 20553529]

[56] Malanchi I, Accardi R, Diehl F, *et al.* Human papillomavirus type 16 E6 promotes retinoblastoma protein phosphorylation and cell cycle progression. J Virol 2004; 78(24): 13769-78.
[http://dx.doi.org/10.1128/JVI.78.24.13769-13778.2004] [PMID: 15564485]

[57] Shai A, Brake T, Somoza C, Lambert PF. The human papillomavirus E6 oncogene dysregulates the cell cycle and contributes to cervical carcinogenesis through two independent activities. Cancer Res 2007; 67(4): 1626-35.
[http://dx.doi.org/10.1158/0008-5472.CAN-06-3344] [PMID: 17308103]

[58] Muench P, Hiller T, Probst S, Florea AM, Stubenrauch F, Iftner T. Binding of PDZ proteins to HPV E6 proteins does neither correlate with epidemiological risk classification nor with the immortalization of foreskin keratinocytes. Virology 2009; 387(2): 380-7.
[http://dx.doi.org/10.1016/j.virol.2009.02.018] [PMID: 19285702]

[59] Javier RT. Cell polarity proteins: common targets for tumorigenic human viruses. Oncogene 2008; 27(55): 7031-46.
[http://dx.doi.org/10.1038/onc.2008.352] [PMID: 19029943]

[60] Culp TD, Cladel NM, Balogh KK, Budgeon LR, Mejia AF, Christensen ND. Papillomavirus particles assembled in 293TT cells are infectious *in vivo*. J Virol 2006; 80(22): 11381-4. [http://dx.doi.org/10.1128/JVI.01328-06] [PMID: 16943284]

[61] Kühne C, Gardiol D, Guarnaccia C, Amenitsch H, Banks L. Differential regulation of human papillomavirus E6 by protein kinase A: conditional degradation of human discs large protein by oncogenic E6. Oncogene 2000; 19(51): 5884-91. [http://dx.doi.org/10.1038/sj.onc.1203988] [PMID: 11127819]

[62] Bodily J, Laimins LA. Persistence of human papillomavirus infection: keys to malignant progression. Trends Microbiol 2011; 19(1): 33-9. [http://dx.doi.org/10.1016/j.tim.2010.10.002] [PMID: 21050765]

[63] Banerjee NS, Wang HK, Broker TR, Chow LT. Human papillomavirus (HPV) E7 induces prolonged G2 following S phase reentry in differentiated human keratinocytes. J Biol Chem 2011; 286(17): 15473-82. [http://dx.doi.org/10.1074/jbc.M110.197574] [PMID: 21321122]

[64] Wang HK, Duffy AA, Broker TR, Chow LT. Robust production and passaging of infectious HPV in squamous epithelium of primary human keratinocytes. Genes Dev 2009; 23(2): 181-94. [http://dx.doi.org/10.1101/gad.1735109] [PMID: 19131434]

[65] Krawczyk E, Suprynowicz FA, Liu X, *et al.* Koilocytosis: a cooperative interaction between the human papillomavirus E5 and E6 oncoproteins. Am J Pathol 2008; 173(3): 682-8. [http://dx.doi.org/10.2353/ajpath.2008.080280] [PMID: 18688031]

[66] Krawczyk E, Suprynowicz FA, Sudarshan SR, Schlegel R. Membrane orientation of the human papillomavirus type 16 E5 oncoprotein. J Virol 2010; 84(4): 1696-703. [http://dx.doi.org/10.1128/JVI.01968-09] [PMID: 19955310]

[67] Suprynowicz FA, Krawczyk E, Hebert JD, *et al.* The human papillomavirus type 16 E5 oncoprotein inhibits epidermal growth factor trafficking independently of endosome acidification. J Virol 2010; 84(20): 10619-29. [http://dx.doi.org/10.1128/JVI.00831-10] [PMID: 20686024]

[68] Yu JH, Lin BY, Deng W, Broker TR, Chow LT. Mitogen-activated protein kinases activate the nuclear localization sequence of human papillomavirus type 11 E1 DNA helicase to promote efficient nuclear import. J Virol 2007; 81(10): 5066-78. [http://dx.doi.org/10.1128/JVI.02480-06] [PMID: 17344281]

[69] Deng W, Lin BY, Jin G, *et al.* Cyclin/CDK regulates the nucleocytoplasmic localization of the human papillomavirus E1 DNA helicase. J Virol 2004; 78(24): 13954-65. [http://dx.doi.org/10.1128/JVI.78.24.13954-13965.2004] [PMID: 15564503]

[70] McIntosh PB, Martin SR, Jackson DJ, *et al.* Structural analysis reveals an amyloid form of the human papillomavirus type 16 E1--E4 protein and provides a molecular basis for its accumulation. J Virol 2008; 82(16): 8196-203. [http://dx.doi.org/10.1128/JVI.00509-08] [PMID: 18562538]

[71] Gulliksen A, Keegan H, Martin C, *et al.* Towards a sample-in, answer-out point-of-care platform for nucleic acid extraction and amplification: Using an HPV E6/E7 mRNA model system. J Oncol 2012; 2012: 1-12.

[72] Wilson R, Ryan GB, Knight GL, Laimins LA, Roberts S. The full-length E1E4 protein of human papillomavirus type 18 modulates differentiation-dependent viral DNA amplification and late gene expression. Virology 2007; 362(2): 453-60. [http://dx.doi.org/10.1016/j.virol.2007.01.005] [PMID: 17303206]

[73] Jones DL, Alani RM, Münger K. The human papillomavirus E7 oncoprotein can uncouple cellular differentiation and proliferation in human keratinocytes by abrogating p21Cip1-mediated inhibition of cdk2. Genes Dev 1997; 11(16): 2101-11.

[http://dx.doi.org/10.1101/gad.11.16.2101] [PMID: 9284049]

[74] Genovese NJ, Banerjee NS, Broker TR, Chow LT. Casein kinase II motif-dependent phosphorylation of human papillomavirus E7 protein promotes p130 degradation and S-phase induction in differentiated human keratinocytes. J Virol 2008; 82(10): 4862-73. [http://dx.doi.org/10.1128/JVI.01202-07] [PMID: 18321970]

[75] Nor Rashid N, Yusof R, Watson RJ. Disruption of repressive p130-DREAM complexes by human papillomavirus 16 E6/E7 oncoproteins is required for cell-cycle progression in cervical cancer cells. J Gen Virol 2011; 92(Pt 11): 2620-7. [http://dx.doi.org/10.1099/vir.0.035352-0] [PMID: 21813705]

[76] McLaughlin-Drubin ME, Huh KW, Münger K. Human papillomavirus type 16 E7 oncoprotein associates with E2F6. J Virol 2008; 82(17): 8695-705. [http://dx.doi.org/10.1128/JVI.00579-08] [PMID: 18579589]

[77] Banerjee NS, Wang HK, Broker TR, Chow LT. Human papillomavirus (HPV) E7 induces prolonged G2 following S phase reentry in differentiated human keratinocytes. J Biol Chem 2011; 286(17): 15473-82. [http://dx.doi.org/10.1074/jbc.M110.197574] [PMID: 21321122]

[78] Genovese NJ, Broker TR, Chow LT. Nonconserved lysine residues attenuate the biological function of the low-risk human papillomavirus E7 protein. J Virol 2011; 85(11): 5546-54. [http://dx.doi.org/10.1128/JVI.02166-10] [PMID: 21411531]

[79] Nguyen CL, Münger K. Human papillomavirus E7 protein deregulates mitosis *via* an association with nuclear mitotic apparatus protein 1. J Virol 2009; 83(4): 1700-7. [http://dx.doi.org/10.1128/JVI.01971-08] [PMID: 19052088]

[80] McCloskey R, Menges C, Friedman A, Patel D, McCance DJ. Human papillomavirus type 16 E6/E7 upregulation of nucleophosmin is important for proliferation and inhibition of differentiation. J Virol 2010; 84(10): 5131-9. [http://dx.doi.org/10.1128/JVI.01965-09] [PMID: 20237089]

[81] Huh KW, DeMasi J, Ogawa H, Nakatani Y, Howley PM, Münger K. Association of the human papillomavirus type 16 E7 oncoprotein with the 600-kDa retinoblastoma protein-associated factor, p600. Proc Natl Acad Sci USA 2005; 102(32): 11492-7. [http://dx.doi.org/10.1073/pnas.0505337102] [PMID: 16061792]

[82] Ozbun MA, Meyers C. Human papillomavirus type 31b E1 and E2 transcript expression correlates with vegetative viral genome amplification. Virology 1998; 248(2): 218-30. [http://dx.doi.org/10.1006/viro.1998.9285] [PMID: 9721231]

[83] Johansson C, Somberg M, Li X, *et al.* HPV-16 E2 contributes to induction of HPV-16 late gene expression by inhibiting early polyadenylation. EMBO J 2012; 31(14): 3212-27. [http://dx.doi.org/10.1038/emboj.2012.147] [PMID: 22617423]

[84] Perea SE, Massimi P, Banks L. Human papillomavirus type 16 E7 impairs the activation of the interferon regulatory factor-1. Int J Mol Med 2000; 5(6): 661-6. [PMID: 10812019]

[85] Matthews K, Leong CM, Baxter L, *et al.* Depletion of Langerhans cells in human papillomavirus type 16-infected skin is associated with E6-mediated down regulation of E-cadherin. J Virol 2003; 77(15): 8378-85. [http://dx.doi.org/10.1128/JVI.77.15.8378-8385.2003] [PMID: 12857907]

[86] Ashrafi GH, Haghshenas M, Marchetti B, Campo MS. E5 protein of human papillomavirus 16 downregulates HLA class I and interacts with the heavy chain *via* its first hydrophobic domain. Int J Cancer 2006; 119(9): 2105-12. [http://dx.doi.org/10.1002/ijc.22089] [PMID: 16823848]

[87] Merad M, Ginhoux F, Collin M. Origin, homeostasis and function of Langerhans cells and other

langerin-expressing dendritic cells. Nat Rev Immunol 2008; 8(12): 935-47.
[http://dx.doi.org/10.1038/nri2455] [PMID: 19029989]

[88] Bedoui S, Whitney PG, Waithman J, *et al.* Cross-presentation of viral and self antigens by skin-derived CD103+ dendritic cells. Nat Immunol 2009; 10(5): 488-95.
[http://dx.doi.org/10.1038/ni.1724] [PMID: 19349986]

[89] Gravitt PE. The known unknowns of HPV natural history. J Clin Invest 2011; 121(12): 4593-9.
[http://dx.doi.org/10.1172/JCI57149] [PMID: 22133884]

[90] Ades S, Koushik A, Duarte-Franco E, *et al.* Selected class I and class II HLA alleles and haplotypes and risk of high-grade cervical intraepithelial neoplasia. Int J Cancer 2008; 122(12): 2820-6.
[http://dx.doi.org/10.1002/ijc.23459] [PMID: 18351579]

[91] Zoodsma M, Nolte IM, Te Meerman GJ, De Vries EG, Van der Zee AG. HLA genes and other candidate genes involved in susceptibility for (pre)neoplastic cervical disease. Int J Oncol 2005; 26(3): 769-84.
[PMID: 15703836]

[92] Heilman SA, Nordberg JJ, Liu Y, Sluder G, Chen JJ. Abrogation of the postmitotic checkpoint contributes to polyploidization in human papillomavirus E7-expressing cells. J Virol 2009; 83(6): 2756-64.
[http://dx.doi.org/10.1128/JVI.02149-08] [PMID: 19129456]

[93] Flores ER, Allen-Hoffmann BL, Lee D, Lambert PF. The human papillomavirus type 16 E7 oncogene is required for the productive stage of the viral life cycle. J Virol 2000; 74(14): 6622-31.
[http://dx.doi.org/10.1128/JVI.74.14.6622-6631.2000] [PMID: 10864676]

[94] Klaes R, Woerner SM, Ridder R, *et al.* Detection of high-risk cervical intraepithelial neoplasia and cervical cancer by amplification of transcripts derived from integrated papillomavirus oncogenes. Cancer Res 1999; 59(24): 6132-6.
[PMID: 10626803]

[95] Khleif SN, DeGregori J, Yee CL, *et al.* Inhibition of cyclin D-CDK4/CDK6 activity is associated with an E2F-mediated induction of cyclin kinase inhibitor activity. Proc Natl Acad Sci USA 1996; 93(9): 4350-4.
[http://dx.doi.org/10.1073/pnas.93.9.4350] [PMID: 8633069]

[96] Klingelhutz AJ, Foster SA, McDougall JK. Telomerase activation by the E6 gene product of human papillomavirus type 16. Nature 1996; 380(6569): 79-82.
[http://dx.doi.org/10.1038/380079a0] [PMID: 8598912]

[97] Sedman J, Stenlund A. Co-operative interaction between the initiator E1 and the transcriptional activator E2 is required for replicator specific DNA replication of bovine papillomavirus *in vivo* and *in vitro*. EMBO J 1995; 14(24): 6218-28.
[PMID: 8557041]

[98] Chiang CM, Broker TR, Chow LT. An E1M--E2C fusion protein encoded by human papillomavirus type 11 is asequence-specific transcription repressor. J Virol 1991; 65(6): 3317-29.
[PMID: 1851879]

[99] Schmitt A, Rochat A, Zeltner R, *et al.* The primary target cells of the high-risk cottontail rabbit papillomavirus colocalize with hair follicle stem cells. J Virol 1996; 70(3): 1912-22.
[PMID: 8627717]

[100] Stünkel W, Bernard HU. The chromatin structure of the long control region of human papillomavirus type 16 represses viral oncoprotein expression. J Virol 1999; 73(3): 1918-30.
[PMID: 9971771]

[101] del Mar Peña LM, Laimins LA. Differentiation-dependent chromatin rearrangement coincides with activation of human papillomavirus type 31 late gene expression. J Virol 2001; 75(20): 10005-13.
[http://dx.doi.org/10.1128/JVI.75.20.10005-10013.2001] [PMID: 11559836]

[102] Wooldridge TR, Laimins LA. Regulation of human papillomavirus type 31 gene expression during the differentiation-dependent life cycle through histone modifications and transcription factor binding. Virology 2008; 374(2): 371-80.
[http://dx.doi.org/10.1016/j.virol.2007.12.011] [PMID: 18237759]

[103] Carson A, Khan SA. Characterization of transcription factor binding to human papillomavirus type 16 DNA during cellular differentiation. J Virol 2006; 80(9): 4356-62.
[http://dx.doi.org/10.1128/JVI.80.9.4356-4362.2006] [PMID: 16611894]

[104] You J, Croyle JL, Nishimura A, Ozato K, Howley PM. Interaction of the bovine papillomavirus E2 protein with Brd4 tethers the viral DNA to host mitotic chromosomes. Cell 2004; 117(3): 349-60.
[http://dx.doi.org/10.1016/S0092-8674(04)00402-7] [PMID: 15109495]

[105] You J, Schweiger MR, Howley PM. Inhibition of E2 binding to Brd4 enhances viral genome loss and phenotypic reversion of bovine papillomavirus-transformed cells. J Virol 2005; 79(23): 14956-61.
[http://dx.doi.org/10.1128/JVI.79.23.14956-14961.2005] [PMID: 16282494]

[106] Abbate EA, Voitenleitner C, Botchan MR. Structure of the papillomavirus DNA-tethering complex E2:Brd4 and a peptide that ablates HPV chromosomal association. Mol Cell 2006; 24(6): 877-89.
[http://dx.doi.org/10.1016/j.molcel.2006.11.002] [PMID: 17189190]

[107] Hirochika H, Hirochika R, Broker TR, Chow LT. Functional mapping of the human papillomavirus type 11 transcriptional enhancer and its interaction with the trans-acting E2 proteins. Genes Dev 1988; 2(1): 54-67.
[http://dx.doi.org/10.1101/gad.2.1.54] [PMID: 2833426]

[108] Schweiger MR, You J, Howley PM. Bromodomain protein 4 mediates the papillomavirus E2 transcriptional activation function. J Virol 2006; 80(9): 4276-85.
[http://dx.doi.org/10.1128/JVI.80.9.4276-4285.2006] [PMID: 16611886]

[109] Lee AY, Chiang CM. Chromatin adaptor Brd4 modulates E2 transcription activity and protein stability. J Biol Chem 2009; 284(5): 2778-86.
[http://dx.doi.org/10.1074/jbc.M805835200] [PMID: 19038968]

[110] Wu SY, Chiang CM. The double bromodomain-containing chromatin adaptor Brd4 and transcriptional regulation. J Biol Chem 2007; 282(18): 13141-5.
[http://dx.doi.org/10.1074/jbc.R700001200] [PMID: 17329240]

[111] Schweiger MR, Ottinger M, You J, Howley PM. Brd4-independent transcriptional repression function of the papillomavirus e2 proteins. J Virol 2007; 81(18): 9612-22.
[http://dx.doi.org/10.1128/JVI.00447-07] [PMID: 17626100]

[112] Jang MK, Mochizuki K, Zhou M, Jeong HS, Brady JN, Ozato K. The bromodomain protein Brd4 is a positive regulatory component of P-TEFb and stimulates RNA polymerase II-dependent transcription. Mol Cell 2005; 19(4): 523-34.
[http://dx.doi.org/10.1016/j.molcel.2005.06.027] [PMID: 16109376]

[113] Yang Z, Yik JH, Chen R, *et al.* Recruitment of P-TEFb for stimulation of transcriptional elongation by the bromodomain protein Brd4. Mol Cell 2005; 19(4): 535-45.
[http://dx.doi.org/10.1016/j.molcel.2005.06.029] [PMID: 16109377]

[114] Bisgrove DA, Mahmoudi T, Henklein P, Verdin E. Conserved P-TEFb-interacting domain of BRD4 inhibits HIV transcription. Proc Natl Acad Sci USA 2007; 104(34): 13690-5.
[http://dx.doi.org/10.1073/pnas.0705053104] [PMID: 17690245]

[115] Cho WK, Zhou M, Jang MK, *et al.* Modulation of the Brd4/P-TEFb interaction by the human T-lymphotropic virus type 1 tax protein. J Virol 2007; 81(20): 11179-86.
[http://dx.doi.org/10.1128/JVI.00408-07] [PMID: 17686863]

[116] Howley PM. Papillomaviruses and their replication, in: D.M. Knipe, P.M. Howley (Eds.), Filelds virology. Lippincott Williams & Wilkins Philadelphia. 2001; 2: 2197.

[117] Thomas JT, Hubert WG, Ruesch MN, Laimins LA. Human papillomavirus type 31 oncoproteins E6 and E7 are required for the maintenance of episomes during the viral life cycle in normal human keratinocytes. Proc Natl Acad Sci USA 1999; 96(15): 8449-54. [http://dx.doi.org/10.1073/pnas.96.15.8449] [PMID: 10411895]

[118] Kadaja M, Silla T, Ustav E, Ustav M. Papillomavirus DNA replication - from initiation to genomic instability. Virology 2009; 384(2): 360-8. [http://dx.doi.org/10.1016/j.virol.2008.11.032] [PMID: 19141359]

[119] Hernandez BY, Shvetsov YB, Goodman MT, *et al.* Reduced clearance of penile human papillomavirus infection in uncircumcised men. J Infect Dis 2010; 201(9): 1340-3. [http://dx.doi.org/10.1086/651607] [PMID: 20350160]

[120] Tolstov Y, Hadaschik B, Pahernik S, Hohenfellner M, Duensing S. Human papillomaviruses in urological malignancies: a critical assessment. In Urologic Oncology: Seminars and Original Investigations 2014; 32 (1): 46-e19.

[121] Mighty KK, Laimins LA. The role of human papillomaviruses in oncogenesis.Viruses and Human Cancer. Springer Berlin Heidelberg 2014; pp. 135-48. [http://dx.doi.org/10.1007/978-3-642-38965-8_8]

[122] Dok R, Nuyts S. HPV positive head and neck cancers: Molecular pathogenesis and evolving treatment strategies. Cancers (Basel) 2016; 8(4): E41. [http://dx.doi.org/10.3390/cancers8040041] [PMID: 27043631]

CHAPTER 5

Natural History of HPV Infections in Cancer Development

Niloofar Naderi, Kimia Kardani and **Azam Bolhassani***

Department of Hepatitis and AIDS, Pasteur Institute of Iran, Tehran, Iran

Department of Pharmaceutical Biotechnology, School of Pharmacy, Shahid Beheshti University of Medical Sciences, Tehran, Iran

Abstract: Cervical infections caused by HPV appear at any age as a benign disorder unless they persist. Different studies on transmission of HPV showed that the rates of transmission between heterosexual couples widely vary dependent on some factors such as intervals between testing points, rates of concordance or discordance at baseline, and difficulty in defining established infections versus contamination. This chapter describes the natural history of (HPV) infection in different stages of cancers in women and men.

Keywords: HPV, Infection, Natural History.

INTRODUCTION

HPV infection is common in both young sexually active women and men [1]. The cervix provides the best model of the natural history of HPV and anogenital neoplasia [2]. The prevalence of cervical HPV peaks at young ages on sexual initiation [3, 4]. Age-specific regional differences in cervical HPV prevalence are not well understood [5]. Given that HPV testing and vaccination have been incorporated into cervical cancer prevention programs based on age of people, it is increasingly important to clarify major issues in the natural history of HPV infection and any potential relationship to pre-cancer and cancer stages [6]. So-called U-shaped HPV prevalence curves characterized by high cervical HPV prevalence at young ages followed by a significant decline and subsequent increase in prevalence beginning at different later ages have been observed in different trials. In other examples, HPV increases in prevalence at young ages and then remains constant with age [6]. Evident potential factors contributing to these age-specific regional HPV prevalence differences at older ages include a) conti-

* **Corresponding author Azam Bolhassani:** Department of Hepatitis and AIDS, Pasteur Institute of Iran, Tehran, Iran; Tel: 66953311-20; E-mails: A_bolhasani@pasteur.ac.ir, azam.bolhassani@yahoo.com

nuing new sexual exposures, b) reappearance of latent HPV; c) changes in immune status, such as decline in immune function and hormonal milieu at older ages or immunosuppression caused by co-infection with other viral or parasitic agents; and d) cofactors including the cervicovaginal microbiota and pH [6]. Most HPV infections are transient and regress spontaneously within 24 months in women. However, persistent HPV infection is strongly associated with precancerous and cancerous lesions [7, 8]. HPV represents a specific tropism for the squamous epithelium of the skin and mucosae [9, 10]. In the absence of a productive viral infection, HPV entry into non-dividing or minimally dividing cervical basal epithelial cells could allow HPV genomes to become as latent states until a triggered replication, division, or differentiation event of the host stem cell occurs [6]. To better understand the natural history of HPV infection, it would be useful to identify markers of declining HPV immunity [6]. Both humoral and cellular immune responses are important for protection against HPV infection and clearance of HPV-infected cells [7 - 11]. The humoral immune response to natural HPV infection is usually slow, weak, and variable. Neutralizing antibodies to HPV specifically recognize L1 capsid protein for inhibition of early infection before viral entry into cells [9, 12]. Among women infected with oncogenic HPV types, only 50% develop antibodies to HPV infection that are not essentially protective against re-infection by the same HPV type [9, 11, 13]. On the other hand, women with cell-mediated immune defects (*e.g.*, HIV infection) are at increased risk of persistent infection caused by HR-HPV [7, 14]. Effective cytotoxic T lymphocytes (CTLs) may be an essential immune response against persistent HPV infections [15, 16]. Regression of HPV infection and CIN is associated with cell-mediated immune response to E6 and E7 oncoproteins [7, 17]. The natural history of HPV showed that persistent HPV infection may lead to CIN2 or CIN3 [2, 9]. It was shown that progression to CIN3 takes 7-15 years and progression to invasive cancer takes 20 years or more [9, 18, 19]. Most HPV infections (*i.e.*, presence of DNA but no detectable lesion) and low-grade CIN (CIN1) resolve due to the development of cell-mediated immunity (CMI) but not certainly by seroconversion and antibody to HPV L1 protein. A minority of women (~10-15%) do not make a successful cell mediated immune response; they remain HPV DNA-positive with a persistent viral infection and also at risk for the development of high-grade intraepithelial disease [1, 20 - 22]. Although most viral infections are cleared by host immune responses, oncogenic HPVs can interfere with immune system by several immune-escaping mechanisms such as down-regulating proliferation of tumor-specific CTL, antigen-processing defects, and defective expression of human leukocyte antigen (HLA) by genomic instability [7, 14]. Briefly, Fig. (**1**) shows natural history of HPV infections in the cervix and progression to cancer.

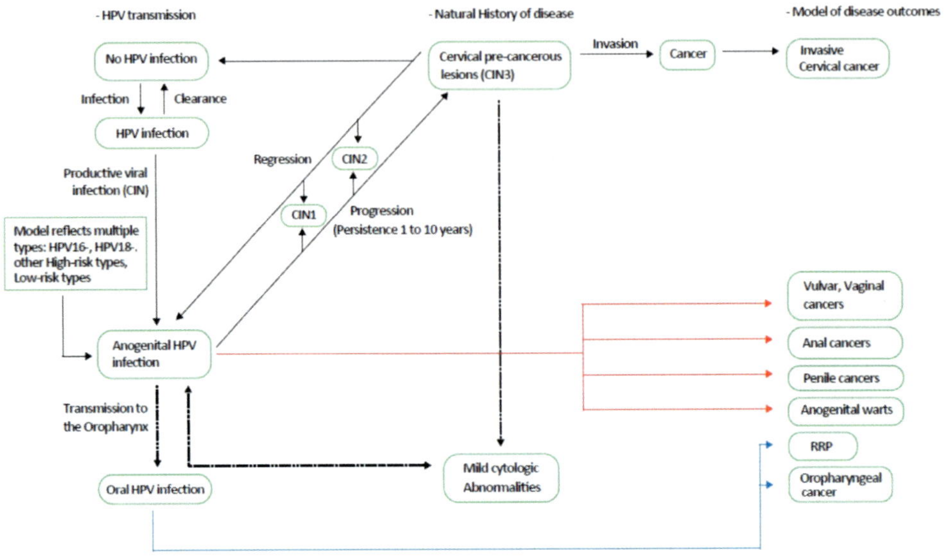

Fig. (1). Schematic diagram of HPV transmission, the natural history of disease, and cervical screening: Most infections are quickly cleared through the innate immune system. Even following establishment, the host immune response can still clear the viral infection. The persistently infected epithelium (1-10 years) will support clonal progression, leading to CIN3. Finally, the lesion progresses into invasive carcinoma [72, 73]. CIN: Cervical intraepithelial neoplasia; RRP: Recurrent respiratory papillomatosis.

Natural History of HPV-Related Neoplasia

Most people encounter genital HPV after the onset of sexual activity [23]. The clinical outcomes of infection will change according to the type of HPVs. Most infections resolve spontaneously by host's immune system [23, 24]; but some individuals do not clear infections caused by oncogenic HPV types leading to an increased risk of dysplasia, intraepithelial neoplasia, and finally invasive carcinomas [23].

Risk of CIN3$^+$ Following a Positive HPV Test

A negative HPV test involves low-risk of CIN3$^+$, and a positive HPV test results in a high risk of CIN3$^+$, although many infections are resolved [2, 25]. Recently, the HPV-16 and -18 DNA positivity has been correlated with increased risk of adenocarcinoma [2, 26]. Indeed, repeated HPV positivity is a sign of HPV persistence and an increased risk of CIN3$^+$ [2, 27]. Although, HPV-16 has the highest risk for CIN3$^+$, rates of HPV16 persistence after an infection are similar to other high risk HPV types [2, 28]. A study showed that the peak of CIN3 was in 25-29 age group in countries where cervical cancer screening was initiated at age 25 years [2, 29].

Risk of CIN3⁺ Following a Negative HPV Test

Several studies confirmed that there is a very low risk of $CIN3^+$ in the years following one or two HPV negative tests at any age. The risk predicted by a negative HPV test has been low for invasive cancer [2, 27]. In a negative HPV test, the cleared infections do not re-appear and do not cause the risk of $CIN3^+$ cases. However, few studies showed the natural history of re-appearing HPV infection. Indeed, young women are likely re-infected with different and the same HPV types after HPV clearance [2, 30, 31]. Because the rate of infections reduces gradually with age, the majority of cancers in a population can be attributed to infections acquired at a young age that do not clear [2, 32].

Non-Viral Co-factors for HPV Persistence

The best established etiologic co-factors for CIN3 or invasive cancer among HPV-infected women are smoking, long-term hormonal contraceptive use, multiparty and human immunodeficiency virus (HIV) infection [2, 33, 34]. Several studies have indicated that HIV infection increases the risk of HPV persistence at all ages [35, 36]. An interesting study indicated that both smoking and oral contraceptives enhance viral persistence in adolescents [37, 38]. The strongest factor resulting in these persistent infections is likely a lack of adequate immune response. The role of *C. trachomatis* infection as a co-factor for $CIN3^+$ is especially controversial [2, 39].

Natural History of CIN2

CIN2 is thought to be an intermediary step from CIN1 to CIN3 [2, 34, 40]. Recent data have shown that regression rates of CIN2 among young women (< 25 years of age, 50-70%) are higher than in older women (30-50%) over a 2-year period [2, 40 - 44]. For all ages, the regression rate for CIN2 appears to be lower than that of CIN1 (~ 90%), and higher than that of CIN3 (~ 20-30%) [2, 27, 34]. Uleberg *et al.* found that several proteins (*e.g.*, cytokeratin 2) can differentiate CIN2 from CIN3 lesions [45, 46]. Cervical cancer is typically the result of a long process that begins with an infection caused by a carcinogenic HPV type [46, 47]. Half of new HPV infections were undetectable within approximately 6-12 months, and more than 90% clear within a few years. The rate of clearance was high within the first months after infection but decreased over time [46, 48]. When a carcinogenic HPV type was detected by HPV testing, a simultaneous cytological abnormality was present about one-quarter to one-third of the time [46, 49]. Most of these abnormalities were not clear. As compared to infection with other carcinogenic HPV types, a woman with an HPV16 infection is most likely to present with serious cytological abnormalities [46, 50]. However, annual screening often lost these slight temporal differences [46, 51]. HPV clearance resulted in long-term humoral and/or cellular protection against re-infection with the same HPV type. Although, the term clearance was used when an HPV infection could no longer be detected using sensitive test methods, HPV might not be completely eliminated (*i.e.,* a latent state of HPV) [46]. Reappearance of HPV from "latency", even in the absence of important immunosuppression is common, but probably benign [46, 52]. In contrast to the cleared HPV infections, the cancer risk increased significantly for the 5% of HPV infections that persist for more than a few years [53 - 55]. However, CIN3 lesions typically grew slowly over many years before invasion. It is clear that the development of CIN3 following a new HPV infection occurs much more quickly than does the development of invasive cancer invasion from CIN3 [56, 57]. The time from infection to invasive cancer is shorter for HPV16 than for other HPV types [58]. Interestingly, clearance of oncogenic HPV infection decreased in men with a high number of female partners and was more rapid with increasing age [59 - 61].

Anal HPV Natural History in Men and Women

Anal intraepithelial neoplasia (AIN) shares similarities in its histologic appearance with CIN and data on its natural history are insignificant on HIV un-infected persons. High-grade AIN (HGAIN) is a true precursor to invasive anal cancer. Most of the studies on AIN have been done in men who have sex with men (MSM). The prevalence of AIN is highest among HIV-infected MSM, followed by HIV-uninfected MSM [2, 62]. A recent analysis of immunocompetent women with CIN, vulvar or vaginal intraepithelial neoplasia showed that 12% and 8% of women had AIN and HGAIN, respectively [2, 36, 63, 64]. The extent to which chronic infection with HIV affects anal HPV persistence in HIV- positive MSM is unclear. Studies in HIV-infected women have shown that detection of cervical HPV is associated with higher HIV viral load and a lower CD4+ T-cell count [65, 66]. This data suggested a direct relationship between immune deficiency and impaired control over HPV clearance [65, 67]. Some researchers have also proposed that the difference may be due to the HIV virus itself. Mucosal cells that cover the anorectal and genital cavities represented the primary site for HIV and HPV entry. It has been suggested that alterations in the local microenvironment caused by infection with HIV may favor HPV entry. The effect of chronic HIV infection on normal immune function leading to HPV persistence, suggests the HIV increases susceptibility to HPV infection and retention. The mechanisms that facilitate this action are still unknown [65, 68 - 71].

CONCLUDING REMARKS

Regarding the studies, most HPV infections regress spontaneously in women, but however, persistent HPV infections do not regress and are strongly associated with precancerous and cancerous lesions. Despite women, prevalence rates of HPV infection are constant at all ages in men suggesting that men do not develop protection against re-infection and these risks are associated with sexual behaviors.

CONFLICT OF INTEREST

The author (editor) declares no conflict of interest, financial or otherwise.

ACKNOWLEDGEMENT

Declare none.

REFERENCES

[1] Stanley M. Pathology and epidemiology of HPV infection in females. Gynecol Oncol 2010; 117(2) (Suppl.): S5-S10.
[http://dx.doi.org/10.1016/j.ygyno.2010.01.024] [PMID: 20304221]

[2] Moscicki AB, Schiffman M, Burchell A, *et al.* Updating the natural history of human papillomavirus and anogenital cancers. Vaccine 2012; 30(5) (Suppl. 5): F24-33.
[http://dx.doi.org/10.1016/j.vaccine.2012.05.089] [PMID: 23199964]

[3] Hariri S, Unger ER, Sternberg M, *et al.* Prevalence of genital human papillomavirus among females in the United States, the National Health And Nutrition Examination Survey, 2003-2006. J Infect Dis 2011; 204(4): 566-73.
[http://dx.doi.org/10.1093/infdis/jir341] [PMID: 21791659]

[4] Wheeler CM, Hunt WC, Cuzick J, *et al.* A population-based study of human papillomavirus genotype prevalence in the United States: baseline measures prior to mass human papillomavirus vaccination. Int J Cancer 2013; 132(1): 198-207.
[http://dx.doi.org/10.1002/ijc.27608] [PMID: 22532127]

[5] Franceschi S, Herrero R, Clifford GM, *et al.* Variations in the age-specific curves of human papillomavirus prevalence in women worldwide. Int J Cancer 2006; 119(11): 2677-84.
[http://dx.doi.org/10.1002/ijc.22241] [PMID: 16991121]

[6] Wheeler CM. The natural history of cervical human papillomavirus infections and cervical cancer: gaps in knowledge and future horizons. Obstet Gynecol Clin North Am 2013; 40(2): 165-76.
[http://dx.doi.org/10.1016/j.ogc.2013.02.004] [PMID: 23732023]

[7] No JH, Kim MK, Jeon YT, Kim YB, Song YS. Human papillomavirus vaccine: widening the scope for cancer prevention. Mol Carcinog 2011; 50(4): 244-53.
[http://dx.doi.org/10.1002/mc.20657] [PMID: 21465574]

[8] Plummer M, Schiffman M, Castle PE, Maucort-Boulch D, Wheeler CM. A 2-year prospective study of human papillomavirus persistence among women with a cytological diagnosis of atypical squamous cells of undetermined significance or low-grade squamous intraepithelial lesion. J Infect Dis 2007; 195(11): 1582-9.
[http://dx.doi.org/10.1086/516784] [PMID: 17471427]

[9] Pandhi D, Sonthalia S. Human papilloma virus vaccines: Current scenario. Indian J Sex Transm Dis 2011; 32(2): 75-85.
[http://dx.doi.org/10.4103/0253-7184.85409] [PMID: 22021967]

[10] Mariani L, Venuti A. HPV vaccine: an overview of immune response, clinical protection, and new

approaches for the future. J Transl Med 2010; 8: 105.
[http://dx.doi.org/10.1186/1479-5876-8-105] [PMID: 20979636]

[11] Carter JJ, Koutsky LA, Hughes JP, *et al.* Comparison of human papillomavirus types 16, 18, and 6 capsid antibody responses following incident infection. J Infect Dis 2000; 181(6): 1911-9.
[http://dx.doi.org/10.1086/315498] [PMID: 10837170]

[12] Stanley M, Lowy DR, Frazer I. Prophylactic HPV vaccines: Underlying mechanisms. Vaccine 2006; 24(6): S3/106-13.

[13] Carter JJ, Madeleine MM, Shera K, *et al.* Human papillomavirus 16 and 18 L1 serology compared across anogenital cancer sites. Cancer Res 2001; 61(5): 1934-40.
[PMID: 11280749]

[14] Sheu BC, Chang WC, Lin HH, Chow SN, Huang SC. Immune concept of human papillomaviruses and related antigens in local cancer milieu of human cervical neoplasia. J Obstet Gynaecol Res 2007; 33(2): 103-13.
[http://dx.doi.org/10.1111/j.1447-0756.2007.00492.x] [PMID: 17441881]

[15] Bontkes HJ, de Gruijl TD, van den Muysenberg AJ, *et al.* Human papillomavirus type 16 E6/E7-specific cytotoxic T lymphocytes in women with cervical neoplasia. Int J Cancer 2000; 88(1): 92-8.
[http://dx.doi.org/10.1002/1097-0215(20001001)88:1<92::AID-IJC15>3.0.CO;2-E] [PMID: 10962445]

[16] Chen L, Mizuno MT, Singhal MC, *et al.* Induction of cytotoxic T lymphocytes specific for a syngeneic tumor expressing the E6 oncoprotein of human papillomavirus type 16. J Immunol 1992; 148(8): 2617-21.
[PMID: 1313847]

[17] Kadish AS, Timmins P, Wang Y, *et al.* Regression of cervical intraepithelial neoplasia and loss of human papillomavirus (HPV) infection is associated with cell-mediated immune responses to an HPV type 16 E7 peptide. Cancer Epidemiol Biomarkers Prev 2002; 11(5): 483-8.
[PMID: 12010863]

[18] Bosch FX, de Sanjosé S. Chapter 1: Human papillomavirus and cervical cancer--burden and assessment of causality. J Natl Cancer Inst Monogr 2003; 31(31): 3-13.
[http://dx.doi.org/10.1093/oxfordjournals.jncimonographs.a003479] [PMID: 12807939]

[19] Koshiol J, Lindsay L, Pimenta JM, Poole C, Jenkins D, Smith JS. Persistent human papillomavirus infection and cervical neoplasia: a systematic review and meta-analysis. Am J Epidemiol 2008; 168(2): 123-37.
[http://dx.doi.org/10.1093/aje/kwn036] [PMID: 18483125]

[20] Moscicki AB, Schiffman M, Kjaer S, Villa LL. Chapter 5: updating the natural history of HPV and anogenital cancer. Vaccine 2006; 24(3): S3/42-51.

[21] Cuschieri KS, Cubie HA, Whitley MW, *et al.* Persistent high risk HPV infection associated with development of cervical neoplasia in a prospective population study. J Clin Pathol 2005; 58(9): 946-50.
[http://dx.doi.org/10.1136/jcp.2004.022863] [PMID: 16126875]

[22] Liaw KL, Hildesheim A, Burk RD, *et al.* A prospective study of human papillomavirus (HPV) type 16 DNA detection by polymerase chain reaction and its association with acquisition and persistence of other HPV types. J Infect Dis 2001; 183(1): 8-15.
[http://dx.doi.org/10.1086/317638] [PMID: 11087198]

[23] Wain G. The human papillomavirus (HPV) vaccine, HPV related diseases and cervical cancer in the post-reproductive years. Maturitas 2010; 65(3): 205-9.
[http://dx.doi.org/10.1016/j.maturitas.2009.12.002] [PMID: 20036786]

[24] Stanley M. A practitioner's guide to understanding immunity to human papillomavirus. US Obstet Gynecol 2009; 4: 2-7.

[25] Sundström K, Eloranta S, Sparén P, *et al.* Prospective study of human papillomavirus (HPV) types, HPV persistence, and risk of squamous cell carcinoma of the cervix. Cancer Epidemiol Biomarkers Prev 2010; 19(10): 2469-78.
[http://dx.doi.org/10.1158/1055-9965.EPI-10-0424] [PMID: 20671136]

[26] Dahlström LA, Ylitalo N, Sundström K, *et al.* Prospective study of human papillomavirus and risk of cervical adenocarcinoma. Int J Cancer 2010; 127(8): 1923-30.
[http://dx.doi.org/10.1002/ijc.25408] [PMID: 20473898]

[27] Bautista OM, Saah A, Muñoz N. Re: Longitudinal study of human papillomavirus persistence and cervical intraepithelial neoplasia grade 2/3: critical role of duration of infection. J Natl Cancer Inst 2011; 103(2): 158-9.
[http://dx.doi.org/10.1093/jnci/djq468] [PMID: 21115883]

[28] Moscicki AB, Widdice L, Ma Y, *et al.* Comparison of natural histories of human papillomavirus detected by clinician- and self-sampling. Int J Cancer 2010; 127(8): 1882-92.
[http://dx.doi.org/10.1002/ijc.25199] [PMID: 20104517]

[29] Winer RL, Kiviat NB, Hughes JP, *et al.* Development and duration of human papillomavirus lesions, after initial infection. J Infect Dis 2005; 191(5): 731-8.
[http://dx.doi.org/10.1086/427557] [PMID: 15688287]

[30] Winer RL, Hughes JP, Feng Q, *et al.* Early natural history of incident, type-specific human papillomavirus infections in newly sexually active young women. Cancer Epidemiol Biomarkers Prev 2011; 20(4): 699-707.
[http://dx.doi.org/10.1158/1055-9965.EPI-10-1108] [PMID: 21173170]

[31] Moscicki AB, Ma Y, Jonte J, *et al.* The role of sexual behavior and human papillomavirus persistence in predicting repeated infections with new human papillomavirus types. Cancer Epidemiol Biomarkers Prev 2010; 19(8): 2055-65.
[http://dx.doi.org/10.1158/1055-9965.EPI-10-0394] [PMID: 20696663]

[32] Rodriguez AC, Schiffman M, Herrero R, *et al.* Low risk of cervical intraepithelial neoplasia grade 2/3 after re-appearance of type-specific carcinogenic HPV. Int J Cancer 2012; 131(8): 1874-81.
[http://dx.doi.org/10.1002/ijc.27418] [PMID: 22213126]

[33] Syrjänen K, Shabalova I, Naud P, *et al.* Co-factors of high-risk human papillomavirus infections display unique profiles in incident CIN1, CIN2 and CIN3. Int J STD AIDS 2011; 22(5): 263-72.
[http://dx.doi.org/10.1258/ijsa.2009.009280] [PMID: 21571974]

[34] Moscicki AB, Ma Y, Wibbelsman C, *et al.* Risks for cervical intraepithelial neoplasia 3 among adolescents and young women with abnormal cytology. Obstet Gynecol 2008; 112(6): 1335-42.
[http://dx.doi.org/10.1097/AOG.0b013e31818c9222] [PMID: 19037044]

[35] Nielsen A, Kjaer SK, Munk C, Osler M, Iftner T. Persistence of high-risk human papillomavirus infection in a population-based cohort of Danish women. J Med Virol 2010; 82(4): 616-23.
[http://dx.doi.org/10.1002/jmv.21750] [PMID: 20166190]

[36] Denny LA, Franceschi S, de Sanjosé S, Heard I, Moscicki AB, Palefsky J. Human papillomavirus, human immunodeficiency virus and immunosuppression. Vaccine 2012; 30(5) (Suppl. 5): F168-74.
[http://dx.doi.org/10.1016/j.vaccine.2012.06.045] [PMID: 23199960]

[37] Hwang LY, Ma Y, Benningfield SM, *et al.* Factors that influence the rate of epithelial maturation in the cervix in healthy young women. J Adolesc Health 2009; 44(2): 103-10.
[http://dx.doi.org/10.1016/j.jadohealth.2008.10.006] [PMID: 19167657]

[38] Louie KS, de Sanjose S, Diaz M, *et al.* Early age at first sexual intercourse and early pregnancy are risk factors for cervical cancer in developing countries. Br J Cancer 2009; 100(7): 1191-7.
[http://dx.doi.org/10.1038/sj.bjc.6604974] [PMID: 19277042]

[39] Safaeian M, Quint K, Schiffman M, *et al.* Chlamydia trachomatis and risk of prevalent and incident cervical premalignancy in a population-based cohort. J Natl Cancer Inst 2010; 102(23): 1794-804.

[http://dx.doi.org/10.1093/jnci/djq436] [PMID: 21098758]

[40] Moscicki AB, Ma Y, Wibbelsman C, *et al.* Rate of and risks for regression of cervical intraepithelial neoplasia 2 in adolescents and young women. Obstet Gynecol 2010; 116(6): 1373-80. [http://dx.doi.org/10.1097/AOG.0b013e3181fe777f] [PMID: 21099605]

[41] McAllum B, Sykes PH, Sadler L, Macnab H, Simcock BJ, Mekhail AK. Is the treatment of CIN 2 always necessary in women under 25 years old? Am J Obstet Gynecol 2011; 205(5): 478.e1-7. [http://dx.doi.org/10.1016/j.ajog.2011.06.069] [PMID: 21872201]

[42] Insinga RP, Dasbach EJ, Elbasha EH. Epidemiologic natural history and clinical management of Human Papillomavirus (HPV) Disease: a critical and systematic review of the literature in the development of an HPV dynamic transmission model. BMC Infect Dis 2009; 9: 119. [http://dx.doi.org/10.1186/1471-2334-9-119] [PMID: 19640281]

[43] Castle PE, Schiffman M, Wheeler CM, Solomon D. Evidence for frequent regression of cervical intraepithelial neoplasia-grade 2. Obstet Gynecol 2009; 113(1): 18-25. [http://dx.doi.org/10.1097/AOG.0b013e31818f5008] [PMID: 19104355]

[44] Matsumoto K, Oki A, Furuta R, *et al.* Predicting the progression of cervical precursor lesions by human papillomavirus genotyping: a prospective cohort study. Int J Cancer 2011; 128(12): 2898-910. [http://dx.doi.org/10.1002/ijc.25630] [PMID: 20734388]

[45] Uleberg KE, Munk AC, Brede C, *et al.* Discrimination of grade 2 and 3 cervical intraepithelial neoplasia by means of analysis of water soluble proteins recovered from cervical biopsies. Proteome Sci 2011; 9: 36. [http://dx.doi.org/10.1186/1477-5956-9-36] [PMID: 21711556]

[46] Schiffman M, Wentzensen N, Wacholder S, Kinney W, Gage JC, Castle PE. Human papillomavirus testing in the prevention of cervical cancer. J Natl Cancer Inst 2011; 103(5): 368-83. [http://dx.doi.org/10.1093/jnci/djq562] [PMID: 21282563]

[47] Muñoz N, Hernandez-Suarez G, Méndez F, *et al.* Persistence of HPV infection and risk of high-grade cervical intraepithelial neoplasia in a cohort of Colombian women. Br J Cancer 2009; 100(7): 1184-90. [http://dx.doi.org/10.1038/sj.bjc.6604972] [PMID: 19293802]

[48] Rodríguez AC, Schiffman M, Herrero R, *et al.* Rapid clearance of human papillomavirus and implications for clinical focus on persistent infections. J Natl Cancer Inst 2008; 100(7): 513-7. [http://dx.doi.org/10.1093/jnci/djn044] [PMID: 18364507]

[49] Kovacic MB, Castle PE, Herrero R, *et al.* Relationships of human papillomavirus type, qualitative viral load, and age with cytologic abnormality. Cancer Res 2006; 66(20): 10112-9. [http://dx.doi.org/10.1158/0008-5472.CAN-06-1812] [PMID: 17047075]

[50] Schiffman M, Wheeler CM, Castle PE. Human papillomavirus DNA remains detectable longer than related cervical cytologic abnormalities. J Infect Dis 2002; 186(8): 1169-72. [http://dx.doi.org/10.1086/343816] [PMID: 12355370]

[51] Stanley M. Immune responses to human papillomavirus. Vaccine 2006; 24(1) (Suppl. 1): S16-22. [http://dx.doi.org/10.1016/j.vaccine.2005.09.002] [PMID: 16219398]

[52] González P, Hildesheim A, Rodríguez AC, *et al.* Behavioral/lifestyle and immunologic factors associated with HPV infection among women older than 45 years. Cancer Epidemiol Biomarkers Prev 2010; 19(12): 3044-54. [http://dx.doi.org/10.1158/1055-9965.EPI-10-0645] [PMID: 20952561]

[53] Castle PE, Solomon D, Schiffman M, Wheeler CM. Human papillomavirus type 16 infections and 2-year absolute risk of cervical precancer in women with equivocal or mild cytologic abnormalities. J Natl Cancer Inst 2005; 97(14): 1066-71. [http://dx.doi.org/10.1093/jnci/dji186] [PMID: 16030304]

[54] Trottier H, Mahmud SM, Lindsay L, *et al.* Persistence of an incident human papillomavirus infection and timing of cervical lesions in previously unexposed young women. Cancer Epidemiol Biomarkers

Prev 2009; 18(3): 854-62.
[http://dx.doi.org/10.1158/1055-9965.EPI-08-1012] [PMID: 19223559]

[55] Schlecht NF, Kulaga S, Robitaille J, *et al.* Persistent human papillomavirus infection as a predictor of cervical intraepithelial neoplasia. JAMA 2001; 286(24): 3106-14.
[http://dx.doi.org/10.1001/jama.286.24.3106] [PMID: 11754676]

[56] Schiffman M, Rodríguez AC. Heterogeneity in CIN3 diagnosis. Lancet Oncol 2008; 9(5): 404-6.
[http://dx.doi.org/10.1016/S1470-2045(08)70110-4] [PMID: 18452848]

[57] McCredie MR, Sharples KJ, Paul C, *et al.* Natural history of cervical neoplasia and risk of invasive cancer in women with cervical intraepithelial neoplasia 3: a retrospective cohort study. Lancet Oncol 2008; 9(5): 425-34.
[http://dx.doi.org/10.1016/S1470-2045(08)70103-7] [PMID: 18407790]

[58] Wheeler CM, Hunt WC, Joste NE, Key CR, Quint WG, Castle PE. Human papillomavirus genotype distributions: implications for vaccination and cancer screening in the United States. J Natl Cancer Inst 2009; 101(7): 475-87.
[http://dx.doi.org/10.1093/jnci/djn510] [PMID: 19318628]

[59] Giuliano AR, Lee JH, Fulp W, *et al.* Incidence and clearance of genital human papillomavirus infection in men (HIM): a cohort study. Lancet 2011; 377(9769): 932-40.
[http://dx.doi.org/10.1016/S0140-6736(10)62342-2] [PMID: 21367446]

[60] Gray RH, Serwadda D, Kong X, *et al.* Male circumcision decreases acquisition and increases clearance of high-risk human papillomavirus in HIV-negative men: a randomized trial in Rakai, Uganda. J Infect Dis 2010; 201(10): 1455-62.
[http://dx.doi.org/10.1086/652184] [PMID: 20370483]

[61] Hernandez BY, Shvetsov YB, Goodman MT, *et al.* Reduced clearance of penile human papillomavirus infection in uncircumcised men. J Infect Dis 2010; 201(9): 1340-3.
[http://dx.doi.org/10.1086/651607] [PMID: 20350160]

[62] Chin-Hong PV, Berry JM, Cheng SC, *et al.* Comparison of patient- and clinician-collected anal cytology samples to screen for human papillomavirus-associated anal intraepithelial neoplasia in men who have sex with men. Ann Intern Med 2008; 149(5): 300-6.
[http://dx.doi.org/10.7326/0003-4819-149-5-200809020-00004] [PMID: 18765699]

[63] Santoso JT, Long M, Crigger M, Wan JY, Haefner HK. Anal intraepithelial neoplasia in women with genital intraepithelial neoplasia. Obstet Gynecol 2010; 116(3): 578-82.
[http://dx.doi.org/10.1097/AOG.0b013e3181ea1834] [PMID: 20733438]

[64] Jacyntho CM, Giraldo PC, Horta AA, *et al.* Association between genital intraepithelial lesions and anal squamous intraepithelial lesions in HIV-negative women. Am J Obstet Gynecol 2011; 205(2): 115.e1-5.
[http://dx.doi.org/10.1016/j.ajog.2011.03.011] [PMID: 21684518]

[65] Machalek DA, Grulich AE, Jin F, Templeton DJ, Poynten IM. The epidemiology and natural history of anal human papillomavirus infection in men who have sex with men. Sex Health 2012; 9(6): 527-37.
[http://dx.doi.org/10.1071/SH12043] [PMID: 23380235]

[66] Strickler HD, Burk RD, Fazzari M, *et al.* Natural history and possible reactivation of human papillomavirus in human immunodeficiency virus-positive women. J Natl Cancer Inst 2005; 97(8): 577-86.
[http://dx.doi.org/10.1093/jnci/dji073] [PMID: 15840880]

[67] Prestage G, Mao L, Fogarty A, *et al.* How has the sexual behaviour of gay men changed since the onset of AIDS: 1986-2003. Aust N Z J Public Health 2005; 29(6): 530-5.
[http://dx.doi.org/10.1111/j.1467-842X.2005.tb00245.x] [PMID: 16370050]

[68] Sapp M, Bienkowska-Haba M. Viral entry mechanisms: human papillomavirus and a long journey

from extracellular matrix to the nucleus. FEBS J 2009; 276(24): 7206-16.
[http://dx.doi.org/10.1111/j.1742-4658.2009.07400.x] [PMID: 19878308]

[69] Haase AT. Targeting early infection to prevent HIV-1 mucosal transmission. Nature 2010; 464(7286): 217-23.
[http://dx.doi.org/10.1038/nature08757] [PMID: 20220840]

[70] Herfs M, Hubert P, Moutschen M, Delvenne P. Mucosal junctions: open doors to HPV and HIV infections? Trends Microbiol 2011; 19(3): 114-20.
[http://dx.doi.org/10.1016/j.tim.2010.12.006] [PMID: 21216598]

[71] Palefsky J. Biology of HPV in HIV infection. Adv Dent Res 2006; 19(1): 99-105.
[http://dx.doi.org/10.1177/154407370601900120] [PMID: 16672559]

[72] Van Doorslaer K, Burk RD. Evolution of human papillomavirus carcinogenicity. Adv Virus Res 2010; 77: 41-62.
[http://dx.doi.org/10.1016/B978-0-12-385034-8.00002-8] [PMID: 20951869]

[73] Bosch FX, Broker TR, Forman D, *et al.* Comprehensive control of human papillomavirus infections and related diseases. Vaccine 2013; 31 (Suppl. 7): H1-H31.
[http://dx.doi.org/10.1016/j.vaccine.2013.10.003] [PMID: 24332295]

CHAPTER 6

HPV-Related Cancers

Kimia Kardani and **Azam Bolhassani***

Department of Pharmaceutical Biotechnology, School of Pharmacy, Shahid Beheshti University of Medical Sciences, Tehran, Iran

Department of Hepatitis and AIDS, Pasteur Institute of Iran, Tehran, Iran

Abstract: Human papillomavirus (HPV)-associated cancers include cervical cancer, vulvar cancer, penile cancer, vaginal and anal cancer and a subset of head and neck cancers. Thus, effective vaccination against HPV infection is recommended to decrease their incidence and progression in the world. The FDA of the USA has approved two preventive vaccines to inhibit the spread of HPV. However, preventive vaccines do not exert therapeutic effects on pre-existing HPV infections, so therapeutic vaccines are being developed to generate a cell-mediated immune response to infected cells. HPV vaccination might be useful not only for prevention of cervical cancer, but also for the reduction of other related cancers. Herein, HPV-related cancers will be explained to consider their preventive and therapeutic pathways in future.

Keywords: Cancer, Genital warts, Infection, HPV, Pathogenesis.

INTRODUCTION

A common risk factor for genital cancers (*i.e.,* cervix, vaginal, vulvar, penile, and anal) is persistent infection with high-risk HPV types [1 - 4]. High-risk HPVs are sexually transmitted leading to the prevalence of several human cancers such as squamous cell carcinomas of the anogenital tract, skin, and the oral cavity. Different studies showed a strong link between high-risk HPV infection and urological malignancies [5]. Among high risk HPV (HR-HPV) types, HPV16 and then HPV18 are the most predominant type associated with genital cancers [6]. In 2014, the reports showed that the proportion of anogenital cancers associated with oncogenic HPV-16/18 was 73%, 38%, 58% and 36% for the anus, penis, vagina, and vulva regions, respectively [6, 7].

Cervical Cancer

Cervical cancer is the fourth most common cancer among women worldwide,

* **Corresponding author Azam Bolhassani:** Department of Hepatitis and AIDS, Pasteur Institute of Iran, Tehran, Iran; Tel: 66953311-20; E-mails: A_bolhasani@pasteur.ac.ir, azam.bolhassani@yahoo.com

with almost 260,000 deaths, annually [8, 9]. Cervical cancer begins in cells on the surface of the cervix and then invades more deeply into the cervix and adjacent tissues [10]. There are four main steps for development of cervical cancer including infection of epithelium at the cervical transformation zone (*i.e.,* the junction of the ectocervix and endocervix), virus persistence, progression of infected epithelium to cervical pre-cancer, and invasion through the basal membrane of the epithelium [8, 11, 12]. The major histologic type of cervical intraepithelial neoplasia (CIN) and cervical cancer is squamous cell carcinoma (SCC) which accounts for up to two thirds of cases [1, 13, 14]. The HPV-16 and -18 genotypes are estimated to account for 70% of all cervical cancers worldwide [1, 15]. Moreover, about 20% of cervical cancers are associated with HPV types 31, 33, 35, 45, 52 and 58 [15 - 17]. In Europe, three grades of CIN lesions are recognized: CIN1, mild; CIN2, moderate; and CIN3, severe. CIN1 can be associated with both high- and low-risk HPV types, although high-risk types predominate [17]. Low-grade CIN lesions likely regress, but high-grade lesions require complete treatment [1, 13].

Anal Cancer

Squamous carcinoma of the anus is a relatively rare malignancy [18]. Variants of SCC include cloacogenic, transitional, basaloid, and epidermoid carcinomas [19]. Several reports indicated that there is little difference between the morphologic variants of SCC. Less common cell types include adenocarcinoma, neuroendocrine neoplasms, malignant melanoma, mesenchymal tumours and lymphoma [19]. The anal canal is histologically divided into three zones: proximal (colorectal), transitional, and distal. The anal membrane represents the junction of the endodermal and ectodermal derivatives, where the anal crypts, ducts and glands are found [19]. Persistent infection with HR-HPV is considered responsible for a large proportion of anal cancers [20]. High-risk HPV serotypes, notably HPV16, provide an environment that allows for the development of dysplasia and subsequently SCC [19]. For anal cancer, HPV 6, 11, 31 and 33 are found in a small proportion of tumors [1, 2]. A strong relationship was shown between development of anal cancer and other genital cancers [21 - 25]. The most important risk factors for anal cancer are human behaviors including receptive anal intercourse and HIV infection. Anal cancer can be often observed in MSM (men who have sex with men), heterosexual men and HIV negative men among the general population. HIV-infected MSM are particularly at high risk of anal HPV infection (95%) [10]. Anal cancer can progress from a pre-invasive condition entitled as anal squamous intraepithelial neoplasia (AIN) [26]. The anal and cervical cancer events are high in HIV-positive women and MSM. The increased risk of HPV-associated diseases in HIV-infected populations is due to a high prevalence of HPV infections and alterations in cell-mediated immunity [26 -

28]. Table **1** shows WHO histologic classification of the anal canal tumors.

Table 1. WHO histologic classification of the anal canal tumors.

-Epithelial tumors	-Premalignant lesions	- Anal intraepithelial neoplasia (dysplasia), low-grade	
		-Anal intraepithelial neoplasia (dysplasia), high-grade	
		-Paget disease	
		-Bowen disease	
		- Perianal squamous intraepithelial neoplasia	
	-Neuroendocrine neoplasms	-Neuroendocrine tumor (NET)	-NET G1 (carcinoid)
			-NET G2
		-Neuroendocrine carcinoma (NEC)	-Small cell NEC
			-Large cell NEC
		-Mixed adenoneuroendocrine carcinoma	
	-Carcinoma	- SCC	
		- Verrucous carcinoma	
		-Undifferentiated carcinoma	
		-Adenocarcinoma	
		- Mucinous adenocarcinoma	
-Mesenchymal tumors			
-Secondary tumors			

Head and Neck Cancer

HPV infection is associated with approximately 85% of squamous cell carcinoma of the head and neck (HNSCC) [29 - 33]. Nearly 25% of HNSCC are associated with high-risk HPVs 16, 18, 31, 33 and 35 worldwide. Moreover, the high-risk HPV types 16, 31, and 33 were detected in oropharyngeal SCC samples. HPV16 accounts for 87% of HPV-positive oropharyngeal cancers [34 - 36]. The HPV-related HNSCCs usually occur in younger male patients [37, 38]. The frequencies of identified HPV positive tumors among HNSCC showed considerable variation ranging from 0% in oral and laryngeal carcinomas to 93% in oropharyngeal carcinomas [39, 40]. Most head and neck cancers are associated with tobacco and alcohol exposures and presented after the age of 60 years. HPV-positive HNSCC seems to be different from HPV-negative HNSCC (*e.g.,* tobacco- and alcohol-associated carcinoma) in its clinical and histopathologic features [10, 37 - 42]. The tonsillar crypts are the most common site of HPV transformation in the head and neck region [3]. Similar to the head and neck, HPV-positivity is more common in non-keratinizing than in keratinizing forms of squamous cell carcinoma involving the sinonasal tract [31, 43]. HPV-negative tumors have higher inhibitory rates of p16INK4a, p15INK4b cyclin D1 overexpression, and also an increased copy number of the epidermal growth factor receptor (EGFR) [44 - 46]. HIV-positive individuals seem to be at moderately increased risk of HPV-associated HNSCC [10].

Penile Cancer

Squamous cell carcinoma of the penis accounts for ~ 0.5% of all cancers in men and affects older men between 50 and 70 years of age [47 - 49]. The prevalence of HPV infection in penile intraepithelial neoplasia (PIN) and penile cancer ranges between 60-100% and 40-100%, respectively [50 - 53]. It seems that HPV types 6 and 11 play a small but significant role in cancer of the penis [10]. The studies demonstrated the presence of HPV-16 and -18 infections in ~70% of penile cancers. In addition, HPV-16 was reported to be the predominant genotype among patients with penile cancer [54 - 56]. HPV types 31 and 33 had a low prevalence among patients with penile cancer (less than 1%) [57]. Davis *et al.* reported that male circumcision decreases high-risk HPV copy number in female partners [58]. Moreover, the incidence of penile cancer is eight-fold higher in HIV-infected men than in non-HIV-infected men [59]. The most important prognostic factor for survival in men with penile cancer is nodal status [10, 60].

Vaginal Cancer

Vaginal cancer is a less frequent cancer in women [10, 61]. Most neoplasms are squamous cell carcinoma, but melanoma and adenocarcinoma also occur. Secondary vaginal cancer is more commonly than primary vaginal cancer, and may occur by direct extension from the cervix, vulva or endometrium [61]. In vaginal and vulvar cancers, HPV types 31, 33, 35 and 45 are found in a small but significant number of cases [1]. Vaginal cancer may be preceded by vaginal intraepithelial neoplasia (VaIN). According to phylogenetic analysis, the most prevalent types of HPV found in vaginal cancer are HPV-66 and -67 [10, 62, 63].

Vulvar Cancer

The vulva cancer constitutes about 4-5% of the genital tract cancers among women younger than 50 years [1, 10, 64, 65]. The majority of tumors are squamous cell carcinoma. The high-risk HPV types 16, 31 and 33 are frequently detected in vulva cancer and its precursor lesions (VIN). Vulva cancer with basaloid histopathology in young women is often associated with HPV-69 [1, 10, 66 - 69].

Adenocarcinoma of Uterine Cervix

The adenocarcinoma of cervix initiates close to the squamous epithelial neoplastic lesions. The higher proportion of adenocarcinoma cases has been observed in those areas where incidence of cervical cancer is low [10].

Ovarian Cancer

Ovarian cancer is the fifth leading cause of death in older women. The actual cause of ovarian cancer is unknown. However, some studies have demonstrated that high-risk HPV types 16 and 18 play an important role in the development of ovarian cancer [10].

Prostate Cancer

Prostate cancer (PCa) is the third most common cancer in men [70]. There is a positive association between the risk of PCa development and sexual activities [71, 72]. Moreover, the association of high-risk HPVs with the risk of prostate cancer may be described by the role of chronic inflammation in genomic oxidative damage to prostate epithelium. The most common types of HPV detected in prostate cancers are HPV types 16, 18, 33 and 31 [70, 73, 74]. The reports showed that HPV18 has high oncogenic potential in some prostate cancers that may be enhanced by the Epstein-Barr virus (EBV) [73].

Lung Cancer

Lung cancer (LC) is the most common cause of cancer morbidity and mortality worldwide [75, 77]. There are several reports on the prevalence rates of HPV infection (0.0-78.3%) in development of lung cancer [78 - 83]. Low- and high-risk HPV prevalence was significantly higher among LC patients than among non-cancer controls. For instance, the mean HPV16/18 incidence was 35.47% in LCs and 9.50% in non-cancer controls [75]. In addition, the studies indicated that HPV infection increases LC risk, especially in SCC. The prevalence of HPV types 16/18 in SCC and adenocarcinoma (AC) was 45.18% and 22.78%, respectively [75].

Bladder Cancer

Bladder cancer accounts for 6% and 2% of all cancers in men and women, respectively [5]. Both genetic and environmental factors are responsible for causing this type of cancer [10]. Moreover, several studies showed a positive association between bladder cancer and high-risk HPV infections, *e.g.,* HPV-16 and HPV-18 [5, 84, 85]. Recently, high-risk HPV-positive SCC was reported in a small group of patients with a long-term history of neurogenic bladder and urinary tract infections [86].

Kidney Cancer

The most common types of kidney cancer are renal cell carcinoma (RCC) and urothelial cell carcinoma. Several groups have indicated a possible association between HPV infection and kidney cancer [5], while others did not detect HPV infection in kidney tumors [87]. In two studies focusing on the prevalence of HPV infection in RCCs among allograft recipients, high-risk HPV-16 and -18 have been identified in 65% and 17.6% of patients, respectively. However, the prevalence of HPV infection was not significantly different among allograft recipients and healthy controls, indicating that HPV do not play a direct role in development of kidney cancer [88, 89].

Testicular Cancer

Testicular cancer represents about 0.1% of cancers worldwide [5]. Serological and molecular studies showed no correlation between HPV infections and testicular cancer [90, 91].

Cancer of Eye

HPV-16 and -18 E6 gene expression was found in intraepithelial neoplasia of the conjunctiva. HPV could be transmitted in utero during vaginal delivery. Therefore, it is important to look for prevalence of HPV infection in retinoblastoma cases [10].

Cancer of Esophagous

Esophageal squamous cell carcinoma (ESCC) is one of the most common cancers worldwide with a rapid progression and a wide regional variation [92, 93]. ESCC occurs mainly due to the HPV serotypes 16 and 18. The most important reasons for ESCC are different food habits, smoking and tobacco chewing [10]. A study indicated a high prevalence of HPV infection (*i.e.,* HPV52) in majority of ESCC patients. The incidence of HPV in ESCC varied widely ranging from 0% to 67% among different populations [92 - 101].

CONCLUDING REMARKS

In general, high-risk HPVs have been implicated in a number of human cancers. However, an association between HPV infections and some cancers such as prostate, bladder, or kidney cancer is still controversial. Thus, the cohort studies with long-term follow-up determine the incidence of persistent HPV infections, the characteristics of infection type and its contribution to carcinogenesis.

CONFLICT OF INTEREST

The author (editor) declares no conflict of interest, financial or otherwise.

ACKNOWLEDGEMENT

Declare none.

REFERENCES

[1] Wakeham K, Kavanagh K. The burden of HPV-associated anogenital cancers. Curr Oncol Rep 2014; 16(9): 402.
[http://dx.doi.org/10.1007/s11912-014-0402-4] [PMID: 25118645]

[2] International Agency for Research on Cancer moteocrth. In: Monograph on human papillomavirus 2007.

[3] Vu HL, Sikora AG, Fu S, Kao J. HPV-induced oropharyngeal cancer, immune response and response to therapy. Cancer Lett 2010; 288(2): 149-55.
[http://dx.doi.org/10.1016/j.canlet.2009.06.026] [PMID: 19628331]

[4] Gillison ML. Human papillomavirus and prognosis of oropharyngeal squamous cell carcinoma: implications for clinical research in head and neck cancers. J Clin Oncol 2006; 24(36): 5623-5.
[http://dx.doi.org/10.1200/JCO.2006.07.1829] [PMID: 17179099]

[5] Tolstov Y, Hadaschik B, Pahernik S, Hohenfellner M, Duensing S. Human papillomaviruses in urological malignancies: a critical assessment. Urol Oncol 2014; 32(1): 46.e19-27.
[http://dx.doi.org/10.1016/j.urolonc.2013.06.012] [PMID: 24140249]

[6] Begum S, Cao D, Gillison M, Zahurak M, Westra WH. Tissue distribution of HPV16 DNA integration in patients with tonsillar carcinoma as visualized by HPV16 *in situ* hybridization and p16 immunohistochemistry. Clin Cancer Res 2005; 11(16): 5694-9.
[http://dx.doi.org/10.1158/1078-0432.CCR-05-0587] [PMID: 16115905]

[7] De Vuyst H, Ndirangu G, Moodley M, *et al.* Prevalence of human papillomavirus in women with invasive cervical carcinoma by HIV status in Kenya and South Africa. Int J Cancer 2012; 131(4): 949-55.
[http://dx.doi.org/10.1002/ijc.26470] [PMID: 21960453]

[8] Mammas IN, Spandidos DA, Sourvinos G. Genomic diversity of human papillomaviruses (HPV) and clinical implications: an overview in adulthood and childhood. Infect Genet Evol 2014; 21: 220-6.
[http://dx.doi.org/10.1016/j.meegid.2013.11.002] [PMID: 24291228]

[9] Castellsagué X. Natural history and epidemiology of HPV infection and cervical cancer. Gynecol Oncol 2008; 110(3) (Suppl. 2): S4-7.
[http://dx.doi.org/10.1016/j.ygyno.2008.07.045] [PMID: 18760711]

[10] Amarakoon GU, Fathima F. An overview of human papillomavirus. World Scientific News 2016; 53(3): 275-308.

[11] Burd EM. Human papillomavirus and cervical cancer. Clin Microbiol Rev 2003; 16(1): 1-17.
[http://dx.doi.org/10.1128/CMR.16.1.1-17.2003] [PMID: 12525422]

[12] Schiffman M, Wentzensen N, Wacholder S, Kinney W, Gage JC, Castle PE. Human papillomavirus testing in the prevention of cervical cancer. J Natl Cancer Inst 2011; 103(5): 368-83.
[http://dx.doi.org/10.1093/jnci/djq562] [PMID: 21282563]

[13] McCredie MR, Sharples KJ, Paul C, *et al.* Natural history of cervical neoplasia and risk of invasive cancer in women with cervical intraepithelial neoplasia 3: a retrospective cohort study. Lancet Oncol 2008; 9(5): 425-34.

[http://dx.doi.org/10.1016/S1470-2045(08)70103-7] [PMID: 18407790]

[14] Herfs M, Yamamoto Y, Laury A, *et al.* A discrete population of squamocolumnar junction cells implicated in the pathogenesis of cervical cancer. Proc Natl Acad Sci USA 2012; 109(26): 10516-21. [http://dx.doi.org/10.1073/pnas.1202684109] [PMID: 22689991]

[15] Clifford G, Franceschi S, Diaz M, Muñoz N, Villa LL. Chapter 3: HPV type-distribution in women with and without cervical neoplastic diseases. Vaccine 2006; 24: S3/26-34.

[16] Kines RC, Thompson CD, Lowy DR, Schiller JT, Day PM. The initial steps leading to papillomavirus infection occur on the basement membrane prior to cell surface binding. Proc Natl Acad Sci USA 2009; 106(48): 20458-63. [http://dx.doi.org/10.1073/pnas.0908502106] [PMID: 19920181]

[17] Stanley M. Pathology and epidemiology of HPV infection in females. Gynecol Oncol 2010; 117(2) (Suppl.): S5-S10. [http://dx.doi.org/10.1016/j.ygyno.2010.01.024] [PMID: 20304221]

[18] Siegel RL, Miller KD, Jemal A. Cancer statistics, 2015. CA Cancer J Clin 2015; 65(1): 5-29. [http://dx.doi.org/10.3322/caac.21254] [PMID: 25559415]

[19] Szmulowicz UM, Wu JS. Squamous cell carcinoma of the anal canal: a review of the aetiology, presentation, staging, prognosis and methods available for treatment. Sex Health 2012; 9(6): 593-609. [http://dx.doi.org/10.1071/SH12010] [PMID: 22951027]

[20] Daling JR, Madeleine MM, Johnson LG, *et al.* Human papillomavirus, smoking, and sexual practices in the etiology of anal cancer. Cancer 2004; 101(2): 270-80. [http://dx.doi.org/10.1002/cncr.20365] [PMID: 15241823]

[21] Frisch M, Glimelius B, van den Brule AJ, *et al.* Sexually transmitted infection as a cause of anal cancer. N Engl J Med 1997; 337(19): 1350-8. [http://dx.doi.org/10.1056/NEJM199711063371904] [PMID: 9358129]

[22] Daling JR, Weiss NS, Hislop TG, *et al.* Sexual practices, sexually transmitted diseases, and the incidence of anal cancer. N Engl J Med 1987; 317(16): 973-7. [http://dx.doi.org/10.1056/NEJM198710153171601] [PMID: 2821396]

[23] Edgren G, Sparén P. Risk of anogenital cancer after diagnosis of cervical intraepithelial neoplasia: a prospective population-based study. Lancet Oncol 2007; 8(4): 311-6. [http://dx.doi.org/10.1016/S1470-2045(07)70043-8] [PMID: 17395104]

[24] Rabkin CS, Biggar RJ, Melbye M, Curtis RE. Second primary cancers following anal and cervical carcinoma: evidence of shared etiologic factors. Am J Epidemiol 1992; 136(1): 54-8. [http://dx.doi.org/10.1093/oxfordjournals.aje.a116420] [PMID: 1329500]

[25] Frisch M, Olsen JH, Melbye M. Malignancies that occur before and after anal cancer: clues to their etiology. Am J Epidemiol 1994; 140(1): 12-9. [http://dx.doi.org/10.1093/oxfordjournals.aje.a117154] [PMID: 8017399]

[26] Palefsky JM, Rubin M. The epidemiology of anal human papillomavirus and related neoplasia. Obstet Gynecol Clin North Am 2009; 36(1): 187-200. [http://dx.doi.org/10.1016/j.ogc.2009.02.003] [PMID: 19344856]

[27] Crum-Cianflone NF, Hullsiek KH, Marconi VC, *et al.* Anal cancers among HIV-infected persons: HAART is not slowing rising incidence. AIDS 2010; 24(4): 535-43. [http://dx.doi.org/10.1097/QAD.0b013e328331f6e2] [PMID: 19926961]

[28] Bower M, Powles T, Newsom-Davis T, *et al.* HIV-associated anal cancer: has highly active antiretroviral therapy reduced the incidence or improved the outcome? J Acquir Immune Defic Syndr 2004; 37(5): 1563-5. [http://dx.doi.org/10.1097/00126334-200412150-00004] [PMID: 15577408]

[29] Wang XI, Thomas J, Zhang S. Changing trends in human papillomavirus-associated head and neck

squamous cell carcinoma. Ann Diagn Pathol 2012; 16(1): 7-12.
[http://dx.doi.org/10.1016/j.anndiagpath.2011.07.003] [PMID: 22001331]

[30] Schiffman M, Castle PE, Jeronimo J, Rodriguez AC, Wacholder S. Human papillomavirus and cervical cancer. Lancet 2007; 370(9590): 890-907.
[http://dx.doi.org/10.1016/S0140-6736(07)61416-0] [PMID: 17826171]

[31] Westra WH. The morphologic profile of HPV-related head and neck squamous carcinoma: implications for diagnosis, prognosis, and clinical management. Head Neck Pathol 2012; 6 (Suppl. 1): S48-54.
[http://dx.doi.org/10.1007/s12105-012-0371-6] [PMID: 22782223]

[32] Gillison ML, Koch WM, Capone RB, *et al.* Evidence for a causal association between human papillomavirus and a subset of head and neck cancers. J Natl Cancer Inst 2000; 92(9): 709-20.
[http://dx.doi.org/10.1093/jnci/92.9.709] [PMID: 10793107]

[33] Adelstein DJ, Ridge JA, Gillison ML, *et al.* Head and neck squamous cell cancer and the human papillomavirus: summary of a National Cancer Institute State of the Science Meeting, November 9-10, 2008, Washington, D.C. Head Neck 2009; 31(11): 1393-422.
[http://dx.doi.org/10.1002/hed.21269] [PMID: 19787782]

[34] zur Hausen H. Papillomaviruses and cancer: from basic studies to clinical application. Nat Rev Cancer 2002; 2(5): 342-50.
[http://dx.doi.org/10.1038/nrc798] [PMID: 12044010]

[35] Kreimer AR, Clifford GM, Boyle P, Franceschi S. Human papillomavirus types in head and neck squamous cell carcinomas worldwide: a systematic review. Cancer Epidemiol Biomarkers Prev 2005; 14(2): 467-75.
[http://dx.doi.org/10.1158/1055-9965.EPI-04-0551] [PMID: 15734974]

[36] Mork J, Lie AK, Glattre E, *et al.* Human papillomavirus infection as a risk factor for squamous-cell carcinoma of the head and neck. N Engl J Med 2001; 344(15): 1125-31.
[http://dx.doi.org/10.1056/NEJM200104123441503] [PMID: 11297703]

[37] Ang KK, Harris J, Wheeler R, *et al.* Human papillomavirus and survival of patients with oropharyngeal cancer. N Engl J Med 2010; 363(1): 24-35.
[http://dx.doi.org/10.1056/NEJMoa0912217] [PMID: 20530316]

[38] Fakhry C, Westra WH, Li S, *et al.* Improved survival of patients with human papillomavirus-positive head and neck squamous cell carcinoma in a prospective clinical trial. J Natl Cancer Inst 2008; 100(4): 261-9.
[http://dx.doi.org/10.1093/jnci/djn011] [PMID: 18270337]

[39] Gallo A, Degener AM, Pagliuca G, *et al.* Detection of human papillomavirus and adenovirus in benign and malignant lesions of the larynx. Otolaryngol Head Neck Surg 2009; 141(2): 276-81.
[http://dx.doi.org/10.1016/j.otohns.2009.04.021] [PMID: 19643265]

[40] Näsman A, Attner P, Hammarstedt L, *et al.* Incidence of human papillomavirus (HPV) positive tonsillar carcinoma in Stockholm, Sweden: an epidemic of viral-induced carcinoma? Int J Cancer 2009; 125(2): 362-6.
[http://dx.doi.org/10.1002/ijc.24339] [PMID: 19330833]

[41] Weinberger PM, Merkley MA, Khichi SS, *et al.* Human papillomavirus-active head and neck cancer and ethnic health disparities. Laryngoscope 2010; 120(8): 1531-7.
[http://dx.doi.org/10.1002/lary.20984] [PMID: 20564751]

[42] Singhi AD, Stelow EB, Mills SE, Westra WH. Lymphoepithelial-like carcinoma of the oropharynx: a morphologic variant of HPV-related head and neck carcinoma. Am J Surg Pathol 2010; 34(6): 800-5.
[http://dx.doi.org/10.1097/PAS.0b013e3181d9ba21] [PMID: 20421782]

[43] El-Mofty SK, Lu DW. Prevalence of high-risk human papillomavirus DNA in nonkeratinizing (cylindrical cell) carcinoma of the sinonasal tract: a distinct clinicopathologic and molecular disease

entity. Am J Surg Pathol 2005; 29(10): 1367-72.
[http://dx.doi.org/10.1097/01.pas.0000173240.63073.fe] [PMID: 16160480]

[44] Poeta ML, Manola J, Goldwasser MA, *et al.* TP53 mutations and survival in squamous-cell carcinoma of the head and neck. N Engl J Med 2007; 357(25): 2552-61.
[http://dx.doi.org/10.1056/NEJMoa073770] [PMID: 18094376]

[45] Haddad RI, Shin DM. Recent advances in head and neck cancer. N Engl J Med 2008; 359(11): 1143-54.
[http://dx.doi.org/10.1056/NEJMra0707975] [PMID: 18784104]

[46] Perrone F, Suardi S, Pastore E, *et al.* Molecular and cytogenetic subgroups of oropharyngeal squamous cell carcinoma. Clin Cancer Res 2006; 12(22): 6643-51.
[http://dx.doi.org/10.1158/1078-0432.CCR-06-1759] [PMID: 17121883]

[47] Hernandez BY, Barnholtz-Sloan J, German RR, *et al.* Burden of invasive squamous cell carcinoma of the penis in the United States, 1998-2003. Cancer 2008; 113(10) (Suppl.): 2883-91.
[http://dx.doi.org/10.1002/cncr.23743] [PMID: 18980292]

[48] Bleeker MC, Heideman DA, Snijders PJ, Horenblas S, Dillner J, Meijer CJ. Penile cancer: epidemiology, pathogenesis and prevention. World J Urol 2009; 27(2): 141-50.
[http://dx.doi.org/10.1007/s00345-008-0302-z] [PMID: 18607597]

[49] Maden C, Sherman KJ, Beckmann AM, *et al.* History of circumcision, medical conditions, and sexual activity and risk of penile cancer. J Natl Cancer Inst 1993; 85(1): 19-24.
[http://dx.doi.org/10.1093/jnci/85.1.19] [PMID: 8380060]

[50] D'Hauwers KW, Depuydt CE, Bogers JJ, *et al.* Human papillomavirus, lichen sclerosus and penile cancer: a study in Belgium. Vaccine 2012; 30(46): 6573-7.
[http://dx.doi.org/10.1016/j.vaccine.2012.08.034] [PMID: 22939906]

[51] Ferrándiz-Pulido C, Masferrer E, de Torres I, *et al.* Identification and genotyping of human papillomavirus in a Spanish cohort of penile squamous cell carcinomas: correlation with pathologic subtypes, p16(INK4a) expression, and prognosis. J Am Acad Dermatol 2013; 68(1): 73-82.
[http://dx.doi.org/10.1016/j.jaad.2012.05.029] [PMID: 22863066]

[52] Afonso LA, Moyses N, Alves G, *et al.* Prevalence of human papillomavirus and Epstein-Barr virus DNA in penile cancer cases from Brazil. Mem Inst Oswaldo Cruz 2012; 107(1): 18-23.
[http://dx.doi.org/10.1590/S0074-02762012000100003] [PMID: 22310531]

[53] Rubin MA, Kleter B, Zhou M, *et al.* Detection and typing of human papillomavirus DNA in penile carcinoma: evidence for multiple independent pathways of penile carcinogenesis. Am J Pathol 2001; 159(4): 1211-8.
[http://dx.doi.org/10.1016/S0002-9440(10)62506-0] [PMID: 11583947]

[54] Carter JJ, Madeleine MM, Shera K, *et al.* Human papillomavirus 16 and 18 L1 serology compared across anogenital cancer sites. Cancer Res 2001; 61(5): 1934-40.
[PMID: 11280749]

[55] Heideman DA, Waterboer T, Pawlita M, *et al.* Human papillomavirus-16 is the predominant type etiologically involved in penile squamous cell carcinoma. J Clin Oncol 2007; 25(29): 4550-6.
[http://dx.doi.org/10.1200/JCO.2007.12.3182] [PMID: 17925550]

[56] zur Hausen H, de Villiers EM. Human papillomaviruses. Annu Rev Microbiol 1994; 48: 427-47.
[http://dx.doi.org/10.1146/annurev.mi.48.100194.002235] [PMID: 7826013]

[57] Bjørge T, Dillner J, Anttila T, *et al.* Prospective seroepidemiological study of role of human papillomavirus in non-cervical anogenital cancers. BMJ 1997; 315(7109): 646-9.
[http://dx.doi.org/10.1136/bmj.315.7109.646] [PMID: 9310566]

[58] Davis MA, Gray RH, Grabowski MK, *et al.* Male circumcision decreases high-risk human papillomavirus viral load in female partners: a randomized trial in Rakai, Uganda. Int J Cancer 2013; 133(5): 1247-52.

[http://dx.doi.org/10.1002/ijc.28100] [PMID: 23400966]

[59] Engels EA, Pfeiffer RM, Goedert JJ, *et al.* Trends in cancer risk among people with AIDS in the United States 1980-2002. AIDS 2006; 20(12): 1645-54.
[http://dx.doi.org/10.1097/01.aids.0000238411.75324.59] [PMID: 16868446]

[60] Ficarra V, Akduman B, Bouchot O, Palou J, Tobias-Machado M. Prognostic factors in penile cancer. Urology 2010; 76(2) (Suppl. 1): S66-73.
[http://dx.doi.org/10.1016/j.urology.2010.04.008] [PMID: 20691887]

[61] Daling JR, Madeleine MM, Schwartz SM, *et al.* A population-based study of squamous cell vaginal cancer: HPV and cofactors. Gynecol Oncol 2002; 84(2): 263-70.
[http://dx.doi.org/10.1006/gyno.2001.6502] [PMID: 11812085]

[62] Gunderson CC, Nugent EK, Elfrink SH, Gold MA, Moore KN. A contemporary analysis of epidemiology and management of vaginal intraepithelial neoplasia. Am J Obstet Gynecol 2013; 208(5): 410.e1-6.
[http://dx.doi.org/10.1016/j.ajog.2013.01.047] [PMID: 23380265]

[63] Gunderson CC, Nugent EK, Yunker AC, *et al.* Vaginal cancer: the experience from 2 large academic centers during a 15-year period. J Low Genit Tract Dis 2013; 17(4): 409-13.
[http://dx.doi.org/10.1097/LGT.0b013e3182800ee2] [PMID: 23609592]

[64] Siegel R, Ma J, Zou Z, Jemal A. Cancer statistics, 2014. CA Cancer J Clin 2014; 64(1): 9-29.
[http://dx.doi.org/10.3322/caac.21208] [PMID: 24399786]

[65] Joura EA, Lösch A, Haider-Angeler MG, Breitenecker G, Leodolter S. Trends in vulvar neoplasia. Increasing incidence of vulvar intraepithelial neoplasia and squamous cell carcinoma of the vulva in young women. J Reprod Med 2000; 45(8): 613-5.
[PMID: 10986677]

[66] Jones RW, Baranyai J, Stables S. Trends in squamous cell carcinoma of the vulva: the influence of vulvar intraepithelial neoplasia. Obstet Gynecol 1997; 90(3): 448-52.
[http://dx.doi.org/10.1016/S0029-7844(97)00298-6] [PMID: 9277660]

[67] van Seters M, van Beurden M, de Craen AJ. Is the assumed natural history of vulvar intraepithelial neoplasia III based on enough evidence? A systematic review of 3322 published patients. Gynecol Oncol 2005; 97(2): 645-51.
[http://dx.doi.org/10.1016/j.ygyno.2005.02.012] [PMID: 15863172]

[68] Judson PL, Habermann EB, Baxter NN, Durham SB, Virnig BA. Trends in the incidence of invasive and *in situ* vulvar carcinoma. Obstet Gynecol 2006; 107(5): 1018-22.
[http://dx.doi.org/10.1097/01.AOG.0000210268.57527.a1] [PMID: 16648405]

[69] Burger MP, Hollema H, Emanuels AG, Krans M, Pras E, Bouma J. The importance of the groin node status for the survival of T1 and T2 vulval carcinoma patients. Gynecol Oncol 1995; 57(3): 327-34.
[http://dx.doi.org/10.1006/gyno.1995.1151] [PMID: 7774836]

[70] Aghakhani A, Hamkar R, Parvin M, *et al.* The role of human papillomavirus infection in prostate carcinoma. Scand J Infect Dis 2011; 43(1): 64-9.
[http://dx.doi.org/10.3109/00365548.2010.502904] [PMID: 20662618]

[71] Adami HO, Kuper H, Andersson SO, Bergström R, Dillner J. Prostate cancer risk and serologic evidence of human papilloma virus infection: a population-based case-control study. Cancer Epidemiol Biomarkers Prev 2003; 12(9): 872-5.
[PMID: 14504197]

[72] Taylor ML, Mainous AG III, Wells BJ. Prostate cancer and sexually transmitted diseases: a meta-analysis. Fam Med 2005; 37(7): 506-12.
[PMID: 15988645]

[73] Whitaker NJ, Glenn WK, Sahrudin A, Orde MM, Delprado W, Lawson JS. Human papillomavirus and Epstein Barr virus in prostate cancer: Koilocytes indicate potential oncogenic influences of human

papillomavirus in prostate cancer. Prostate 2013; 73(3): 236-41.
[http://dx.doi.org/10.1002/pros.22562] [PMID: 22851253]

[74] Lin Y, Mao Q, Zheng X, *et al.* Human papillomavirus 16 or 18 infection and prostate cancer risk: a meta-analysis. Ir J Med Sci 2011; 180(2): 497-503.
[http://dx.doi.org/10.1007/s11845-011-0692-6] [PMID: 21400096]

[75] Zhai K, Ding J, Shi HZ. HPV and lung cancer risk: a meta-analysis. J Clin Virol 2015; 63: 84-90.
[http://dx.doi.org/10.1016/j.jcv.2014.09.014] [PMID: 25315992]

[76] Sun S, Schiller JH, Gazdar AF. Lung cancer in never smokers--a different disease. Nat Rev Cancer 2007; 7(10): 778-90.
[http://dx.doi.org/10.1038/nrc2190] [PMID: 17882278]

[77] Spyratos D, Zarogoulidis P, Porpodis K, *et al.* Occupational exposure and lung cancer. J Thorac Dis 2013; 5 (Suppl. 4): S440-5.
[PMID: 24102018]

[78] Syrjänen K. Detection of human papillomavirus in lung cancer: systematic review and meta-analysis. Anticancer Res 2012; 32(8): 3235-50.
[PMID: 22843898]

[79] Hobbs CG, Sterne JA, Bailey M, Heyderman RS, Birchall MA, Thomas SJ. Human papillomavirus and head and neck cancer: a systematic review and meta-analysis. Clin Otolaryngol 2006; 31(4): 259-66.
[http://dx.doi.org/10.1111/j.1749-4486.2006.01246.x] [PMID: 16911640]

[80] Syrjänen S, Lodi G, von Bültzingslöwen I, *et al.* Human papillomaviruses in oral carcinoma and oral potentially malignant disorders: a systematic review. Oral Dis 2011; 17(1) (Suppl. 1): 58-72.
[http://dx.doi.org/10.1111/j.1601-0825.2011.01792.x] [PMID: 21382139]

[81] Srinivasan M, Taioli E, Ragin CC. Human papillomavirus type 16 and 18 in primary lung cancers--a meta-analysis. Carcinogenesis 2009; 30(10): 1722-8.
[http://dx.doi.org/10.1093/carcin/bgp177] [PMID: 19620233]

[82] Krikelis D, Tzimagiorgis G, Georgiou E, *et al.* Frequent presence of incomplete HPV16 E7 ORFs in lung carcinomas: memories of viral infection. J Clin Virol 2010; 49(3): 169-74.
[http://dx.doi.org/10.1016/j.jcv.2010.07.020] [PMID: 20850378]

[83] Sagerup CM, Nymoen DA, Halvorsen AR, Lund-Iversen M, Helland A, Brustugun OT. Human papilloma virus detection and typing in 334 lung cancer patients. Acta Oncol 2014; 53(7): 952-7.
[http://dx.doi.org/10.3109/0284186X.2013.879608] [PMID: 24446743]

[84] Moonen PM, Bakkers JM, Kiemeney LA, Schalken JA, Melchers WJ, Witjes JA. Human papilloma virus DNA and p53 mutation analysis on bladder washes in relation to clinical outcome of bladder cancer. Eur Urol 2007; 52(2): 464-8.
[http://dx.doi.org/10.1016/j.eururo.2006.11.017] [PMID: 17116360]

[85] Badawi H, Ahmed H, Ismail A, *et al.* Role of human papillomavirus types 16, 18, and 52 in recurrent cystitis and urinary bladder cancer among Egyptian patients. Medscape J Med 2008; 10(10): 232.
[PMID: 19099026]

[86] Blochin EB, Park KJ, Tickoo SK, Reuter VE, Al-Ahmadie H. Urothelial carcinoma with prominent squamous differentiation in the setting of neurogenic bladder: role of human papillomavirus infection. Mod Pathol 2012; 25(11): 1534-42.
[http://dx.doi.org/10.1038/modpathol.2012.112] [PMID: 22766788]

[87] Salehipoor M, Khezri A, Behzad-Behbahani A, *et al.* Role of viruses in renal cell carcinoma. Saudi J Kidney Dis Transpl 2012; 23(1): 53-7.
[PMID: 22237219]

[88] Brown MR, Noffsinger A, First MR, Penn I, Husseinzadeh N. HPV subtype analysis in lower genital tract neoplasms of female renal transplant recipients. Gynecol Oncol 2000; 79(2): 220-4.

[http://dx.doi.org/10.1006/gyno.2000.5942] [PMID: 11063648]

[89] Paternoster DM, Cester M, Resente C, *et al.* Human papilloma virus infection and cervical intraepithelial neoplasia in transplanted patients. Transplant Proc 2008; 40(6): 1877-80. [http://dx.doi.org/10.1016/j.transproceed.2008.05.074] [PMID: 18675077]

[90] Kondoh G, Murata Y, Aozasa K, Yutsudo M, Hakura A. Very high incidence of germ cell tumorigenesis (seminomagenesis) in human papillomavirus type 16 transgenic mice. J Virol 1991; 65(6): 3335-9.
[PMID: 1851881]

[91] Strickler HD, Schiffman MH, Shah KV, *et al.* A survey of human papillomavirus 16 antibodies in patients with epithelial cancers. Eur J Cancer Prev 1998; 7(4): 305-13.
[http://dx.doi.org/10.1097/00008469-199808000-00006] [PMID: 9806119]

[92] Vaiphei K, Kochhar R, Bhardawaj S, Dutta U, Singh K. High prevalence of human papillomavirus in esophageal squamous cell carcinoma: a study in paired samples. Dis Esophagus 2013; 26(3): 282-7.
[http://dx.doi.org/10.1111/j.1442-2050.2012.01365.x] [PMID: 22676445]

[93] Parkin DM, Bray F, Ferlay J, Pisani P. Global cancer statistics, 2002. CA Cancer J Clin 2005; 55(2): 74-108.
[http://dx.doi.org/10.3322/canjclin.55.2.74] [PMID: 15761078]

[94] Herrera-Goepfert R, Lizano M, Akiba S, Carrillo-García A, Becker-D'Acosta M. Human papilloma virus and esophageal carcinoma in a Latin-American region. World J Gastroenterol 2009; 15(25): 3142-7.
[http://dx.doi.org/10.3748/wjg.15.3142] [PMID: 19575494]

[95] Berumen-Campos J. [Human papilloma virus and cervical cancer]. Gac Med Mex 2006; 142 (Suppl. 2): 51-9.
[PMID: 19031679]

[96] Syrjänen K, Pyrhönen S, Aukee S, Koskela E. Squamous cell papilloma of the esophagus: a tumour probably caused by human papilloma virus (HPV). Diagn Histopathol 1982; 5(4): 291-6.
[PMID: 6188592]

[97] Khurshid A, Kazuya N, Hanae I, Manabu I. Infection of human papillomavirus (HPV) and Epstein-Barr virus (EBV) and p53 expression in human esophageal carcinoma. J Pak Med Assoc 1998; 48(5): 138-42.
[PMID: 9813975]

[98] Benamouzig R, Jullian E, Chang F, *et al.* Absence of human papillomavirus DNA detected by polymerase chain reaction in French patients with esophageal carcinoma. Gastroenterology 1995; 109(6): 1876-81.
[http://dx.doi.org/10.1016/0016-5085(95)90754-8] [PMID: 7498652]

[99] Bjørge T, Hakulinen T, Engeland A, *et al.* A prospective, seroepidemiological study of the role of human papillomavirus in esophageal cancer in Norway. Cancer Res 1997; 57(18): 3989-92.
[PMID: 9307283]

[100] Van Doornum GJ, Korse CM, Buning-Kager JC, *et al.* Reactivity to human papillomavirus type 16 L1 virus-like particles in sera from patients with genital cancer and patients with carcinomas at five different extragenital sites. Br J Cancer 2003; 88(7): 1095-100.
[http://dx.doi.org/10.1038/sj.bjc.6600870] [PMID: 12671710]

[101] Kamangar F, Qiao YL, Schiller JT, *et al.* Human papillomavirus serology and the risk of esophageal and gastric cancers: results from a cohort in a high-risk region in China. Int J Cancer 2006; 119(3): 579-84.
[http://dx.doi.org/10.1002/ijc.21871] [PMID: 16496409]

[102] Bosman FT, Carneiro F, Hruban RH, *et al.* WHO classification of tumours of the digestive system No. 4th ed., World Health Organization 2010.

CHAPTER 7

The Epidemiology of HPV-Related Cancer Types

Kimia Kardani, Afshin Khavari and **Azam Bolhassani***

Department of Pharmaceutical Biotechnology, School of Pharmacy, Shahid Beheshti University of Medical Sciences, Tehran, Iran

Department of Hepatitis and AIDS, Pasteur Institute of Iran, Tehran, Iran

Abstract: Differences in prevalence rates of HPV infections are observed worldwide. Cervical cancer remains a major public health concern, especially in developing countries. Cancers of the anus, penis, vagina, and vulva are relatively uncommon cancers, but their incidence is gradually increasing in the world. Indeed, the epidemiology of HPV-associated anogenital cancers of the cervix, anus, penis, vagina and vulva is changing, likely due to increasing HPV transmission secondary to changes in sexual behaviour. Molecular epidemiologic studies indicate that certain HPV types were highly prevalent among women aged below 30 years with a peak in the 21-25 year age group and those who are above 30 years. Thus, screening programs and the HPV vaccines are required to prevent the anogenital cancers. In this chapter, the epidemiology of HPV-related cancer types will be studied based on new data.

Keywords: Cancer, Epidemiology, HPV types.

INTRODUCTION

HPV is a public health problem for its role in developing various types of cancers. Differences in prevalence rates of HPV infections are observed worldwide [1]. Molecular epidemiologic studies indicate that certain HPV types were highly prevalent among women aged below 30 years with a peak in the 21-25 year age group and those who are above 30 years [1]. Cervical cancer is a main health problem, especially in developing countries, but screening and vaccination programs are hopeful for prevention or treatment of this cancer [2]. Other HPV-associated anogenital cancers, *e.g.*, the anus and vulva cancers are increasing in incidence [2]. A study showed that the most common HPV type was HPV16 (~3.6% of the population) in Costa Rica [3]. Other reports demonstrated that oncogenic and non-oncogenic types were detected in 13.7%, and 17.5% of the women, respectively. The age-specific prevalence of oncogenic HPV types was

* **Corresponding author Azam Bolhassani:** Department of Hepatitis and AIDS, Pasteur Institute of Iran, Tehran, Iran; Tel: 66953311-20; E-mails: A_bolhasani@pasteur.ac.ir, azam.bolhassani@yahoo.com

decreased from 24.4% in the women aged < 25 years to 9.7% and 9.8% in the women aged 35-44 and 45-54 years, respectively [4]. In addition, the prevalence of HPV DNA among cytologically normal middle-aged women in Spain, Colombia, and Brazil, was positively associated with the number of lifetime sexual partners and inversely related to the levels of family income and with age at first sexual intercourse [5]. On the other hand, women with normal cervical cytology who are infected with high-risk HPV have an approximately 100 fold increased risk of developing CIN3 compared with uninfected women [1]. Prevalence estimates show persons that have detectable infections with one of 37 HPV types. These studies represented that 21.6% of women are infected with more than one HPV type [6 - 9]. Among women aged 15-59 years, the annual probability of acquiring a new infection ranged from 25% among 20-24-year-olds to 2% among 50-59-year-olds [6, 10]. Currently, there is a constant increase in the incidence of malignant tumors [11, 12]. Tables **1** and **2** show the general epidemiological data in 2012.

Table 1. New cancer cases and ASR in some countries.

	Population in thousands	Annual number of new cancer cases	Age-standardized incidence rate *	Cumulative risk (%) at 75 years old **
United states of America	321,773.6	12,966	6.6	0.6
Australia	23,969.0	793	5.5	0.5
Canada	35,939.9	1,408	6.3	0.6
Brazil	207,847.5	18,503	16.3	1.7
China	1,376,048.8	69,691	7.5	0.7
Iran	79,109.3	947	2.8	0.3
Saudi Arabia	31,540.4	241	2.7	0.3
United Kingdom	64,715.8	2,659	7.1	0.6
Sweden	9,779.4	451	7.4	0.7
Ethiopia	99,390.7	7,095	26.4	3.0

* Rates per 100,000 women per year

** Cumulative risk (incidence) is the probability or risk of individuals getting from the disease during ages 0-74 years. For cancer, it is expressed as the % of new born children who would be expected to develop from a particular cancer before the age of 75 if they had the rates of cancer observed in the period in the absence of competing causes

Data sources: Ferlay J, Soerjomataram I, Ervik M, Dikshit R, Eser S, Mathers C, Rebelo M, Parkin DM, Forman D, Bray F. GLOBOCAN 2012 v1.2, Cancer Incidence and Mortality Worldwide: IARC CancerBase No. 11 [Internet]. Lyon, France: International Agency for Research on Cancer; 2013. Available from: http://globocan.iarc.fr

Cervical Cancer

For cervical cancer, more than 85% of the global burden occurs in developing countries. There is marked geographical variation in the incidence of cervical cancer [2]. High-risk regions include Eastern, Western, Southern and Middle Africa, South Central Asia and South America. Rates were found to be the lowest in Western Asia, Northern America and Australia/New Zealand [13 - 18]. To compare the burden of cervical cancer between countries, GLOBOCAN in 2012 has estimated the age-standardized incidence rate (ASR) by country and region [2]. Crude HPV prevalence estimates in 576,281 women with normal and abnormal cytology stratified by 35 world regions. The crude HPV prevalence among women was 32.1% worldwide. The highest HPV prevalence (57.7%) was observed in Asia, particularly Eastern Asia. The lowest HPV prevalence was detected in Europe, especially Western Europe (3.7%) and Southern Europe (15.1%). Prevalence of HPV was higher in developing countries (~ 42.2%) than in developed countries (~ 22.6%) [13]. Moreover, the most common HPV types were HPV-16 (9.5%), HPV-18 (6.2%), and HPV-33, -52 and -58 (0.3%). HPV-16 was found to be the predominant type in the world with the exception of South Africa (common type: HPV-52) [13]. The geographical variation in the incidence of cervical cancer shows the importance of a national cervical screening program [18 - 20]. Disease stage is the most important prognostic indicator for survival from cervical cancer [21]. For example, in low-income countries, the majority of women diagnosed with cervical cancer will die due to limitation of cancer treatment modalities and extensive transmission of virus [22]. Increased prevalence of high-risk HPV infection (~ 54.4%) was observed in China among women aged < 20 [23, 24]. The presence of HPV DNA in cervical tissue (~ 75%) as well as in placental tissue (~ 47.2%) of pregnant Mexican women determined that HPV-18 was the most frequently identified HPV type in both tissues [25].

Table 2. Annual cancer deaths and ASR in some countries.

	Annual number of deaths	Age-standardized mortality rate *	Cumulative risk (%) at 75 years old **
United states of America	6,605	2.7	0.3
Australia	303	1.6	0.2
Canada	503	1.7	0.2
Brazil	8,414	7.3	0.8
China	29,562	3.4	0.3
Iran	370	1.2	0.1
Saudi Arabia	84	1.1	0.1
United Kingdom	979	1.8	0.2
Sweden	187	1.9	0.2
Ethiopia	4,732	18.4	2.1

* Rates per 100,000 women per year

** Cumulative risk (mortality) is the probability or risk of dying from the disease during ages 0-74 years. For cancer, it is expressed as the % of new born children who would be expected to develop from a particular cancer before the age of 75 if they had the rates of cancer observed in the period in the absence of competing causes

Data sources: Ferlay J, Soerjomataram I, Ervik M, Dikshit R, Eser S, Mathers C, Rebelo M, Parkin DM, Forman D, Bray F. GLOBOCAN 2012 v1.2, Cancer Incidence and Mortality Worldwide: IARC CancerBase No. 11 [Internet]. Lyon, France: International Agency for Research on Cancer; 2013. Available from: http://globocan.iarc.fr

Briefly, cervical cancer is the 4th most common cancer among women worldwide, with an estimated 527,624 new cases and 265,672 deaths in 2012 (GLOBOCAN). The majority of cases are squamous cell carcinoma followed by adenocarcinomas. About 947 and 145,946 new cervical cancer cases are diagnosed annually in Iran and Southern Asia, respectively. Crude incidence rates are 2.5, 17.1 and 15.1 in Iran, Southern Asia and worldwide, respectively. Age-standardized incidence rates are 2.8, 19.3, and 14 in Iran, Southern Asia and worldwide, respectively. On the other hand, about 370 and 79,958 cervical cancer deaths occur annually in Iran and Southern Asia, respectively. Crude mortality rates are 1.0, 9.4 and 7.6 in Iran, Southern Asia and worldwide, respectively. Age-standardized mortality rates are 1.2, 11.0, and 6.8 in Iran, Southern Asia and worldwide, respectively based on ICO Information Centre on HPV and Cancer. Fig. (**1**) shows Age-standardized incidence rates (ASR) of cervical cancer in the World.

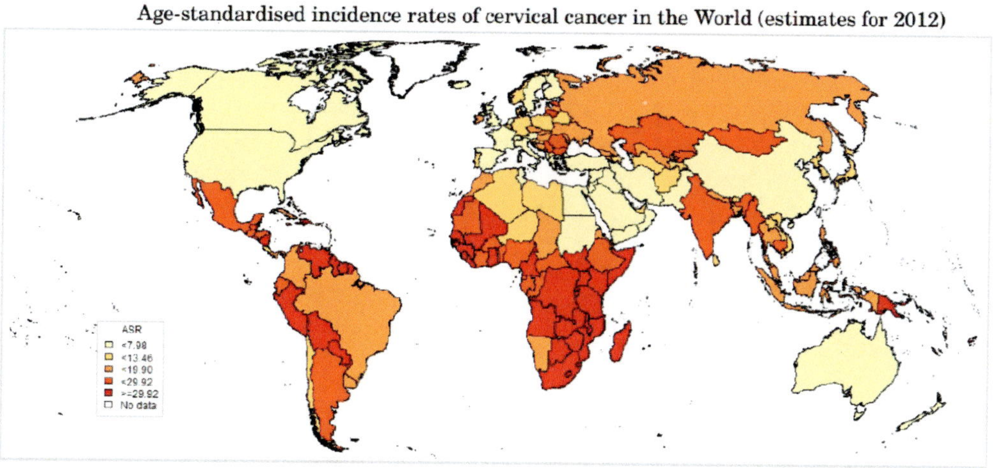

Fig. (1). Age-standardized incidence rates (ASR) of cervical cancer in the World (estimates for 2012): Standardized rates have been estimated using the direct method and the World population as the reference; Rates per 100,000 women per year [Data sources: FerlayJ, SoerjomataramI, ErvikM, DikshitR, EserS, Mathers C, RebeloM, ParkinDM, Forman D, Bray F. GLOBOCAN 2012 v1.2, Cancer Incidence and Mortality Worldwide: IARC CancerBaseNo. 11 [Internet]. Lyon, France: International Agency for Research on Cancer; 2013. Available from: http://globocan.iarc.fr].

Head and Neck Cancer

The prevalence of HPV in oropharyngeal squamous cell carcinoma (OPSCC) was estimated to be present in 70% of all newly diagnosed cases [26 - 28]. On the other hand, a prevalence of HPV-positive OPSCCs and tonsillar cancers was reported to be ~ 36% and ~ 51%, respectively [29, 30]. HPV-16 accounts for the majority of HPV-positive OPSCCs (~ 86.7%) whereas HPV18 accounts for ~ 2.8% of these cases [29, 31]. Biron *et al* found a significant increase in the overall incidence of cervical cancer in women with OPSCC in the province of Alberta, Canada suggesting a possible association of HPV-related cancers secondary to HPV co-infection [32]. Moreover, very little data was found on the association between HPV-related OPSCC and anogenital cancers [33]. In 2010, in Poland 2709 men were diagnosed with lip, mouth or throat cancer (~ 9.84% of all cancers) and 1763 died (~ 3.4%). At the same time 960 women were diagnosed (~ 1.4%) and 464 (~ 1.1%) died. Moreover, the incidence of larynx cancer was ~ 2.75% of all cancers in men, and the mortality among men was 2.62% [11, 12]. Oral cancers represented 2.4% and 1.1% of cancers in men and women, respectively which in turn accounts for approximately 30% of all malignant neoplasms of head and neck, in comparison with malignant tumors of the mouth and neck (~ 12% of all malignant tumors) [11, 34].

Anal Cancer

The reported rate of anal cancer incidence (ASR) is about 1.0 per 100,000 worldwide [35]. Although anal cancer is relatively uncommon, but the incidence has been reported to be increasing in Scotland, Denmark, the USA and Australia and also in HIV-infected men in the North America [36 - 40]. HPV infection in the external genital tract of men has been detected in a range of 1.8-73% of healthy men. Furthermore, the age range of men in whom infection is detected is higher than in women, and serological evidence of infection appears later in men than in women [41 - 43].

Penile Cancer

Squamous cell carcinoma of the penis is a rare malignancy in Europe and North America (< 1% of all cancers in men) [2, 20, 44]. The reported rate of penile cancer incidence (ASR) is about 0.1-0.5 per 100,000 in developed countries and more than 2.0 per 100,000 in developing countries such as Uganda, Brazil, Vietnam, Columbia, Malawi, Paraguay and India (*i.e.,* ~ 10% of reported cancers) [2, 35].

Vaginal Cancer

Vaginal cancer is a relatively uncommon cancer, with an ASR of 0.2-0.7 per 100,000 in most countries [2, 45]. The median age at diagnosis of squamous cell carcinoma (SCC) is 69 years old, although it is sometimes observed in the third and fourth decades [2, 46].

Vulvar Cancer

Vulvar cancer constitutes ~ 4-5% of cancers in the female genital tract with an

ASR of 1.0-1.8 per 100,000 worldwide [2, 20, 47]. The peak incidence of HPV-related vulva cancer (about 50%) was reported in menopause, although a decline was observed in the median age of vulval cancers related to HPV [4]. A 10% increase in the incidence of vulvar cancer was reported among women younger than 50 years, *e.g.,* in Scotland [2, 20, 48].

CONCLUDING REMARKS

Generally, the rates of HPV infection in young women are high following first sexual intercourse. The incidence of HPV-associated cancers in women usually decreases with age, although the second peak is sometimes observed in older women. Moreover, the incidence rates of cancers are generally higher for high-risk HPV types than for low-risk types. It was confirmed that incidence rates for HPV-16 is higher than those observed for other HPV types. Co-infection with multiple HPV types and the next infection with new types are common, and the risk of acquiring novel HPV types is independent of previous infection with other types.

CONFLICT OF INTEREST

The author (editor) declares no conflict of interest, financial or otherwise.

ACKNOWLEDGEMENT

Declare none.

REFERENCES

[1] Forcier M, Musacchio N. An overview of Human Papilloma Virus. WSN 2016; 53(3): 275-308.

[2] Wakeham K, Kavanagh K. The burden of HPV-associated anogenital cancers. Curr Oncol Rep 2014; 16(9): 402.
[http://dx.doi.org/10.1007/s11912-014-0402-4] [PMID: 25118645]

[3] Herrero R, Castle PE, Schiffman M, *et al.* Epidemiologic profile of type-specific human papillomavirus infection and cervical neoplasia in Guanacaste, Costa Rica. J Infect Dis 2005; 191(11): 1796-807.
[http://dx.doi.org/10.1086/428850] [PMID: 15871111]

[4] Wain G. The human papillomavirus (HPV) vaccine, HPV related diseases and cervical cancer in the post-reproductive years. Maturitas 2010; 65(3): 205-9.
[http://dx.doi.org/10.1016/j.maturitas.2009.12.002] [PMID: 20036786]

[5] Muñoz N, Kato I, Bosch FX, *et al.* Risk factors for HPV DNA detection in middle-aged women. Sex Transm Dis 1996; 23(6): 504-10.
[http://dx.doi.org/10.1097/00007435-199611000-00012] [PMID: 8946637]

[6] Satterwhite CL, Torrone E, Meites E, *et al.* Sexually transmitted infections among US women and men: prevalence and incidence estimates, 2008. Sex Transm Dis 2013; 40(3): 187-93.
[http://dx.doi.org/10.1097/OLQ.0b013e318286bb53] [PMID: 23403598]

[7] Hariri S, Unger ER, Sternberg M, *et al.* Prevalence of genital human papillomavirus among females in

the United States, the National Health And Nutrition Examination Survey, 2003-2006. J Infect Dis 2011; 204(4): 566-73.
[http://dx.doi.org/10.1093/infdis/jir341] [PMID: 21791659]

[8] Hariri S, Lucena-Silva N, Unger E, *et al.* HPV coinfection among females in the United States. International Papillomavirus Conference and Clinical Workshop. Berlin. 2011.

[9] Dunne EF, Nielson CM, Stone KM, Markowitz LE, Giuliano AR. Prevalence of HPV infection among men: A systematic review of the literature. J Infect Dis 2006; 194(8): 1044-57.
[http://dx.doi.org/10.1086/507432] [PMID: 16991079]

[10] Partridge JM, Hughes JP, Feng Q, *et al.* Genital human papillomavirus infection in men: incidence and risk factors in a cohort of university students. J Infect Dis 2007; 196(8): 1128-36.
[http://dx.doi.org/10.1086/521192] [PMID: 17955430]

[11] Morshed K, Polz-Gruszka D, Szymański M, Polz-Dacewicz M. Human Papillomavirus (HPV) - structure, epidemiology and pathogenesis. Otolaryngol Pol 2014; 68(5): 213-9.
[http://dx.doi.org/10.1016/j.otpol.2014.06.001] [PMID: 25283316]

[12] Wojciechowska U, Didkowska J, Zatoński W. Nowotwory złośliwe w Polsce w 2010 roku. Warszawa: Centrum Onkologii–Instytut im M Skłodowskiej-Curie 2012; pp. 3-4.

[13] Vinodhini K, Shanmughapriya S, Das BC, Natarajaseenivasan K. Prevalence and risk factors of HPV infection among women from various provinces of the world. Arch Gynecol Obstet 2012; 285(3): 771-7.
[http://dx.doi.org/10.1007/s00404-011-2155-8] [PMID: 22159694]

[14] Curado MP, Edwards B, Shin HR, Eds. Cancer incidence in five continents.IARC ScientiWc Publications. 9th ed., Lyon, France: International Agency for Research on Cancer 2007.

[15] Parkin DM, Pisani P, Ferlay J. Estimates of the worldwide incidence of 25 major cancers in 1990. Int J Cancer 1999; 80(6): 827-41.
[http://dx.doi.org/10.1002/(SICI)1097-0215(19990315)80:6<827::AID-IJC6>3.0.CO;2-P] [PMID: 10074914]

[16] Parkin DM, Pisani P, Ferlay J. Estimates of the worldwide incidence of eighteen major cancers in 1985. Int J Cancer 1993; 54(4): 594-606.
[http://dx.doi.org/10.1002/ijc.2910540413] [PMID: 8514451]

[17] Ferlay J, Pisani P. GLOBOCAN 1: cancer incidence and mortality worldwide IARC Cancer Base no 3. Lyon: IARC Press 1998.

[18] Parkin DM, Bray F. Chapter 2: the burden of HPV-related cancers. Vaccine 2006; 24(3): S3/11-25.

[19] Information Service Division S. Scottish Cervical Screening Programme. 2014.

[20] Information Service Division S. Cancer incidence and mortality in Scotland by site/type of cancer, sex and year of diagnosis/registration of death: 2002-2011; 2014.

[21] Quinn MA, Benedet JL, Odicino F, *et al.* Carcinoma of the cervix uteri. FIGO 26th annual report on the results of treatment in gynecological cancer. Int J Gynaecol Obstet 2006; 95(1) (Suppl. 1): S43-S103.
[http://dx.doi.org/10.1016/S0020-7292(06)60030-1] [PMID: 17161167]

[22] Sankaranarayanan R, Swaminathan R, Jayant K, Brenner H. An overview of cancer survival in Africa, Asia, the Caribbean and Central America: the case for investment in cancer health services. IARC Sci Publ 2011; 162(162): 257-91.
[PMID: 21675431]

[23] Li LK, Dai M, Clifford GM, *et al.* Human papillomavirus infection in Shenyang City, People's Republic of China: A population-based study. Br J Cancer 2006; 95(11): 1593-7.
[http://dx.doi.org/10.1038/sj.bjc.6603450] [PMID: 17088908]

[24] Zhang WY, Xue YZ, Chen M, Han L, Luo M. Prevalence of high-risk human papillomavirus infection

in different cervical lesion among organized health-examination women in Shanghai, China. Chin Med J (Engl) 2008; 121(16): 1578-82.
[PMID: 18982872]

[25] Uribarren-Berrueta O, Sánchez-Corona J, Montoya-Fuentes H, Trujillo-Hernández B, Vásquez C. Presence of HPV DNA in placenta and cervix of pregnant Mexican women. Arch Gynecol Obstet 2012; 285(1): 55-60.
[http://dx.doi.org/10.1007/s00404-011-1911-0] [PMID: 21538009]

[26] Marzouki HZ, Biron VL, Harris J, O'Connell D, Seikaly H. Human papillomavirus-associated oropharyngeal squamous cell carcinoma and anogenital cancers in men: Epidemiologic evaluation of association. Head Neck 2016; 38(1) (Suppl. 1): E2100-2.
[http://dx.doi.org/10.1002/hed.24388] [PMID: 26849535]

[27] Jemal A, Siegel R, Ward E, *et al.* Cancer statistics, 2008. CA Cancer J Clin 2008; 58(2): 71-96.
[http://dx.doi.org/10.3322/CA.2007.0010] [PMID: 18287387]

[28] D'Souza G, Kreimer AR, Viscidi R, *et al.* Case-control study of human papillomavirus and oropharyngeal cancer. N Engl J Med 2007; 356(19): 1944-56.
[http://dx.doi.org/10.1056/NEJMoa065497] [PMID: 17494927]

[29] Kreimer AR, Clifford GM, Boyle P, Franceschi S. Human papillomavirus types in head and neck squamous cell carcinomas worldwide: a systematic review. Cancer Epidemiol Biomarkers Prev 2005; 14(2): 467-75.
[http://dx.doi.org/10.1158/1055-9965.EPI-04-0551] [PMID: 15734974]

[30] Syrjänen S. HPV infections and tonsillar carcinoma. J Clin Pathol 2004; 57(5): 449-55.
[http://dx.doi.org/10.1136/jcp.2003.008656] [PMID: 15113849]

[31] Nichols AC, Dhaliwal SS, Palma DA, *et al.* Does HPV type affect outcome in oropharyngeal cancer? J Otolaryngol Head Neck Surg 2013; 42: 9.
[http://dx.doi.org/10.1186/1916-0216-42-9] [PMID: 23663293]

[32] Biron VL, Côté DW, Seikaly H. Oropharyngeal squamous cell carcinoma and human papillomavirus-associated cancers in women: epidemiologic evaluation of association. J Otolaryngol Head Neck Surg 2011; 40(1) (Suppl. 1): S65-9.
[PMID: 21453664]

[33] Sikora AG, Morris LG, Sturgis EM. Bidirectional association of anogenital and oral cavity/pharyngeal carcinomas in men. Arch Otolaryngol Head Neck Surg 2009; 135(4): 402-5.
[http://dx.doi.org/10.1001/archoto.2009.19] [PMID: 19380365]

[34] Parkin DM, Bray F, Ferlay J, Pisani P. Global cancer statistics, 2002. CA Cancer J Clin 2005; 55(2): 74-108.
[http://dx.doi.org/10.3322/canjclin.55.2.74] [PMID: 15761078]

[35] Boyle P, Levin B. World Cancer Report 2008. 2014.

[36] Silverberg MJ, Lau B, Justice AC, *et al.* Risk of anal cancer in HIV-infected and HIV-uninfected individuals in North America. Clin Infect Dis 2012; 54(7): 1026-34.
[http://dx.doi.org/10.1093/cid/cir1012] [PMID: 22291097]

[37] Johnson LG, Madeleine MM, Newcomer LM, Schwartz SM, Daling JR. Anal cancer incidence and survival: the surveillance, epidemiology, and end results experience, 1973-2000. Cancer 2004; 101(2): 281-8.
[http://dx.doi.org/10.1002/cncr.20364] [PMID: 15241824]

[38] Brewster DH, Bhatti LA. Increasing incidence of squamous cell carcinoma of the anus in Scotland, 1975-2002. Br J Cancer 2006; 95(1): 87-90.
[http://dx.doi.org/10.1038/sj.bjc.6603175] [PMID: 16721368]

[39] Frisch M, Melbye M, Møller H. Trends in incidence of anal cancer in Denmark. BMJ 1993; 306(6875): 419-22.

[http://dx.doi.org/10.1136/bmj.306.6875.419] [PMID: 8461721]

[40] Jin F, Stein AN, Conway EL, *et al.* Trends in anal cancer in Australia, 1982-2005. Vaccine 2011; 29(12): 2322-7.
[http://dx.doi.org/10.1016/j.vaccine.2011.01.015] [PMID: 21255682]

[41] Newall AT, Brotherton JM, Quinn HE, *et al.* Population seroprevalence of human papillomavirus types 6, 11, 16, and 18 in men, women, and children in Australia. Clin Infect Dis 2008; 46(11): 1647-55.
[http://dx.doi.org/10.1086/587895] [PMID: 18444790]

[42] Nielsen A, Munk C, Kjaer SK. Trends in incidence of anal cancer and high-grade anal intraepithelial neoplasia in Denmark, 1978-2008. Int J Cancer 2012; 130(5): 1168-73.
[http://dx.doi.org/10.1002/ijc.26115] [PMID: 21469144]

[43] Robinson D, Coupland V, Møller H. An analysis of temporal and generational trends in the incidence of anal and other HPV-related cancers in Southeast England. Br J Cancer 2009; 100(3): 527-31.
[http://dx.doi.org/10.1038/sj.bjc.6604871] [PMID: 19156144]

[44] Hernandez BY, Barnholtz-Sloan J, German RR, *et al.* Burden of invasive squamous cell carcinoma of the penis in the United States, 1998-2003. Cancer 2008; 113(10) (Suppl.): 2883-91.
[http://dx.doi.org/10.1002/cncr.23743] [PMID: 18980292]

[45] Human papillomavirus and related diseases report. L'Hospitalet de Llobregat: ICO Information Centre on HPV and Cancer, 2014.

[46] Daling JR, Madeleine MM, Schwartz SM, *et al.* A population-based study of squamous cell vaginal cancer: HPV and cofactors. Gynecol Oncol 2002; 84(2): 263-70.
[http://dx.doi.org/10.1006/gyno.2001.6502] [PMID: 11812085]

[47] Siegel R, Ma J, Zou Z, Jemal A. Cancer statistics, 2014. CA Cancer J Clin 2014; 64(1): 9-29.
[http://dx.doi.org/10.3322/caac.21208] [PMID: 24399786]

[48] Judson PL, Habermann EB, Baxter NN, Durham SB, Virnig BA. Trends in the incidence of invasive and in situ vulvar carcinoma. Obstet Gynecol 2006; 107(5): 1018-22.
[http://dx.doi.org/10.1097/01.AOG.0000210268.57527.a1] [PMID: 16648405]

CHAPTER 8

Immunity against HPV-Related Cancers

Afshin Khavari, Kimia Kardani and **Azam Bolhassani***

Department of Hepatitis and AIDS, Pasteur Institute of Iran, Tehran, Iran

Department of Pharmaceutical Biotechnology, School of Pharmacy, Shahid Beheshti University of Medical Sciences, Tehran, Iran

Abstract: The induction of immunotolerance of the host's immune system by the persistent infection of HPV is one of the most important mechanisms for cervical lesions. The immune system modifications induced by HPV infection include tumor-associated macrophage differentiation, a compromised cellular immune response, an abnormal imbalance between type 1 T-helper cells (Th1) and Th2 cells, regulatory T cell infiltration, and down-regulated DC activation. In this chapter, the effects of HPV and its mechanism of action will be discussed on immune system.

Keywords: Adaptive immune system, HPV, Immunobiology, Innate immune system.

INTRODUCTION

Human papillomaviruses (HPVs) are infectious agents that have no systemic sequelae and avoid the host defense systems [1]. HPV viruses possess an ability to evade resistance with human immune system [2]. As known, the expression of the viral oncogenes is kept at low levels throughout the initial life cycle, and highly immunogenic products including L1 and L2 capsid proteins are synthesized only in superficial layers of the epithelium [1 - 5]. It is a replication strategy in which viral DNA replication and virus assembly occur in a cell that will terminally differentiate and die by natural causes. Thus, there is no viral-induced cytolysis or necrosis, and therefore no inflammation [1]. For most of the duration of the HPV infectious cycle, there is little or no release into the local milieu of pro-inflammatory cytokines, which is important for APC activation and migration. The central signals to start the immune responses in squamous epithelia are absent [1, 4]. There is no blood-borne or viremic phase of the HPV life cycle, and only minimal amounts of replicating virus are exposed to immune defenses; in fact, the virus is practically invisible in the host for long periods of time [1].

* **Corresponding author Azam Bolhassani:** Department of Hepatitis and AIDS, Pasteur Institute of Iran, Tehran, Iran; Tel: 66953311-20; E-mails: A_bolhasani@pasteur.ac.ir, azam.bolhassani@yahoo.com

The incidence of some cancers is higher in immunocompromised patients. Immune suppression after organ transplantation is connected with increased risk of virus-associated cancers including HPV-associated cancers. For example, individuals with acquired immunodeficiency syndrome (AIDS) are at higher risk of HPV-associated cancers [6 - 11]. HPV-induced anal cancer in an HIV-positive population is most commonly associated with HPV-16 infection (75%) followed by HPV-18 (less than 10%). A low CD4 T-cell count measured at AIDS onset was associated with significantly increased risks of HPV-associated invasive cancers, including anal cancers among men and vaginal or vulvar cancers among women. In contrast to the high risk of anal and other HPV-associated cancers, the risk of invasive oropharyngeal cancer was moderately elevated among individuals with HIV [6, 11].

Immune Responses to HPV-Related Cancer

Most HPV infections are transient and undetectable within the first two years in immunocompetent individuals. It was shown that lesions often regress spontaneously in young women [6]. Indeed, a number of CIN2-3 lesions can regress spontaneously to CIN1 or less [12]. However, different spontaneous regression rates depend on the type of HPVs [13, 14]. The spontaneous regression of HPV lesions is associated with the local presence of a range of adaptive immune cells (B cells and $CD8^+$, $CD4^+$ and $CD25^+$ T cells) [12, 15]. The results obtained from immuno-deficient or -competent individuals suggest that the immune system is highly involved in the success or failure of spontaneous HPV clearance. Indeed, boosting such immune responses by therapeutic vaccine could enhance clearance rates [6].

Innate Immunity *Versus* HPV

The innate immunity is the non-specific part of the immune system that is mediated by epithelial barrier, the complement system, and a variety of cells that phagocytose antigens and present them to other cells or destroy them [2]. Once HPV enters a host cell, HPV DNA can be recognized by innate pathogen sensors. The cytosolic DNA sensors include the absent in melanoma 2 (AIM2), IFN-γ inducible protein 16 (IFI16), and cyclic guanosine monophosphate-adenosine monophosphate synthase (cGAS). IFI16 also detects foreign DNA in the nucleus [16 - 20]. Triggering of the AIM2 inflammasome by viral DNA leads to the maturation of caspase-1 and interleukin-1β (IL-1β), which are commonly activated in HPV16-infected lesions and keratinocytes [16, 21]. IFI16 restricts HPV genome replication and gene transcription by enhancing heterochromatin association with the early and late promoters [22]. Furthermore, there is a significant correlation between clearance of initial HPV infection and higher expression of nucleic acid-sensing toll-like receptors (TLR3, TLR7, TLR8, and TLR9) as well as TLR2 in women [23]. One of the downstream effects of pathogen recognition by pattern recognition receptors (PRRs) is the production of type I interferons (IFN-α and -β). IFN-β treatment hinders HPV entry and promotes clearance of latent HPV episomes in persistently infected cells [24 - 26]. HPV genomes in HPV-positive cervical lesions and IFN-β-treated cervical keratinocytes are edited by several IFN-inducible cytidine deaminase APOBEC3 family members. The studies indicated that one of these family members, APOBEC3A, significantly restricts HPV infection [27 - 29]. Innate immune cells are also involved in early host responses against HPV infection. HPV infection recruits Langerhans (LC), dendritic (DC), natural killer T (NKT), and natural killer (NK) cells to the HPV-infected microenvironment [30]. The immunosurveillance of squamous epithelium of the cervix is managed by Langerhans cells which are abundant in the skin and mucosa eliciting both innate and adaptive immunity against the virus [31]. Dendritic cells recognize special patterns on the pathogens using their toll-like receptors and present the antigens to the T cells through MHC I and II. Langerhans cells of the epidermis do not produce a sufficient T-cell response compared to the dendritic cells of the dermis, due to the lack of appropriate co-stimulatory microenvironment. Consequently, Langerhans cells may be unable to elicit a successful immune response and become a part of the virus tolerance tactics [32]. Moreover, the activation of toll-like receptors (TLRs) elicits a pro-inflammatory expression profile which promotes innate immunity. The double stranded HPV DNA is recognized mainly by TLR-9 inducing a cascade of interferons [33]. The studies showed that the tumorigenic E6 and E7 genes in HPV-16 are responsible for the down-regulation of TLR9. Decreased expression of IFN-γ is considered to be originated from the direct down-regulation by the HPV oncogenes [34 - 37]. Thus, the up-regulation of certain TLRs is considered to be an attractive target for novel treatments in cervical cancer [38, 39].

On the other hand, macrophages have an important role in both innate and adaptive immune responses by digesting pathogens and stimulating lymphocytes and other immune cells. Certain proteins such as monocyte chemotactic protein-1 (MCP-1) and macrophage inflammatory protein (MIPa3) help the aggregation of macrophages. Both of these proteins are down-regulated directly or indirectly by HPV [40 - 42]. In addition, tumor-associated macrophages (TAMs) promote cancer cell proliferation and migration, angiogenesis and restriction of immune defenses [43]. This can be explained by the identification of two distinct macrophage phenotypes: M1 pro-inflammatory and M2 immunomodulatory [44, 45]. As cervical lesions progress, M2 macrophages are the main population in HPV-associated tumors that promote the differentiation of naïve T cells to T-regulatory cells through IL-10 and subsequently tumor growth. Depletion of TAM can be considered as a possible target of immunotherapy [46 - 48]. Another important part of innate immune response against viral attack is attributed to natural killer cells (NK cells), without the need of MHC system. In cervical cancer caused by HPV16, the NK-activating receptors NKp30 and NKp45 (and NKG2D only in cancer) are significantly decreased, affecting the cytolytic functionality [49]. On the other hand, plasmacytoid dendritic cells (pDC) have been shown to respond to the presence of HPV16 virus-like particles (VLPs) in cervical cancer tissue and secrete various cytokines including IFN-α, IL-6, TNF-α and IL-8 following activation of MyD88-dependent signaling. Furthermore, the incidence of HPV infection and HPV-associated cancer has been increased in individuals with various functional NK cell deficiencies [16, 50 - 53]. Generally, the early inflammatory response might be critical for initiating a robust host defense against HPV infection [16].

Adaptive Immunity *Versus* HPV

Adaptive immunity consists of B cells and T cells. B cells are responsible for the humoral immune response and T cells which are divided in CD4 helper T cells, CD8 cytotoxic T cells (CTLs), and regulatory T cells (Tregs) are responsible for a variety of functions [2]. T-helper cells determine the direction of the immune response. Both IFN-γ and IL-12 are required for the differentiation of Th0 (naïve lymphocyte) to Th1, which produces IFN-γ, lymphotoxin, and IL2 (and IL10, TNF-α) and leads to the activation of cell-mediated immunity. On the other hand, for the Th2 phenotype, IL4 and IL2 are prerequisite, and the cytokine products consist of IL4, IL5, IL13, IL25, IL10, and amphiregulin, contributing to the development of humoral immune response [2, 54, 55]. T-helper cells are suggested as the dominant response required for clearance of an HPV infection [2, 56]. The HPV life cycle is strictly intraepithelial and virions are produced only from the fully differentiated upper layer of skin. Thus, there is no virus-induced cytolysis or viremia, which limits the exposure of HPV to systemic immune responses. However, many studies indicated that host T-cell responses are required to eliminate HPV-infected cells. The regression rate of cervical precancerous lesions strongly correlates with the presence of intraepithelial granzyme B-positive cytotoxic T cells [16, 57]. The reduced Th1 (*e.g.,* low levels of IL-2 and TNF-α cytokines) and increased Th2 responses lead to suppression of cellular immunity and progression of intraepithelial and invasive cervical HPV lesions [2, 58 - 60]. Although, the level of IL4 seems to increase in low grade squamous intraepithelial lesion (LSIL), it slightly decreases with development of lesion. Generally, in HPV lesions, both Th1 and Th2 phenotypes are suppressed, especially Th1, likely due to the activity of the Treg cells [2]. On the other hand, the cytotoxic T lymphocytes (CTLs) are the main agent in antigen-specific immunity, and recognize the antigens with the assistance of MHC class I [2, 61,

62]. T-cell activation is caused by HPV E6 and E7 oncoproteins, and the destruction is promoted by the up-regulation of adhesion molecules like ICAM-1, VCAM-1, and E-selectin in infected cells and down-regulates the expression of antigen peptide transporter-1 (TAP-1) [63 - 65]. Moreover, HPV16 E5 down-regulates MHCI [2, 66]. T-regulatory cells are a subset of T cells expressing CD4, CD25, and transcription factor Foxp3, that is normally necessary in the induction of tolerance and their increase may suppress the proliferation of T-helper and CTLs, and anti-tumor effects through inhibiting cytokines. Their activation is induced by TGF-β and IL-2 [67 - 74]. The studies showed that the levels of TGF-1 and TGF-2 increase while the lesion progresses from LSIL to invasive cervical cancer; in contrast, the levels of IL-12 and TNF-α significantly decrease. Also, IL-10 cytokine is rising as the disease declines, especially in high squamous intraepithelial lesion (HSIL) [59, 75].

B-cells are responsible for humoral response which neutralize and opsonize viral agents. The HPV L1 protein assembles into capsids and is completely immunogenic *in vivo* [6, 76, 77]. The natural antibody response to L1 is poor, likely because of its expression in the squamous epithelium. However, these capsids are a major tool for serological responses to HPV [6, 78]. Humoral immunity is stimulated by Th2 cytokines and depends on CD4 helper T cells that help B cells to mature and generate antibodies [2, 79]. The kinetic of IgG antibody development is slow (~ 6-12 months), but antibodies can persist for decades unless HPV-associated lesions resolve. Secretory IgA antibodies can also be detected in the cervical secretions of HPV-positive women with a similar time course to IgG antibodies, but with a shorter persistence time [6, 80 - 82]. Antibodies against HPV16 and HPV18 non-structural E2, E6 and E7 proteins were detected in only half of patients. A stronger correlation was demonstrated between E7 antibodies and advanced cervical cancer [6, 83 - 86]. In a study performed by our group, the ELISA and western blot analyses indicated that patients suffering from cervical cancer with high antibody response to HPV16E7 had significant seroreactivity to the C-terminal fragment of glycoprotein 96 (CT-gp96) known as a heat shock protein (HSP). In adenocarcinoma, no significant difference was observed in seroreactivities between normal and patients [87]. There are two types of neutralizing L1 antibodies. The first class inhibits cell surface binding, while the second class prevents binding to the basal membrane (*e.g.*, VLPs in prophylactic vaccine) [1, 2, 88]. Fig. (**1**) shows simple summary of immunological responses to HPV infection.

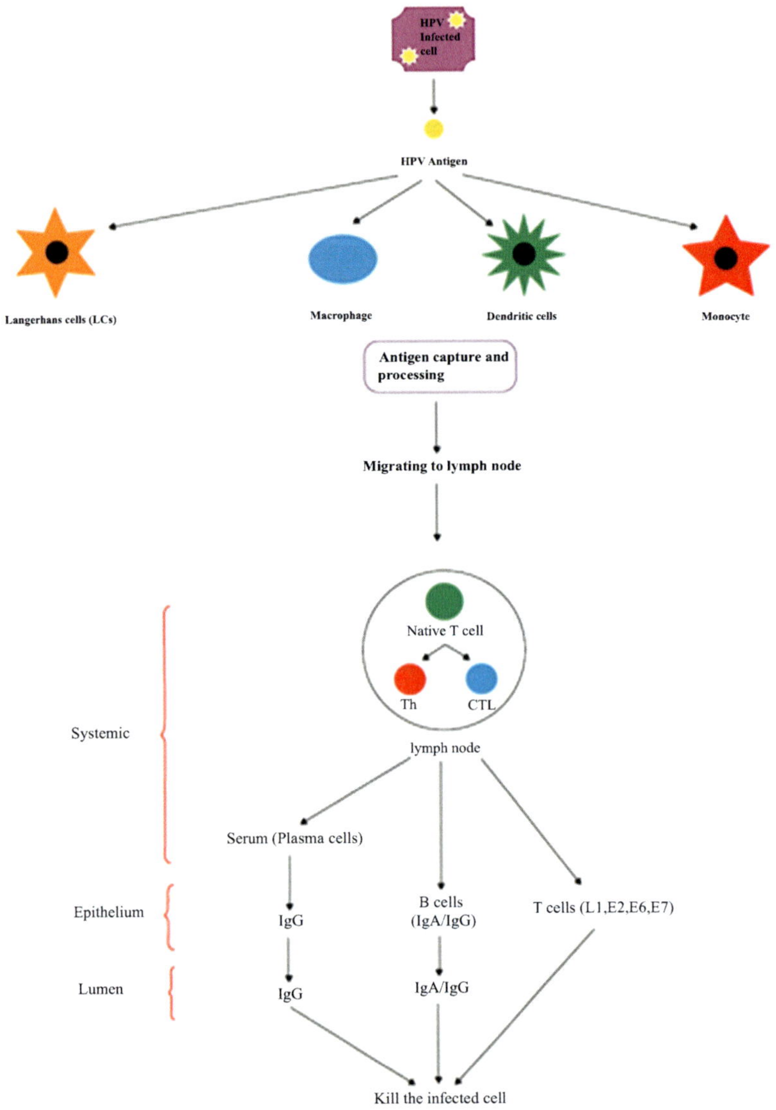

Fig. (1). Simple summary of immunological responses to HPV infection: Free virus particles are shed from the surface of squamous epithelial with poor access to vascular and lymphatic channels and to lymph nodes where immune responses are initiated [1]. Both innate and adaptive immune systems work to prevent viral infection. The innate immunity is the first line of defense and acts non-specifically on the infection, whereas the adaptive immunity is the second line of defense and prevents re-infection. Adaptive immunity specifically reacts to certain HPV proteins. Adaptive immunity is composed of two systems: Th1and Th2 responses. Th1 cells promote cell-mediated immunity (CMI) [*i.e.,* these cells induce cytotoxic T lymphocytes (CTLs) to kill virus-infected cells], whereas Th2 cells stimulate humoral immunity (*i.e.,* these cells stimulate B cells to produce antibodies). During HPV infection, Th1 immunity against HPV16 E2 and E6 proteins plays an essential role in eliminating HPV infection. Despite such a great defense system, several mechanisms of immune evasion exist in HPV infection, and may facilitate cancer development [1, 177].

High-Risk HPVs Hinder LC Activity

HPV infections should be detected by the professional APC of squamous epithelia. Virus capsids usually activate DCs, but not Langerhans cells (LCs) [1, 89]. In addition, stromal DCs are activated by VLPs and stimulate HPV-specific T-cells, but since the virus remains in the epithelium, the stromal DCs are disabling to induce immune responses [1, 90].

High-Risk HPVs Down-Regulate Interferon Responses

The type 1 interferons (*i.e.,* IFN-α, and IFN-β) have immunostimulatory properties that act as a bridge between innate and adaptive immunity [1, 91]. High-risk HPV infection down-regulates IFN-α inducible gene expression and the HPV16 E6 and E7 oncoproteins directly interact with components of the interferon signaling pathways [3, 92, 93].

Immune Response to HPV in Natural Infections

Anogenital warts and low-grade intraepithelial lesions are usually cleared by an effective cell-mediated immune response directed against early HPV proteins especially E2 and E6 [94 - 97]. However, the levels of antibody in animals and humans are low, and many women do not seroconvert [98 - 100]. Although 80-90% of genital HPV infections resolve with time, about 10-20% of individuals do not become HPV DNA negative and develop persistent infection, and progress to CIN2/3. It was observed that the episomal HPV is cleared from cells after exposure to IFN-β, but cells with integrated HPV-DNA are resistant to this anti-viral effect [101, 102]. T-cell responses to E2 and E6 are reduced in CIN3 and invasive carcinoma. Even if HPV antigen-specific CTLs are generated, the regulatory T-cells significantly abrogate the killer defense response [103, 104]. Recently, the challenge for development of HPV therapeutic vaccine is to reverse this immunologically suppressive microenvironment and access the cytotoxic killers to the infected and neoplastic cells [1].

Altering Host Gene Expression by HPV Infection

In order to evade host immune defenses and establish persistence, HPV modulates host gene expression by deregulating host DNA methylation, histone modification, and transcription factors as described in following [16].

Deregulation of DNA Methylation

Epigenetic regulation by DNA methylation provides distinct gene expression patterns in different developmental stages, organ tissue types, and disease states [105 - 107]. DNA methylation also functions as a host defense mechanism. By methylating CpG residues of foreign DNA in eukaryotic cells, pathogen activity can be shut down due to alterations in pathogen transcriptional profiles [108, 109]. HPV DNA is also frequently methylated and viral gene transcription is repressed following DNA methylation [16, 110, 111]. Previous studies have shown that several pathogens hijack the host DNA methylation machinery to manipulate host transcription to their benefit [16, 112 - 114]. Interestingly, the HPV oncoprotein E7 interacts with the DNA methyltransferase DNMT1, and stimulates its methyltransferase activity. This may partially explain the global changes in HPV-positive keratinocytes [115, 116]. Recently, expression of the chemokine CXCL14 was down-regulated during HPV-associated cancer progression by promoter hypermethylation in an E7-dependent manner [116]. Since restoration of CXCL14 expression in HPV-positive HNC cells significantly suppresses tumor growth *in vivo*, methylation of HPV E7-mediated CXCL14 promoter may represent an immune evasion strategy during HPV persistence. Other studies indicated that CXCL14 induces direct chemotaxis of various immune cells including DCs, LCs, NK, and T cells [116 - 118]. Furthermore, it has been demonstrated that HPV16 E7 expression in the epidermis creates a strong immunosuppressive area where LC and $CD8^+$ T cell functions are significantly suppressed in transgenic mouse models [119 - 121]. This immune suppression appears to be mediated by an influx of HPV16 E7-induced regulatory T (Treg) cells and tolerization of cytotoxic T cells. In addition to HPV E7, HPV E6 is also involved in deregulation of host DNA methylation. High-risk HPV E6 represses Interferon kappa (IFN-κ), which is constitutively expressed in keratinocytes and serves to reinforce IFN-stimulated gene expression. E6-mediated repression of IFN-κ can be reversed by treatment with a DNA methyltransferase inhibitor [120, 122]. These findings suggest that HPV manipulates host DNA methylation to evade host immune defenses [16].

Deregulation of Histone Modification

Histone modification is another mechanism of epigenetic reprogramming altered by HPV. Cellular gene expression is tightly regulated by chromosome remodeling through histone methylation, phosphorylation, acetylation, ubiquitination, and sumoylation. HPV16 E7 binds to E2F6 (E2F Transcription Factor 6) and interferes with the formation of E2F6-containing polycomb transcriptional repressor complexes. HPV-mediated modulation of host histone methylation has been well described. Interestingly, HPV38 E7 recruits polycomb protein enhancer of zeste homolog 2 (EZH2) to the TLR9 promoter region, resulting in histone 3 trimethylation at lysine 27 (H3K27me3) and repression of TLR9 transcription [123 - 126]. Another study has shown that HPV16 E7 recruits histone deacetylase HDAC1 and histone demethylase JARID1B (also known as KDM5B) to the regulatory region upstream of the TLR9 transcriptional start site and reduces H4 acetylation and H3K4me3, leading to down-regulation of TLR9 expression. Since TLR9 recognizes viral DNA and induces innate immune responses, TLR9 repression may represent an important host immune response pathway antagonized by HPV. In addition, both high-risk and low-risk HPVE7 proteins inhibit the transcriptional activity of IRF1 by recruiting HDAC1 to promoters that contain IRF1 response elements [127, 128]. Consequently, IRF1 responsive genes, including the ATP-binding cassette (ABC) peptide transporter associated with antigen processing 1 (TAP1), IFN-β, and CCL2 are significantly down-regulated in HPV16 E7 expressing cells and mice. Consistently, treatment of HPV-positive tumor cells with an HDAC inhibitor increased the surface expression of MHCI molecules and subsequently the susceptibility of tumor cells to E7-specific $CD8^+$ T cells [129 - 131].

Modulation of NF-κB

HPV deregulates the activity of transcription factors to repress pro-inflammatory cytokine production. Nuclear factor-κB (NF-κB) is one of the most important transcription factors involved in immune signaling. Accordingly, NF-κB is frequently targeted by many different viruses (*e.g.,* HPV) [132 - 137]. High-risk HPVs decrease K310 acetylation of NF-κB in keratinocytes by enhancing IFN-related developmental regulator 1 (IFRD1) expression, resulting in down-regulation of proinflammatory cytokines [138]. E7 alone is capable of inhibiting imiquimod-induced NF-κB transactivation of IFN-α, IL-6, and TNF-α. Impairing the acetylation at K310 in the p65 subunit of NF-κB requires the CR1 and CR3 domains of E7 and leads to the reduced nuclear translocation of NF-κB [139]. A study has shown that HPV16 E6 and E7 also bind to p300/CBP-associated factor (PCAF) and inhibits NF-κB activation, resulting in IL-8 down-regulation [140].

Deregulation of Protein Functions

HPV infections influence different functions of proteins such as protein-protein interaction/sequestration, posttranslational modification, and protein degradation as follows.

Protein-Protein Interaction/Sequestration

The HPV oncoproteins E6 and E7 lack enzymatic activity. Instead, they act as adaptor proteins that interact with multiple host proteins, recruit them to desired locations, and hijack their activities to enhance virus replication and persistence, and induce malignancy [141, 142]. HPV E6 and E7 frequently inhibit host protein functions by direct binding. The HPV18 E6 protein directly interacts with non-receptor tyrosine-protein kinase 2 (TYK2), resulting in a reduction of IFN-α-induced phosphorylation in TYK2 and Signal Transducer and Activator of

Transcription 2 (STAT2) proteins [143]. TYK2 is a member of the JAK family and is important for signal transduction following receptor binding by various cytokines including IL-6, IL-12, and type I IFNs. The IFN regulatory transcription factor IRF3 is selectively bound and inhibited by HPV16 E6 protein, while HPV6, HPV11, and HPV18 E6 proteins bind poorly to IRF3. IRF3 plays a central role in inducing innate immune response against viral infections [144, 145]. The interaction of HPV16 E6 to IRF3 does not lead to ubiquitination or degradation of IRF3, but significantly represses its activity on target gene transcription and IFN-β production. This data suggests that HPV16 E6 binding is sufficient for inhibition of IRF3 functions. Cytosolic DNA can be detected by cGAS, which initiates innate immune signaling through the adapter proteins STING and IRF3 [146, 147]. Interestingly, HPV18 E7 antagonizes the activation of the cGAS-STING pathway and limits the production of type I IFNs by binding with STING through its LXCXE motif [148]. Furthermore, HPV16 E7 protein interacts with IRF1, probably at its N-terminal DNA-binding domain, resulting in decreased expression of IRF1 responsive genes, including TAP1, IFN-β, and CCL2 [128, 129, 149]. IFN signaling is further repressed by HPV16 E7 as it also binds to IRF9, another IFN regulatory factor [150]. IFN signaling lies at the core of anti-viral innate immune responses and appears to be greatly targeted by the HPV oncoproteins E6 and E7. The studies have shown that IFN-β treatment significantly inhibits HPV infection in primary and immortalized keratinocytes [16, 26, 29]. These findings indicated that evasion of IFN signaling mediated through HPV E6 and E7 interactions with host proteins might be critical for HPV persistence [16].

Post-translational Modification and Protein Degradation

The mechanisms of host protein degradation by the HPV oncoproteins E6 and E7 are well established, but, posttranslational modification of immunoregulatory proteins is relatively understood. Karim *et al.* have shown that high-risk HPVs up-regulate the cellular protein ubiquitin carboxyl-terminal hydrolase L1 (UCHL1) in keratinocytes [151, 152]. UCHL1 inhibits K63-linked ubiquitination of tumor necrosis factor receptor-associated factor 3 (TRAF3) resulting in decreased TRAF3- TBK1 complex formation and IRF3 phosphorylation. UCHL1 also mediates degradation of the essential modulator of NF-κB, NEMO, and suppresses p65 phosphorylation and NF-κB signaling. HPV16 E6 also induces degradation of pro-IL1β in a proteasome-dependent manner [153]. E6-mediated pro-IL-1β degradation is independent from caspase-1 activation, autophagy, or lysosomal degradation, but requires E6AP expression and poly-ubiquitination of pro-IL-1β. Since the proinflammatory cytokine IL-1β plays important roles in antiviral defense, these results suggest that high-risk HPV suppresses the proinflammatory response by inducing proteasome-mediated degradation of intracellular cytokines. Interestingly, the reports have shown that polymorphism in the IL-1β gene cluster is tightly linked to cervical cancer [154 - 157]. Specifically, women with IL-1β T-allele containing genotypes showed an increased risk of cervical cancer. Indeed, IL-1β expression is significantly down-regulated in HPV-positive normal keratinocytes but up-regulated in cervical cancer tissues. These results suggest that IL-1β may play dual roles in inhibiting HPV infection by its antiviral function in early stages of disease, but facilitating cancer progression through chronic inflammation in late stages [16, 116, 158].

Varied Cytoplasmic Trafficking of Host Proteins

Antigen presentation of viral epitopes by MHC-I molecules is critical to elicit cell-mediated immune responses that eliminate virus-infected cells. In order to escape host recognition, many viruses such as HPV have different strategies to suppress surface expression of MHC-I molecules. HPV bovine papillomavirus (BPV) E5 proteins are small transmembrane proteins that bind to several host transmembrane proteins, including MHCI. E5 binding to MHC-I leads to its down-regulation at the host cell surface [159 - 165]. Upon binding of antigenic peptides delivered by TAP1 in the ER, MHC-I molecules, composed of a heavy α chain and a soluble subunit β2-microglobulin (β2m), traffic through the secretary pathway and imbed within the cell membrane [166]. Indeed, HPV16 E5 physically interacts with the heavy chain of the MHC-I molecule through the hydrophobic region of E5 protein and retains MHC-I in the Golgi and ER. Moreover, HPV16 E5 specifically down-regulates HLA-A and -B expression, but not HLA-C and HLA-E [162, 163]. The studies indicated that HLA-C and HLA-E are the two most transcriptionally down-regulated MHC-I molecules in HPV-positive keratinocytes, and this down-regulation is dependent on HPV16 E7 expression [116]. Furthermore, down-regulation of MHC-I molecules at the cell surface by HPV E5 correlates with poor CD8+ T cell responses in E5 expressing cells [66]. An additional study has described a correlation between surface expression of MHC-I molecules and decreased TAP1 expression, suggesting that TAP1 down-regulation by E7 may also interfere with MHC-I trafficking [167]. HPV16 E5 also down-regulates the surface expression of MHC-II molecules by preventing degradation of the invariant chain that blocks peptide loading. Both high-risk HPV16 and low-risk HPV6 E5 proteins also down-regulate surface expression of the non-classical MHC molecule CD1d. HPV E5 directly interacts with calnexin in the ER and redirects CD1d to the cytosolic proteolytic pathway. CD1d expression on the cell surface activates NKT cell responses to various viral, bacterial, and fungal infections. Thus, HPV may evade host immune responses by down-regulating the surface expression of CD1d. Further investigation is necessary to determine if CD1d presents HPV-related antigens to induce protective antiviral activity [168 - 170]. The HPV minor structural protein L2 disrupts normal endocytic trafficking of virus particles in DCs and LCs. LCs, which are skin resident DCs, uptake L1-only virus-like particles (VLPs) and efficiently induce expression of pro-inflammatory cytokines and co-stimulatory molecules leading to the activation of cytotoxic T cell responses [171 - 173]. In contrast, HPV VLPs containing both L1 and L2 proteins do not activate LCs to present viral antigens. Interestingly, HPV16 L2 facilitates internalization of VLPs through interaction with the annexin A2 (ANXA2) heterotetramer. ANXA2 is associated with S100A10 as a heterotetramer and critical for HPV16 VLP internalization [171 - 174]. Thus, it is likely that HPV16 L2 blocks LC maturation and viral antigen presentation by modulating intracellular trafficking of viral particles. According to the previous study, overexpression of the interferon-inducible transmembrane protein 1 (IFITM) delays viral capsid protein degradation and significantly enhances HPV16 VLP entry into primary keratinocytes [16, 26]. IFITMs, induced by IFN treatment, inhibit a series of RNA viruses by redirecting virus particles to low-pH late endosomes and lysosomes during intracellular trafficking [175, 176]. These results implied that HPV not only bypasses IFITM restriction but also may utilize certain IFN-inducible proteins to facilitate virus infection [16].

CONCLUDING REMARKS

HPV infection can lead to lethal cancers such as cervical cancer especially in developing countries. The immunological aspects of HPV infection including HPV evasion and defense tactics are a significant issue for development of novel preventive and therapeutic pathways. Effective innate and adaptive immune responses are necessary to clear the virus despite its significant evasion tactics. In particular, the clearance of HPV infections depends on a strong Th1 immune response, limitation of Treg cells, and generation of stimulating cytokines. This cell-mediated response is the main concern of the developing vaccines. Novel therapeutic vaccines are designed to eradicate existing lesions and subsequently, the impact upon the prevalence of HPV-associated malignancies.

CONFLICT OF INTEREST

The author (editor) declares no conflict of interest, financial or otherwise.

ACKNOWLEDGEMENT

Declare none.

REFERENCES

[1] Stanley M. Immunobiology of HPV and HPV vaccines. Gynecol Oncol 2008; 109(2) (Suppl.): S15-21. [http://dx.doi.org/10.1016/j.ygyno.2008.02.003] [PMID: 18474288]

[2] Deligeoroglou E, Giannouli A, Athanasopoulos N, *et al.* HPV infection: Immunological aspects and their utility in future therapy. Infect dis obstet gynecol 2013; 2013: 540850.

[3] Kanodia S, Fahey LM, Kast WM. Mechanisms used by human papillomaviruses to escape the host immune response. Curr Cancer Drug Targets 2007; 7(1): 79-89. [http://dx.doi.org/10.2174/156800907780006869] [PMID: 17305480]

[4] Stanley M. Immune responses to human papillomavirus. Vaccine 2006; 24(1) (Suppl. 1): S16-22. [http://dx.doi.org/10.1016/j.vaccine.2005.09.002] [PMID: 16219398]

[5] Doorbar J. The papillomavirus life cycle. J Clin Virol 2005; 32(1) (Suppl. 1): S7-S15. [http://dx.doi.org/10.1016/j.jcv.2004.12.006] [PMID: 15753007]

[6] Bergot AS, Kassianos A, Frazer IH, Mittal D. New approaches to immunotherapy for HPV associated cancers. Cancers (Basel) 2011; 3(3): 3461-95. [http://dx.doi.org/10.3390/cancers3033461] [PMID: 24212964]

[7] Vajdic CM, McDonald SP, McCredie MR, *et al.* Cancer incidence before and after kidney transplantation. JAMA 2006; 296(23): 2823-31. [http://dx.doi.org/10.1001/jama.296.23.2823] [PMID: 17179459]

[8] Grulich AE, van Leeuwen MT, Falster MO, Vajdic CM. Incidence of cancers in people with HIV/AIDS compared with immunosuppressed transplant recipients: a meta-analysis. Lancet 2007; 370(9581): 59-67. [http://dx.doi.org/10.1016/S0140-6736(07)61050-2] [PMID: 17617273]

[9] Frisch M, Biggar RJ, Engels EA, Goedert JJ. Association of cancer with AIDS-related immunosuppression in adults. JAMA 2001; 285(13): 1736-45. [http://dx.doi.org/10.1001/jama.285.13.1736] [PMID: 11277828]

[10] Harris TG, Burk RD, Palefsky JM, *et al.* Incidence of cervical squamous intraepithelial lesions associated with HIV serostatus, CD4 cell counts, and human papillomavirus test results. JAMA 2005; 293(12): 1471-6. [http://dx.doi.org/10.1001/jama.293.12.1471] [PMID: 15784870]

[11] Chaturvedi AK, Madeleine MM, Biggar RJ, Engels EA. Risk of human papillomavirus-associated cancers among persons with AIDS. J Natl Cancer Inst 2009; 101(16): 1120-30. [http://dx.doi.org/10.1093/jnci/djp205] [PMID: 19648510]

[12] Øvestad IT, Gudlaugsson E, Skaland I, *et al.* Local immune response in the microenvironment of CIN2-3 with and without spontaneous regression. Mod Pathol 2010; 23(9): 1231-40. [http://dx.doi.org/10.1038/modpathol.2010.109] [PMID: 20512116]

[13] Molano M, Van den Brule A, Plummer M, *et al.* Determinants of clearance of human papillomavirus infections in Colombian women with normal cytology: a population-based, 5-year follow-up study. Am J Epidemiol 2003; 158(5): 486-94. [http://dx.doi.org/10.1093/aje/kwg171] [PMID: 12936904]

[14] Richardson H, Kelsall G, Tellier P, *et al.* The natural history of type-specific human papillomavirus infections in female university students. Cancer Epidemiol Biomarkers Prev 2003; 12(6): 485-90. [PMID: 12814991]

[15] Monnier-Benoit S, Mauny F, Riethmuller D, *et al.* Immunohistochemical analysis of CD4+ and CD8+ T-cell subsets in high risk human papillomavirus-associated pre-malignant and malignant lesions of the uterine cervix. Gynecol Oncol 2006; 102(1): 22-31. [http://dx.doi.org/10.1016/j.ygyno.2005.11.039] [PMID: 16427684]

[16] Westrich JA, Warren CJ, Pyeon D. Evasion of host immune defenses by human papillomavirus. Virus Res 2017; 231: 21-33. [http://dx.doi.org/10.1016/j.virusres.2016.11.023] [PMID: 27890631]

[17] Hornung V, Ablasser A, Charrel-Dennis M, *et al.* AIM2 recognizes cytosolic dsDNA and forms a

caspase-1-activating inflammasome with ASC. Nature 2009; 458(7237): 514-8. [http://dx.doi.org/10.1038/nature07725] [PMID: 19158675]

[18] Kerur N, Veettil MV, Sharma-Walia N, *et al.* IFI16 acts as a nuclear pathogen sensor to induce the inflammasome in response to Kaposi Sarcoma-associated herpesvirus infection. Cell Host Microbe 2011; 9(5): 363-75. [http://dx.doi.org/10.1016/j.chom.2011.04.008] [PMID: 21575908]

[19] Li X, Shu C, Yi G, *et al.* Cyclic GMP-AMP synthase is activated by double-stranded DNA-induced oligomerization. Immunity 2013; 39(6): 1019-31. [http://dx.doi.org/10.1016/j.immuni.2013.10.019] [PMID: 24332030]

[20] Unterholzner L, Keating SE, Baran M, *et al.* IFI16 is an innate immune sensor for intracellular DNA. Nat Immunol 2010; 11(11): 997-1004. [http://dx.doi.org/10.1038/ni.1932] [PMID: 20890285]

[21] Reinholz M, Kawakami Y, Salzer S, *et al.* HPV16 activates the AIM2 inflammasome in keratinocytes. Arch Dermatol Res 2013; 305(8): 723-32. [http://dx.doi.org/10.1007/s00403-013-1375-0] [PMID: 23764897]

[22] Lo Cigno I, De Andrea M, Borgogna C, *et al.* The nuclear DNA sensor IFI16 acts as a restriction factor for human papillomavirus replication through epigenetic modifications of the viral promoters. J Virol 2015; 89(15): 7506-20. [http://dx.doi.org/10.1128/JVI.00013-15] [PMID: 25972554]

[23] Daud II, Scott ME, Ma Y, Shiboski S, Farhat S, Moscicki AB. Association between toll-like receptor expression and human papillomavirus type 16 persistence. Int J Cancer 2011; 128(4): 879-86. [http://dx.doi.org/10.1002/ijc.25400] [PMID: 20473890]

[24] Chang YE, Pena L, Sen GC, Park JK, Laimins LA. Long-term effect of interferon on keratinocytes that maintain human papillomavirus type 31. J Virol 2002; 76(17): 8864-74. [http://dx.doi.org/10.1128/JVI.76.17.8864-8874.2002] [PMID: 12163606]

[25] Herdman MT, Pett MR, Roberts I, *et al.* Interferon-β treatment of cervical keratinocytes naturally infected with human papillomavirus 16 episomes promotes rapid reduction in episome numbers and emergence of latent integrants. Carcinogenesis 2006; 27(11): 2341-53. [http://dx.doi.org/10.1093/carcin/bgl172] [PMID: 16973673]

[26] Warren CJ, Griffin LM, Little AS, Huang IC, Farzan M, Pyeon D. The antiviral restriction factors IFITM1, 2 and 3 do not inhibit infection of human papillomavirus, cytomegalovirus and adenovirus. PLoS One 2014; 9(5): e96579. [http://dx.doi.org/10.1371/journal.pone.0096579] [PMID: 24827144]

[27] Vartanian JP, Guétard D, Henry M, Wain-Hobson S. Evidence for editing of human papillomavirus DNA by APOBEC3 in benign and precancerous lesions. Science 2008; 320(5873): 230-3. [http://dx.doi.org/10.1126/science.1153201] [PMID: 18403710]

[28] Wang Z, Wakae K, Kitamura K, *et al.* APOBEC3 deaminases induce hypermutation in human papillomavirus 16 DNA upon beta interferon stimulation. J Virol 2014; 88(2): 1308-17. [http://dx.doi.org/10.1128/JVI.03091-13] [PMID: 24227842]

[29] Warren CJ, Xu T, Guo K, *et al.* APOBEC3A functions as a restriction factor of human papillomavirus. J Virol 2015; 89(1): 688-702. [http://dx.doi.org/10.1128/JVI.02383-14] [PMID: 25355878]

[30] Amador-Molina A, Hernández-Valencia JF, Lamoyi E, Contreras-Paredes A, Lizano M. Role of innate immunity against human papillomavirus (HPV) infections and effect of adjuvants in promoting specific immune response. Viruses 2013; 5(11): 2624-42. [http://dx.doi.org/10.3390/v5112624] [PMID: 24169630]

[31] Manickam A, Sivanandham M, Tourkova IL. Immunological role of dendritic cells in cervical cancer. Adv Exp Med Biol 2007; 601: 155-62.

[http://dx.doi.org/10.1007/978-0-387-72005-0_16] [PMID: 17713002]

[32] Fausch SC, Da Silva DM, Kast WM. Differential uptake and cross-presentation of human papillomavirus virus-like particles by dendritic cells and Langerhans cells. Cancer Res 2003; 63(13): 3478-82.
[PMID: 12839929]

[33] Akira S, Takeda K. Toll-like receptor signalling. Nat Rev Immunol 2004; 4(7): 499-511.
[http://dx.doi.org/10.1038/nri1391] [PMID: 15229469]

[34] DeCarlo CA, Rosa B, Jackson R, Niccoli S, Escott NG, Zehbe I. Toll-like receptor transcriptome in the HPV-positive cervical cancer microenvironment. Clin Dev Immunol 2012; 2012: 1-9.

[35] Hasan UA, Bates E, Takeshita F, *et al.* TLR9 expression and function is abolished by the cervical cancer-associated human papillomavirus type 16. J Immunol 2007; 178(5): 3186-97.
[http://dx.doi.org/10.4049/jimmunol.178.5.3186] [PMID: 17312167]

[36] DeCarlo CA, Severini A, Edler L, *et al.* IFN-κ, a novel type I IFN, is undetectable in HPV-positive human cervical keratinocytes. Lab Invest 2010; 90(10): 1482-91.
[http://dx.doi.org/10.1038/labinvest.2010.95] [PMID: 20479716]

[37] Rincon-Orozco B, Halec G, Rosenberger S, *et al.* Epigenetic silencing of interferon-κ in human papillomavirus type 16-positive cells. Cancer Res 2009; 69(22): 8718-25.
[http://dx.doi.org/10.1158/0008-5472.CAN-09-0550] [PMID: 19887612]

[38] Zhu J, Mohan C. Toll-like receptor signaling pathways-therapeutic opportunities. Mediators of Inflammation 2010; 2010: 1-7.

[39] So EY, Ouchi T. The application of Toll like receptors for cancer therapy. Int J Biol Sci 2010; 6(7): 675-81.
[http://dx.doi.org/10.7150/ijbs.6.675] [PMID: 21060729]

[40] Hacke K, Rincon-Orozco B, Buchwalter G, *et al.* Regulation of MCP-1 chemokine transcription by p53. Mol Cancer 2010; 9: 82.
[http://dx.doi.org/10.1186/1476-4598-9-82] [PMID: 20406462]

[41] Guess JC, McCance DJ. Decreased migration of Langerhans precursor-like cells in response to human keratinocytes expressing human papillomavirus type 16 E6/E7 is related to reduced macrophage inflammatory protein-3α production. J Virol 2005; 79(23): 14852-62.
[http://dx.doi.org/10.1128/JVI.79.23.14852-14862.2005] [PMID: 16282485]

[42] Martinez FO, Helming L, Gordon S. Alternative activation of macrophages: an immunologic functional perspective. Annu Rev Immunol 2009; 27: 451-83.
[http://dx.doi.org/10.1146/annurev.immunol.021908.132532] [PMID: 19105661]

[43] Mazibrada J, Rittà M, Mondini M, *et al.* Interaction between inflammation and angiogenesis during different stages of cervical carcinogenesis. Gynecol Oncol 2008; 108(1): 112-20.
[http://dx.doi.org/10.1016/j.ygyno.2007.08.095] [PMID: 17936343]

[44] Quatromoni JG, Eruslanov E. Tumor-associated macrophages: function, phenotype, and link to prognosis in human lung cancer. Am J Transl Res 2012; 4(4): 376-89.
[PMID: 23145206]

[45] Tang X, Mo C, Wang Y, Wei D, Xiao H. Anti-tumour strategies aiming to target tumour-associated macrophages. Immunology 2013; 138(2): 93-104.
[http://dx.doi.org/10.1111/imm.12023] [PMID: 23113570]

[46] Hammes LS, Tekmal RR, Naud P, *et al.* Macrophages, inflammation and risk of cervical intraepithelial neoplasia (CIN) progression--clinicopathological correlation. Gynecol Oncol 2007; 105(1): 157-65.
[http://dx.doi.org/10.1016/j.ygyno.2006.11.023] [PMID: 17229459]

[47] Lepique AP, Daghastanli KR, Cuccovia IM, Villa LL. HPV16 tumor associated macrophages suppress

antitumor T cell responses. Clin Cancer Res 2009; 15(13): 4391-400.
[http://dx.doi.org/10.1158/1078-0432.CCR-09-0489] [PMID: 19549768]

[48] Bolpetti A, Silva JS, Villa LL, Lepique AP. Interleukin-10 production by tumor infiltrating macrophages plays a role in Human Papillomavirus 16 tumor growth. BMC Immunol 2010; 11: 27.
[http://dx.doi.org/10.1186/1471-2172-11-27] [PMID: 20525400]

[49] Garcia-Iglesias T, Del Toro-Arreola A, Albarran-Somoza B, *et al.* Low NKp30, NKp46 and NKG2D expression and reduced cytotoxic activity on NK cells in cervical cancer and precursor lesions. BMC Cancer 2009; 9: 186.
[http://dx.doi.org/10.1186/1471-2407-9-186] [PMID: 19531227]

[50] Bontkes HJ, Ruizendaal JJ, Kramer D, Meijer CJ, Hooijberg E. Plasmacytoid dendritic cells are present in cervical carcinoma and become activated by human papillomavirus type 16 virus-like particles. Gynecol Oncol 2005; 96(3): 897-901.
[http://dx.doi.org/10.1016/j.ygyno.2004.10.040] [PMID: 15721448]

[51] Lenz P, Lowy DR, Schiller JT. Papillomavirus virus-like particles induce cytokines characteristic of innate immune responses in plasmacytoid dendritic cells. Eur J Immunol 2005; 35(5): 1548-56.
[http://dx.doi.org/10.1002/eji.200425547] [PMID: 15832296]

[52] Yang R, Murillo FM, Cui H, *et al.* Papillomavirus-like particles stimulate murine bone marrow-derived dendritic cells to produce alpha interferon and Th1 immune responses via MyD88. J Virol 2004; 78(20): 11152-60.
[http://dx.doi.org/10.1128/JVI.78.20.11152-11160.2004] [PMID: 15452235]

[53] Orange JS. Natural killer cell deficiency. J Allergy Clin Immunol 2013; 132(3): 515-25.
[http://dx.doi.org/10.1016/j.jaci.2013.07.020] [PMID: 23993353]

[54] Mosmann TR, Cherwinski H, Bond MW, Giedlin MA, Coffman RL. Two types of murine helper T cell clone. I. Definition according to profiles of lymphokine activities and secreted proteins. J Immunol 1986; 136(7): 2348-57.
[PMID: 2419430]

[55] Zhu J, Paul WE. CD4 T cells: fates, functions, and faults. Blood 2008; 112(5): 1557-69.
[http://dx.doi.org/10.1182/blood-2008-05-078154] [PMID: 18725574]

[56] Steele JC, Mann CH, Rookes S, *et al.* T-cell responses to human papillomavirus type 16 among women with different grades of cervical neoplasia. Br J Cancer 2005; 93(2): 248-59.
[http://dx.doi.org/10.1038/sj.bjc.6602679] [PMID: 15986031]

[57] Woo YL, Sterling J, Damay I, *et al.* Characterising the local immune responses in cervical intraepithelial neoplasia: a cross-sectional and longitudinal analysis. BJOG 2008; 115(13): 1616-21.
[http://dx.doi.org/10.1111/j.1471-0528.2008.01936.x] [PMID: 19035938]

[58] Clerici M, Merola M, Ferrario E, *et al.* Cytokine production patterns in cervical intraepithelial neoplasia: association with human papillomavirus infection. J Natl Cancer Inst 1997; 89(3): 245-50.
[http://dx.doi.org/10.1093/jnci/89.3.245] [PMID: 9017005]

[59] Peghini BC, Abdalla DR, Barcelos AC, Teodoro Ld, Murta EF, Michelin MA. Local cytokine profiles of patients with cervical intraepithelial and invasive neoplasia. Hum Immunol 2012; 73(9): 920-6.
[http://dx.doi.org/10.1016/j.humimm.2012.06.003] [PMID: 22749886]

[60] Kobayashi A, Weinberg V, Darragh T, Smith-McCune K. Evolving immunosuppressive microenvironment during human cervical carcinogenesis. Mucosal Immunol 2008; 1(5): 412-20.
[http://dx.doi.org/10.1038/mi.2008.33] [PMID: 19079205]

[61] Chirgwin KD, Feldman J, Augenbraun M, Landesman S, Minkoff H. Incidence of venereal warts in human immunodeficiency virus-infected and uninfected women. J Infect Dis 1995; 172(1): 235-8.
[http://dx.doi.org/10.1093/infdis/172.1.235] [PMID: 7797919]

[62] Fruchter RG, Maiman M, Arrastia CD, Matthews R, Gates EJ, Holcomb K. Is HIV infection a risk factor for advanced cervical cancer? J Acquir Immune Defic Syndr Hum Retrovirol 1998; 18(3): 241-

5.
[http://dx.doi.org/10.1097/00042560-199807010-00007] [PMID: 9665501]

[63] Scott M, Nakagawa M, Moscicki AB. Cell-mediated immune response to human papillomavirus infection. Clin Diagn Lab Immunol 2001; 8(2): 209-20.
[PMID: 11238198]

[64] Vambutas A, DeVoti J, Pinn W, Steinberg BM, Bonagura VR. Interaction of human papillomavirus type 11 E7 protein with TAP-1 results in the reduction of ATP-dependent peptide transport. Clin Immunol 2001; 101(1): 94-9.
[http://dx.doi.org/10.1006/clim.2001.5094] [PMID: 11580231]

[65] Keating PJ, Cromme FV, Duggan-Keen M, *et al.* Frequency of down-regulation of individual HLA-A and -B alleles in cervical carcinomas in relation to TAP-1 expression. Br J Cancer 1995; 72(2): 405-11.
[http://dx.doi.org/10.1038/bjc.1995.346] [PMID: 7640226]

[66] Campo MS, Graham SV, Cortese MS, *et al.* HPV-16 E5 down-regulates expression of surface HLA class I and reduces recognition by CD8 T cells. Virology 2010; 407(1): 137-42.
[http://dx.doi.org/10.1016/j.virol.2010.07.044] [PMID: 20813390]

[67] Correll A, Tuettenberg A, Becker C, Jonuleit H. Increased regulatory T-cell frequencies in patients with advanced melanoma correlate with a generally impaired T-cell responsiveness and are restored after dendritic cell-based vaccination. Exp Dermatol 2010; 19(8): e213-21.
[http://dx.doi.org/10.1111/j.1600-0625.2009.01055.x] [PMID: 20500773]

[68] French JD, Weber ZJ, Fretwell DL, Said S, Klopper JP, Haugen BR. Tumor-associated lymphocytes and increased FoxP3+ regulatory T cell frequency correlate with more aggressive papillary thyroid cancer. J Clin Endocrinol Metab 2010; 95(5): 2325-33.
[http://dx.doi.org/10.1210/jc.2009-2564] [PMID: 20207826]

[69] Fu J, Xu D, Liu Z, *et al.* Increased regulatory T cells correlate with CD8 T-cell impairment and poor survival in hepatocellular carcinoma patients. Gastroenterology 2007; 132(7): 2328-39.
[http://dx.doi.org/10.1053/j.gastro.2007.03.102] [PMID: 17570208]

[70] Oderup C, Cederbom L, Makowska A, Cilio CM, Ivars F. Cytotoxic T lymphocyte antigen-4-dependent down-modulation of costimulatory molecules on dendritic cells in CD4+ CD25+ regulatory T-cell-mediated suppression. Immunology 2006; 118(2): 240-9.
[http://dx.doi.org/10.1111/j.1365-2567.2006.02362.x] [PMID: 16771859]

[71] Nakamura K, Kitani A, Strober W. Cell contact-dependent immunosuppression by CD4(+)CD25(+) regulatory T cells is mediated by cell surface-bound transforming growth factor β. J Exp Med 2001; 194(5): 629-44.
[http://dx.doi.org/10.1084/jem.194.5.629] [PMID: 11535631]

[72] Collison LW, Workman CJ, Kuo TT, *et al.* The inhibitory cytokine IL-35 contributes to regulatory T-cell function. Nature 2007; 450(7169): 566-9.
[http://dx.doi.org/10.1038/nature06306] [PMID: 18033300]

[73] Garín MI, Chu CC, Golshayan D, Cernuda-Morollón E, Wait R, Lechler RI. Galectin-1: a key effector of regulation mediated by CD4+CD25+ T cells. Blood 2007; 109(5): 2058-65.
[http://dx.doi.org/10.1182/blood-2006-04-016451] [PMID: 17110462]

[74] Lee SS, Gao W, Mazzola S, *et al.* Heme oxygenase-1, carbon monoxide, and bilirubin induce tolerance in recipients toward islet allografts by modulating T regulatory cells. FASEB J 2007; 21(13): 3450-7.
[http://dx.doi.org/10.1096/fj.07-8472com] [PMID: 17551098]

[75] Mocellin S, Marincola FM, Young HA. Interleukin-10 and the immune response against cancer: a counterpoint. J Leukoc Biol 2005; 78(5): 1043-51.
[http://dx.doi.org/10.1189/jlb.0705358] [PMID: 16204623]

[76] Christensen ND, Höpfl R, DiAngelo SL, *et al.* Assembled baculovirus-expressed human papillomavirus type 11 L1 capsid protein virus-like particles are recognized by neutralizing monoclonal antibodies and induce high titres of neutralizing antibodies. J Gen Virol 1994; 75(Pt 9): 2271-6.
[http://dx.doi.org/10.1099/0022-1317-75-9-2271] [PMID: 7521393]

[77] Kirnbauer R, Booy F, Cheng N, Lowy DR, Schiller JT. Papillomavirus L1 major capsid protein self-assembles into virus-like particles that are highly immunogenic. Proc Natl Acad Sci USA 1992; 89(24): 12180-4.
[http://dx.doi.org/10.1073/pnas.89.24.12180] [PMID: 1334560]

[78] Kirnbauer R, Hubbert NL, Wheeler CM, Becker TM, Lowy DR, Schiller JT. A virus-like particle enzyme-linked immunosorbent assay detects serum antibodies in a majority of women infected with human papillomavirus type 16. J Natl Cancer Inst 1994; 86(7): 494-9.
[http://dx.doi.org/10.1093/jnci/86.7.494] [PMID: 8133532]

[79] Viscidi RP, Schiffman M, Hildesheim A, *et al.* Seroreactivity to human papillomavirus (HPV) types 16, 18, or 31 and risk of subsequent HPV infection: results from a population-based study in Costa Rica. Cancer Epidemiol Biomarkers Prev 2004; 13(2): 324-7.
[http://dx.doi.org/10.1158/1055-9965.EPI-03-0166] [PMID: 14973086]

[80] Galloway DA. Papillomavirus vaccines in clinical trials. Lancet Infect Dis 2003; 3(8): 469-75.
[http://dx.doi.org/10.1016/S1473-3099(03)00720-5] [PMID: 12901889]

[81] af Geijersstam V, Kibur M, Wang Z, *et al.* Stability over time of serum antibody levels to human papillomavirus type 16. J Infect Dis 1998; 177(6): 1710-4.
[http://dx.doi.org/10.1086/517428] [PMID: 9607854]

[82] Andersson K, Waterboer T, Kirnbauer R, *et al.* Seroreactivity to cutaneous human papillomaviruses among patients with nonmelanoma skin cancer or benign skin lesions. Cancer Epidemiol Biomarkers Prev 2008; 17(1): 189-95.
[http://dx.doi.org/10.1158/1055-9965.EPI-07-0405] [PMID: 18199724]

[83] Rosales R, López-Contreras M, Cortes RR. Antibodies against human papillomavirus (HPV) type 16 and 18 E2, E6 and E7 proteins in sera: correlation with presence of papillomavirus DNA. J Med Virol 2001; 65(4): 736-44.
[http://dx.doi.org/10.1002/jmv.2098] [PMID: 11745939]

[84] Jochmus-Kudielka I, Schneider A, Braun R, *et al.* Antibodies against the human papillomavirus type 16 early proteins in human sera: correlation of anti-E7 reactivity with cervical cancer. J Natl Cancer Inst 1989; 81(22): 1698-704.
[http://dx.doi.org/10.1093/jnci/81.22.1698] [PMID: 2553991]

[85] Müller M, Gausepohl H, de Martynoff G, Frank R, Brasseur R, Gissmann L. Identification of seroreactive regions of the human papillomavirus type 16 protein E4, E6, E7 and L1. J Gen Virol 1990; 71(Pt 11): 2709-17.
[http://dx.doi.org/10.1099/0022-1317-71-11-2709] [PMID: 1701482]

[86] Köchel HG, Monazahian M, Sievert K, *et al.* Occurrence of antibodies to L1, L2, E4 and E7 gene products of human papillomavirus types 6b, 16 and 18 among cervical cancer patients and controls. Int J Cancer 1991; 48(5): 682-8.
[http://dx.doi.org/10.1002/ijc.2910480509] [PMID: 1649138]

[87] Bolhassani A, Zahedifard F, Taslimi Y, Taghikhani M, Nahavandian B, Rafati S. Antibody detection against HPV16 E7 & GP96 fragments as biomarkers in cervical cancer patients. Indian J Med Res 2009; 130(5): 533-41.
[PMID: 20090101]

[88] Carter JJ, Koutsky LA, Hughes JP, *et al.* Comparison of human papillomavirus types 16, 18, and 6 capsid antibody responses following incident infection. J Infect Dis 2000; 181(6): 1911-9.
[http://dx.doi.org/10.1086/315498] [PMID: 10837170]

[89] Fausch SC, Da Silva DM, Rudolf MP, Kast WM. Human papillomavirus virus-like particles do not activate Langerhans cells: a possible immune escape mechanism used by human papillomaviruses. J Immunol 2002; 169(6): 3242-9.
[http://dx.doi.org/10.4049/jimmunol.169.6.3242] [PMID: 12218143]

[90] Da Silva DM, Fausch SC, Verbeek JS, Kast WM. Uptake of human papillomavirus virus-like particles by dendritic cells is mediated by Fcgamma receptors and contributes to acquisition of T cell immunity. J Immunol 2007; 178(12): 7587-97.
[http://dx.doi.org/10.4049/jimmunol.178.12.7587] [PMID: 17548594]

[91] Le Bon A, Tough DF. Links between innate and adaptive immunity via type I interferon. Curr Opin Immunol 2002; 14(4): 432-6.
[http://dx.doi.org/10.1016/S0952-7915(02)00354-0] [PMID: 12088676]

[92] Chang YE, Laimins LA. Microarray analysis identifies interferon-inducible genes and Stat-1 as major transcriptional targets of human papillomavirus type 31. J Virol 2000; 74(9): 4174-82.
[http://dx.doi.org/10.1128/JVI.74.9.4174-4182.2000] [PMID: 10756030]

[93] Nees M, Geoghegan JM, Hyman T, Frank S, Miller L, Woodworth CD. Papillomavirus type 16 oncogenes downregulate expression of interferon-responsive genes and upregulate proliferation-associated and NF-kappaB-responsive genes in cervical keratinocytes. J Virol 2001; 75(9): 4283-96.
[http://dx.doi.org/10.1128/JVI.75.9.4283-4296.2001] [PMID: 11287578]

[94] Coleman N, Birley HD, Renton AM, *et al.* Immunological events in regressing genital warts. Am J Clin Pathol 1994; 102(6): 768-74.
[http://dx.doi.org/10.1093/ajcp/102.6.768] [PMID: 7801889]

[95] de Jong A, van der Burg SH, Kwappenberg KM, *et al.* Frequent detection of human papillomavirus 16 E2-specific T-helper immunity in healthy subjects. Cancer Res 2002; 62(2): 472-9.
[PMID: 11809698]

[96] Welters MJ, de Jong A, van den Eeden SJ, *et al.* Frequent display of human papillomavirus type 16 E6-specific memory t-Helper cells in the healthy population as witness of previous viral encounter. Cancer Res 2003; 63(3): 636-41.
[PMID: 12566307]

[97] Nicholls PK, Moore PF, Anderson DM, *et al.* Regression of canine oral papillomas is associated with infiltration of $CD4^+$ and $CD8^+$ lymphocytes. Virology 2001; 283(1): 31-9.
[http://dx.doi.org/10.1006/viro.2000.0789] [PMID: 11312659]

[98] Carter JJ, Wipf GC, Hagensee ME, *et al.* Use of human papillomavirus type 6 capsids to detect antibodies in people with genital warts. J Infect Dis 1995; 172(1): 11-8.
[http://dx.doi.org/10.1093/infdis/172.1.11] [PMID: 7797899]

[99] Carter JJ, Koutsky LA, Wipf GC, *et al.* The natural history of human papillomavirus type 16 capsid antibodies among a cohort of university women. J Infect Dis 1996; 174(5): 927-36.
[http://dx.doi.org/10.1093/infdis/174.5.927] [PMID: 8896492]

[100] Dillner J. The serological response to papillomaviruses. Semin Cancer Biol 1999; 9(6): 423-30.
[http://dx.doi.org/10.1006/scbi.1999.0146] [PMID: 10712889]

[101] Pett M, Coleman N. Integration of high-risk human papillomavirus: a key event in cervical carcinogenesis? J Pathol 2007; 212(4): 356-67.
[http://dx.doi.org/10.1002/path.2192] [PMID: 17573670]

[102] Pett MR, Herdman MT, Palmer RD, *et al.* Selection of cervical keratinocytes containing integrated HPV16 associates with episome loss and an endogenous antiviral response. Proc Natl Acad Sci USA 2006; 103(10): 3822-7.
[http://dx.doi.org/10.1073/pnas.0600078103] [PMID: 16505361]

[103] de Jong A, van Poelgeest MI, van der Hulst JM, *et al.* Human papillomavirus type 16-positive cervical cancer is associated with impaired CD4+ T-cell immunity against early antigens E2 and E6. Cancer

Res 2004; 64(15): 5449-55.
[http://dx.doi.org/10.1158/0008-5472.CAN-04-0831] [PMID: 15289354]

[104] Kobayashi A, Greenblatt RM, Anastos K, *et al.* Functional attributes of mucosal immunity in cervical intraepithelial neoplasia and effects of HIV infection. Cancer Res 2004; 64(18): 6766-74.
[http://dx.doi.org/10.1158/0008-5472.CAN-04-1091] [PMID: 15374995]

[105] Hochedlinger K, Plath K. Epigenetic reprogramming and induced pluripotency. Development 2009; 136(4): 509-23.
[http://dx.doi.org/10.1242/dev.020867] [PMID: 19168672]

[106] Kim KC, Friso S, Choi SW. DNA methylation, an epigenetic mechanism connecting folate to healthy embryonic development and aging. J Nutr Biochem 2009; 20(12): 917-26.
[http://dx.doi.org/10.1016/j.jnutbio.2009.06.008] [PMID: 19733471]

[107] Robertson KD. DNA methylation and human disease. Nat Rev Genet 2005; 6(8): 597-610.
[http://dx.doi.org/10.1038/nrg1655] [PMID: 16136652]

[108] Shalginskikh N, Poleshko A, Skalka AM, Katz RA. Retroviral DNA methylation and epigenetic repression are mediated by the antiviral host protein Daxx. J Virol 2013; 87(4): 2137-50.
[http://dx.doi.org/10.1128/JVI.02026-12] [PMID: 23221555]

[109] Waterhouse PM, Wang MB, Lough T. Gene silencing as an adaptive defence against viruses. Nature 2001; 411(6839): 834-42.
[http://dx.doi.org/10.1038/35081168] [PMID: 11459066]

[110] Badal V, Chuang LS, Tan EH, *et al.* CpG methylation of human papillomavirus type 16 DNA in cervical cancer cell lines and in clinical specimens: genomic hypomethylation correlates with carcinogenic progression. J Virol 2003; 77(11): 6227-34.
[http://dx.doi.org/10.1128/JVI.77.11.6227-6234.2003] [PMID: 12743279]

[111] Kalantari M, Calleja-Macias IE, Tewari D, *et al.* Conserved methylation patterns of human papillomavirus type 16 DNA in asymptomatic infection and cervical neoplasia. J Virol 2004; 78(23): 12762-72.
[http://dx.doi.org/10.1128/JVI.78.23.12762-12772.2004] [PMID: 15542628]

[112] Liu X, Wang Y, Wang X, *et al.* Epigenetic silencing of WNT5A in Epstein-Barr virus-associated gastric carcinoma. Arch Virol 2013; 158(1): 123-32.
[http://dx.doi.org/10.1007/s00705-012-1481-x] [PMID: 23001722]

[113] Hino R, Uozaki H, Murakami N, *et al.* Activation of DNA methyltransferase 1 by EBV latent membrane protein 2A leads to promoter hypermethylation of PTEN gene in gastric carcinoma. Cancer Res 2009; 69(7): 2766-74.
[http://dx.doi.org/10.1158/0008-5472.CAN-08-3070] [PMID: 19339266]

[114] Silmon de Monerri NC, Kim K. Pathogens hijack the epigenome: a new twist on host-pathogen interactions. Am J Pathol 2014; 184(4): 897-911.
[http://dx.doi.org/10.1016/j.ajpath.2013.12.022] [PMID: 24525150]

[115] Burgers WA, Blanchon L, Pradhan S, de Launoit Y, Kouzarides T, Fuks F. Viral oncoproteins target the DNA methyltransferases. Oncogene 2007; 26(11): 1650-5.
[http://dx.doi.org/10.1038/sj.onc.1209950] [PMID: 16983344]

[116] Cicchini L, Westrich JA, Xu T, *et al.* Suppression of antitumor immune responses by human papillomavirus through epigenetic down-regulation of CXCL14. MBio 2016; 7(3): e00270-16.
[http://dx.doi.org/10.1128/mBio.00270-16] [PMID: 27143385]

[117] Schaerli P, Willimann K, Ebert LM, Walz A, Moser B. Cutaneous CXCL14 targets blood precursors to epidermal niches for Langerhans cell differentiation. Immunity 2005; 23(3): 331-42.
[http://dx.doi.org/10.1016/j.immuni.2005.08.012] [PMID: 16169505]

[118] Shurin GV, Ferris RL, Tourkova IL, *et al.* Loss of new chemokine CXCL14 in tumor tissue is associated with low infiltration by dendritic cells (DC), while restoration of human CXCL14

expression in tumor cells causes attraction of DC both *in vitro* and *in vivo*. J Immunol 2005; 174(9): 5490-8.
[http://dx.doi.org/10.4049/jimmunol.174.9.5490] [PMID: 15843547]

[119] Tindle RW, Herd K, Doan T, *et al.* Nonspecific down-regulation of CD8+ T-cell responses in mice expressing human papillomavirus type 16 E7 oncoprotein from the keratin-14 promoter. J Virol 2001; 75(13): 5985-97.
[http://dx.doi.org/10.1128/JVI.75.13.5985-5997.2001] [PMID: 11390600]

[120] Doan T, Herd K, Street M, *et al.* Human papillomavirus type 16 E7 oncoprotein expressed in peripheral epithelium tolerizes E7-directed cytotoxic T-lymphocyte precursors restricted through human (and mouse) major histocompatibility complex class I alleles. J Virol 1999; 73(7): 6166-70.
[PMID: 10364377]

[121] Abd Warif NM, Stoitzner P, Leggatt GR, Mattarollo SR, Frazer IH, Hibma MH. Langerhans cell homeostasis and activation is altered in hyperplastic human papillomavirus type 16 E7 expressing epidermis. PLoS One 2015; 10(5): e0127155.
[http://dx.doi.org/10.1371/journal.pone.0127155] [PMID: 25992642]

[122] Narayan S, Choyce A, Linedale R, *et al.* Epithelial expression of human papillomavirus type 16 E7 protein results in peripheral CD8 T-cell suppression mediated by CD4+CD25+ T cells. Eur J Immunol 2009; 39(2): 481-90.
[http://dx.doi.org/10.1002/eji.200838527] [PMID: 19180468]

[123] Kouzarides T. Chromatin modifications and their function. Cell 2007; 128(4): 693-705.
[http://dx.doi.org/10.1016/j.cell.2007.02.005] [PMID: 17320507]

[124] McLaughlin-Drubin ME, Huh KW, Münger K. Human papillomavirus type 16 E7 oncoprotein associates with E2F6. J Virol 2008; 82(17): 8695-705.
[http://dx.doi.org/10.1128/JVI.00579-08] [PMID: 18579589]

[125] McLaughlin-Drubin ME, Crum CP, Münger K. Human papillomavirus E7 oncoprotein induces KDM6A and KDM6B histone demethylase expression and causes epigenetic reprogramming. Proc Natl Acad Sci USA 2011; 108(5): 2130-5.
[http://dx.doi.org/10.1073/pnas.1009933108] [PMID: 21245294]

[126] Pacini L, Savini C, Ghittoni R, *et al.* Down-regulation of toll-like receptor 9 expression by beta human papillomavirus 38 and implications for cell cycle control. J Virol 2015; 89(22): 11396-405.
[http://dx.doi.org/10.1128/JVI.02151-15] [PMID: 26339055]

[127] Hasan UA, Zannetti C, Parroche P, *et al.* The human papillomavirus type 16 E7 oncoprotein induces a transcriptional repressor complex on the Toll-like receptor 9 promoter. J Exp Med 2013; 210(7): 1369-87.
[http://dx.doi.org/10.1084/jem.20122394] [PMID: 23752229]

[128] Park JS, Kim EJ, Kwon HJ, Hwang ES, Namkoong SE, Um SJ. Inactivation of interferon regulatory factor-1 tumor suppressor protein by HPV E7 oncoprotein. Implication for the E7-mediated immune evasion mechanism in cervical carcinogenesis. J Biol Chem 2000; 275(10): 6764-9.
[http://dx.doi.org/10.1074/jbc.275.10.6764] [PMID: 10702232]

[129] Um SJ, Rhyu JW, Kim EJ, Jeon KC, Hwang ES, Park JS. Abrogation of IRF-1 response by high-risk HPV E7 protein *in vivo*. Cancer Lett 2002; 179(2): 205-12.
[http://dx.doi.org/10.1016/S0304-3835(01)00871-0] [PMID: 11888675]

[130] Georgopoulos NT, Proffitt JL, Blair GE. Transcriptional regulation of the major histocompatibility complex (MHC) class I heavy chain, TAP1 and LMP2 genes by the human papillomavirus (HPV) type 6b, 16 and 18 E7 oncoproteins. Oncogene 2000; 19(42): 4930-5.
[http://dx.doi.org/10.1038/sj.onc.1203860] [PMID: 11039910]

[131] Lee SY, Huang Z, Kang TH, *et al.* Histone deacetylase inhibitor AR-42 enhances E7-specific $CD8^+$ T cell-mediated antitumor immunity induced by therapeutic HPV DNA vaccination. J Mol Med (Berl) 2013; 91(10): 1221-31.

[http://dx.doi.org/10.1007/s00109-013-1054-9] [PMID: 23715898]

[132] Lee MS, Kim YJ. Signaling pathways downstream of pattern-recognition receptors and their cross talk. Annu Rev Biochem 2007; 76: 447-80. [http://dx.doi.org/10.1146/annurev.biochem.76.060605.122847] [PMID: 17328678]

[133] Ghosh S, May MJ, Kopp EB. NF-κ B and Rel proteins: evolutionarily conserved mediators of immune responses. Annu Rev Immunol 1998; 16: 225-60. [http://dx.doi.org/10.1146/annurev.immunol.16.1.225] [PMID: 9597130]

[134] Brady G, Bowie AG. Innate immune activation of NFκB and its antagonism by poxviruses. Cytokine Growth Factor Rev 2014; 25(5): 611-20. [http://dx.doi.org/10.1016/j.cytogfr.2014.07.004] [PMID: 25081317]

[135] Correia S, Ventura S, Parkhouse RM. Identification and utility of innate immune system evasion mechanisms of ASFV. Virus Res 2013; 173(1): 87-100. [http://dx.doi.org/10.1016/j.virusres.2012.10.013] [PMID: 23165138]

[136] Qu L, Lemon SM. Hepatitis A and hepatitis C viruses: divergent infection outcomes marked by similarities in induction and evasion of interferon responses. Semin Liver Dis 2010; 30(4): 319-32. [http://dx.doi.org/10.1055/s-0030-1267534] [PMID: 20960373]

[137] Vandermark ER, Deluca KA, Gardner CR, *et al.* Human papillomavirus type 16 E6 and E 7 proteins alter NF-kB in cultured cervical epithelial cells and inhibition of NF-kB promotes cell growth and immortalization. Virology 2012; 425(1): 53-60. [http://dx.doi.org/10.1016/j.virol.2011.12.023] [PMID: 22284893]

[138] Tummers B, Goedemans R, Pelascini LP, *et al.* The interferon-related developmental regulator 1 is used by human papillomavirus to suppress NFκB activation. Nat Commun 2015; 6: 6537. [http://dx.doi.org/10.1038/ncomms7537] [PMID: 26055519]

[139] Richards KH, Wasson CW, Watherston O, *et al.* The human papillomavirus (HPV) E7 protein antagonises an Imiquimod-induced inflammatory pathway in primary human keratinocytes. Sci Rep 2015; 5: 12922. [http://dx.doi.org/10.1038/srep12922] [PMID: 26268216]

[140] Huang SM, McCance DJ. Down regulation of the interleukin-8 promoter by human papillomavirus type 16 E6 and E7 through effects on CREB binding protein/p300 and P/CAF. J Virol 2002; 76(17): 8710-21. [http://dx.doi.org/10.1128/JVI.76.17.8710-8721.2002] [PMID: 12163591]

[141] Roman A, Munger K. The papillomavirus E7 proteins. Virology 2013; 445(1-2): 138-68. [http://dx.doi.org/10.1016/j.virol.2013.04.013] [PMID: 23731972]

[142] Vande Pol SB, Klingelhutz AJ. Papillomavirus E6 oncoproteins. Virology 2013; 445(1-2): 115-37. [http://dx.doi.org/10.1016/j.virol.2013.04.026] [PMID: 23711382]

[143] Li S, Labrecque S, Gauzzi MC, *et al.* The human papilloma virus (HPV)-18 E6 oncoprotein physically associates with Tyk2 and impairs Jak-STAT activation by interferon-alpha. Oncogene 1999; 18(42): 5727-37. [http://dx.doi.org/10.1038/sj.onc.1202960] [PMID: 10523853]

[144] Ronco LV, Karpova AY, Vidal M, Howley PM. Human papillomavirus 16 E6 oncoprotein binds to interferon regulatory factor-3 and inhibits its transcriptional activity. Genes Dev 1998; 12(13): 2061-72. [http://dx.doi.org/10.1101/gad.12.13.2061] [PMID: 9649509]

[145] Haller O, Kochs G, Weber F. The interferon response circuit: induction and suppression by pathogenic viruses. Virology 2006; 344(1): 119-30. [http://dx.doi.org/10.1016/j.virol.2005.09.024] [PMID: 16364743]

[146] Cai X, Chiu YH, Chen ZJ. The cGAS-cGAMP-STING pathway of cytosolic DNA sensing and signaling. Mol Cell 2014; 54(2): 289-96.

[http://dx.doi.org/10.1016/j.molcel.2014.03.040] [PMID: 24766893]

[147] Sun L, Wu J, Du F, Chen X, Chen ZJ. Cyclic GMP-AMP synthase is a cytosolic DNA sensor that activates the type I interferon pathway. Science 2013; 339(6121): 786-91. [http://dx.doi.org/10.1126/science.1232458] [PMID: 23258413]

[148] Lau L, Gray EE, Brunette RL, Stetson DB. DNA tumor virus oncogenes antagonize the cGAS-STING DNA-sensing pathway. Science 2015; 350(6260): 568-71. [http://dx.doi.org/10.1126/science.aab3291] [PMID: 26405230]

[149] Perea SE, Massimi P, Banks L. Human papillomavirus type 16 E7 impairs the activation of the interferon regulatory factor-1. Int J Mol Med 2000; 5(6): 661-6. [PMID: 10812019]

[150] Antonsson A, Payne E, Hengst K, McMillan NA. The human papillomavirus type 16 E7 protein binds human interferon regulatory factor-9 via a novel PEST domain required for transformation. J Interferon Cytokine Res 2006; 26(7): 455-61. [http://dx.doi.org/10.1089/jir.2006.26.455] [PMID: 16800784]

[151] Howley PM. Warts, cancer and ubiquitylation: lessons from the papillomaviruses. Trans Am Clin Climatol Assoc 2006; 117: 113-26. [PMID: 18528468]

[152] Karim R, Tummers B, Meyers C, *et al.* Human papillomavirus (HPV) upregulates the cellular deubiquitinase UCHL1 to suppress the keratinocyte's innate immune response. PLoS Pathog 2013; 9(5): e1003384. [http://dx.doi.org/10.1371/journal.ppat.1003384] [PMID: 23717208]

[153] Niebler M, Qian X, Höfler D, *et al.* Post-translational control of IL-1β via the human papillomavirus type 16 E6 oncoprotein: a novel mechanism of innate immune escape mediated by the E3-ubiquitin ligase E6-AP and p53. PLoS Pathog 2013; 9(8): e1003536. [http://dx.doi.org/10.1371/journal.ppat.1003536] [PMID: 23935506]

[154] Gram AM, Frenkel J, Ressing ME. Inflammasomes and viruses: cellular defence *versus* viral offence. J Gen Virol 2012; 93(Pt 10): 2063-75. [http://dx.doi.org/10.1099/vir.0.042978-0] [PMID: 22739062]

[155] Poeck H, Ruland J. From virus to inflammation: mechanisms of RIG-I-induced IL-1β production. Eur J Cell Biol 2012; 91(1): 59-64. [http://dx.doi.org/10.1016/j.ejcb.2011.01.013] [PMID: 21481488]

[156] Wu S, Hu G, Chen J, Xie G. Interleukin 1β and interleukin 1 receptor antagonist gene polymorphisms and cervical cancer: a meta-analysis. Int J Gynecol Cancer 2014; 24(6): 984-90. [http://dx.doi.org/10.1097/IGC.0000000000000165] [PMID: 24905619]

[157] Xu J, Yin Z, Cao S, *et al.* Systematic review and meta-analysis on the association between IL-1B polymorphisms and cancer risk. PLoS One 2013; 8(5): e63654. [http://dx.doi.org/10.1371/journal.pone.0063654] [PMID: 23704929]

[158] Dutta S, Chakraborty C, Mandal RK, *et al.* Persistent HPV16/18 infection in Indian women with the A-allele (rs6457617) of HLA-DQB1 and T-allele (rs16944) of IL-1β -511 is associated with development of cervical carcinoma. Cancer Immunol Immunother 2015; 64(7): 843-51. [http://dx.doi.org/10.1007/s00262-015-1693-5] [PMID: 25893807]

[159] Blagoveshchenskaya AD, Thomas L, Feliciangeli SF, Hung CH, Thomas G. HIV-1 Nef downregulates MHC-I by a PACS-1- and PI3K-regulated ARF6 endocytic pathway. Cell 2002; 111(6): 853-66. [http://dx.doi.org/10.1016/S0092-8674(02)01162-5] [PMID: 12526811]

[160] Hewitt EW. The MHC class I antigen presentation pathway: strategies for viral immune evasion. Immunology 2003; 110(2): 163-9. [http://dx.doi.org/10.1046/j.1365-2567.2003.01738.x] [PMID: 14511229]

[161] Jackson SE, Mason GM, Wills MR. Human cytomegalovirus immunity and immune evasion. Virus

Res 2011; 157(2): 151-60.
[http://dx.doi.org/10.1016/j.virusres.2010.10.031] [PMID: 21056604]

[162] Ashrafi GH, Haghshenas M, Marchetti B, Campo MS. E5 protein of human papillomavirus 16 downregulates HLA class I and interacts with the heavy chain via its first hydrophobic domain. Int J Cancer 2006; 119(9): 2105-12.
[http://dx.doi.org/10.1002/ijc.22089] [PMID: 16823848]

[163] Ashrafi GH, Haghshenas MR, Marchetti B, O'Brien PM, Campo MS. E5 protein of human papillomavirus type 16 selectively downregulates surface HLA class I. Int J Cancer 2005; 113(2): 276-83.
[http://dx.doi.org/10.1002/ijc.20558] [PMID: 15386416]

[164] Ashrafi GH, Tsirimonaki E, Marchetti B, *et al.* Down-regulation of MHC class I by bovine papillomavirus E5 oncoproteins. Oncogene 2002; 21(2): 248-59.
[http://dx.doi.org/10.1038/sj.onc.1205008] [PMID: 11803468]

[165] DiMaio D, Petti LM. The E5 proteins. Virology 2013; 445(1-2): 99-114.
[http://dx.doi.org/10.1016/j.virol.2013.05.006] [PMID: 23731971]

[166] Donaldson JG, Williams DB. Intracellular assembly and trafficking of MHC class I molecules. Traffic 2009; 10(12): 1745-52.
[http://dx.doi.org/10.1111/j.1600-0854.2009.00979.x] [PMID: 19761542]

[167] Li W, Deng XM, Wang CX, *et al.* Down-regulation of HLA class I antigen in human papillomavirus type 16 E7 expressing HaCaT cells: correlate with TAP-1 expression. Int J Gynecol Cancer 2010; 20(2): 227-32.
[http://dx.doi.org/10.1111/IGC.0b013e3181cceec5] [PMID: 20134267]

[168] Zhang B, Li P, Wang E, *et al.* The E5 protein of human papillomavirus type 16 perturbs MHC class II antigen maturation in human foreskin keratinocytes treated with interferon-gamma. Virology 2003; 310(1): 100-8.
[http://dx.doi.org/10.1016/S0042-6822(03)00103-X] [PMID: 12788634]

[169] Miura S, Kawana K, Schust DJ, *et al.* CD1d, a sentinel molecule bridging innate and adaptive immunity, is downregulated by the human papillomavirus (HPV) E5 protein: a possible mechanism for immune evasion by HPV. J Virol 2010; 84(22): 11614-23.
[http://dx.doi.org/10.1128/JVI.01053-10] [PMID: 20810727]

[170] Brigl M, Brenner MB. CD1: antigen presentation and T cell function. Annu Rev Immunol 2004; 22: 817-90.
[http://dx.doi.org/10.1146/annurev.immunol.22.012703.104608] [PMID: 15032598]

[171] Fahey LM, Raff AB, Da Silva DM, Kast WM. A major role for the minor capsid protein of human papillomavirus type 16 in immune escape. J Immunol 2009; 183(10): 6151-6.
[http://dx.doi.org/10.4049/jimmunol.0902145] [PMID: 19864613]

[172] Lenz P, Day PM, Pang YY, *et al.* Papillomavirus-like particles induce acute activation of dendritic cells. J Immunol 2001; 166(9): 5346-55.
[http://dx.doi.org/10.4049/jimmunol.166.9.5346] [PMID: 11313370]

[173] Rudolf MP, Fausch SC, Da Silva DM, Kast WM. Human dendritic cells are activated by chimeric human papillomavirus type-16 virus-like particles and induce epitope-specific human T cell responses in vitro. J Immunol 2001; 166(10): 5917-24.
[http://dx.doi.org/10.4049/jimmunol.166.10.5917] [PMID: 11342606]

[174] Woodham AW, Raff AB, Raff LM, *et al.* Inhibition of Langerhans cell maturation by human papillomavirus type 16: a novel role for the annexin A2 heterotetramer in immune suppression. J Immunol 2014; 192(10): 4748-57.
[http://dx.doi.org/10.4049/jimmunol.1303190] [PMID: 24719459]

[175] Woodham AW, Da Silva DM, Skeate JG, *et al.* The S100A10 subunit of the annexin A2

heterotetramer facilitates L2-mediated human papillomavirus infection. PLoS One 2012; 7(8): e43519. [http://dx.doi.org/10.1371/journal.pone.0043519] [PMID: 22927980]

[176] Dziduszko A, Ozbun MA. Annexin A2 and S100A10 regulate human papillomavirus type 16 entry and intracellular trafficking in human keratinocytes. J Virol 2013; 87(13): 7502-15. [http://dx.doi.org/10.1128/JVI.00519-13] [PMID: 23637395]

[177] Sasagawa T, Takagi H, Makinoda S. Immune responses against human papillomavirus (HPV) infection and evasion of host defense in cervical cancer. J Infect Chemother 2012; 18(6): 807-15. [http://dx.doi.org/10.1007/s10156-012-0485-5] [PMID: 23117294]

CHAPTER 9

Risk Factors and Symptoms for HPV-Related Cancers

Kimia Kardani and **Azam Bolhassani***

Department of Pharmaceutical Biotechnology, School of Pharmacy, Shahid Beheshti University of Medical Sciences, Tehran, Iran

Department of Hepatitis and AIDS, Pasteur Institute of Iran, Tehran, Iran

Abstract: Up to now, the major environmental risk factors have been reported to develop cervical cancer such as smoking, parity, nutrition, and HPV infections. However, it is not clear whether the association of these environmental factors with cervical cancer leads to further sensitivity against HPV infection (*i.e.*, as cofactors to HPV infection) or they may act as independent risk factors in cervical carcinogenesis. In this chapter, the correlation of HPV infections and risk factors with various cancers will be described.

Keywords: Cancer, HPV infection, Risk factor, Symptom.

INTRODUCTION

There are several factors which contribute to facilitate HPV infection leading to the progression of cancer. Some of those factors are tobacco smoking, parity fertility, oral contraceptive use, immunosuppression, and certain dietary deficiencies [1]. Some of the studies suggested that HPV infections are highly prevalent in almost every country and at least 50 percent of sexually active women are infected with one or more types of HPV [1]. The potential risk of infection from non-penetrative sexual contact remains uncertain but there is a possible association between oral and penile contact [1]. HPV co-infection with HIV has also been identified as an established cofactor which increases the risk of cancer and HPV co-infection with *Chlamydia trachomatis* and Herpes simplex virus-2. Although, the biological factors including genetic, immunological factors and viral factors (*e.g.*, type, viral load and viral integration) are important, but their exact mechanism has not been clearly identified [1 - 3]. The studies showed that first coitus at a younger age (<15), a large number of sexual partners and/ or

* **Corresponding author Azam Bolhassani:** Department of Hepatitis and AIDS, Pasteur Institute of Iran, Tehran, Iran; Tel: 66953311-20; E-mails: A_bolhasani@pasteur.ac.ir, azam.bolhassani@yahoo.com

pregnancies, use of contraceptives, smoking and early age at marriage can be considered as the significant risk factors for HPV infection [4]. Table **1** shows some risk factors for various types of cancers.

Table 1. Risk factors for various types of cancers.

	Risk Factors	Ref.
Anal cancer	-HPV infection -HIV infection -High number of sexual partners -Anoreceptive intercourse -Chronic immunosuppression -Cigarette smoking - Cervical dysplasia or cancer	51
Cervical cancer	-HPV infection -Immunosuppression -High number of sexual partners -Sex at early age -High parity -History of abnormal Papanicolaou (Pap) test Results -Low socioeconomic class -Cigarette smoking	52
Vulvar cancer	-HPV infection -Vulvar dystrophy -Cigarette smoking -Immunosuppression	4
Penile cancer	-HPV infection -chronic inflammation -Genital hygiene -Lack of circumcision -High number of sexual partners -Having a sexual partner with CIN -History of other sexually transmitted diseases -Cigarette smoking	4
Head and neck carcinoma	-HPV infection -Alcohol drinking -Age at first intercourse -High number of sexual partners -History of sexually transmitted infections	16

Risk Factors

The risk factors for various cancer types are mentioned in below.

• Cervical Cancer

Risk factors for invasive cervical carcinoma (ICC) and pre-invasive disease include early onset of sexual activity, multiple sexual partners, increased frequency of alcohol consumption, smoking, high frequency of vaginal sex, a history of sexually transmitted diseases, early age at first pregnancy, chronic immunosuppression (*e.g.,* HIV infection), and an increase in duration of contraceptive use [4 - 15].

• Anal Cancer

Similar to cervical cancer, anal cancer may progress from a pre-invasive condition called anal squamous intraepithelial neoplasia (AIN) [5]. Most of the risk factors for development of anal cancer are associated with sexual activity [12 - 14]. The most important risk factors include HIV infection, high-risk sexual behavior and a history of other HPV-associated genital cancers [2, 5]. The increased risk of HPV-associated disease in HIV-infected populations is due to a high prevalence of HPV infections and alterations in cell-mediated immunity among individuals co-infected with HIV [16]. The studies showed that the use of anti-retroviral therapy (ART) has not decreased the incidence of anal cancer in England [17, 18].

• Head and Neck Cancer

The studies showed that HPV DNA-negative tumor cases have a significantly higher risk of head and neck carcinoma (HNC) associated with tobacco and alcohol as compared to HPV DNA-positive tumor cases. Indeed, risk factors including an HPV infection, age at first intercourse, number of sex partners and history of sexually transmitted infections lead to increase the risk of an HPV-related head and neck tumor [19].

• Penile and Vaginal Cancers

The incidence rates of penile cancer show the presence of main risk factors for the disease including chronic inflammation and persistent HPV infection. Penile cancer is typically a disease of older men, and is associated with low socioeconomic status. High grade penile intraepithelial neoplasia (PIN) can be developed to invasive cancer by the risk factors such as HPV infections [5, 20 - 22]. Risk factors for penile HPV infection include a high number of sexual partners, a sexual partner with CIN, a history of other sexually transmitted diseases, lack of circumcision, and a history of smoking [5, 23 - 25]. On the other hand, the studies indicated that women previously treated for high-grade CIN are at a four-fold increased risk of developing invasive vaginal cancer. Moreover, immunosuppression increased the risk of vaginal cancer among women with HIV and also after solid organ transplant [5, 26 - 29].

• Vulvar Cancer

Risk factors for vulvar cancer include smoking, vulvar dystrophy, HPV infection, a history of high-grade CIN, VIN, and immunodeficiency syndromes (HIV infection) [30 - 33]. The rate of VIN progression to invasive vulvar carcinoma is low [34 - 36]. Definitive surgery is the first treatment for early-stage vulvar cancer [37 - 40]. The studies indicated that the use of condom and really circumcision reduces the risk of HPV infections, and subsequently CIN and VIN in women and penile lesions in men [41 - 47].

HPV and Smoking

Cigarette smoking was found to increase the risk of CIN3 and cervical cancer among women infected with oncogenic HPVs as compared to women who do not smoke. A synergistic effect was reported between cigarette smoking and HPV16 DNA load for development of cervical cancer in Sweden women [48]. The impact of cigarette smoking has focused on humoral immune responses to HPV and on the prevalence, incidence, and persistence of HPV infections [48]. A recent *in vitro* study demonstrated that exposure of cervical cells to Benzo[*a*]pyrene, a major carcinogen in cigarette smoke, stimulates higher levels of virion synthesis in HPV-infected cells. On the other hand, the researchers showed that among smokers, the viral load did not change significantly by the intensity and duration of cigarette smoking, suggesting a low threshold for the effect of smoke on HPV DNA load [48].

Symptoms

Sign and symptoms for cervical cancer include vaginal discharge, intermenstrual, postcoital bleeding, lower abdominal pain, and bleeding after menopause having periods that are longer or heavier than usual pain during intercourse. When women are infected with this virus, never show the symptoms. But when the pre-cancerous stage occurs or changes into cancer, then the symptoms are shown [11]. When the high risk of HPV occurs, and then the DNA of HPV is mixed into host DNA, it develops into pre-cancer or cancer. For instance, oropharyngeal cancer can share symptoms such as sore throat, earaches and enlarged lymph nodes with benign conditions [49]. On the other hand, the clinical symptoms of penile carcinoma can also vary from a slight swelling or a small lump to an extensive carcinoma with peeling. Macroscopically, it may present vegetative or ulcerated lesions [50].

CONCLUDING REMARKS

Persistent infection with an oncogenic HPV in the presence of risk factors is essential to develop cervical cancer and other HPV-associated cancers. While, the majority of sexually active women are infected with HPV, only about 50% develop an effective antibody response to this natural infection. In some cases, this may not be sufficient to protect against further infections as well as antibody responses are HPV type-specific.

CONFLICT OF INTEREST

The author (editor) declares no conflict of interest, financial or otherwise.

ACKNOWLEDGEMENT

Declare none.

REFERENCES

[1] Amarakoon GU, Daulagala SW, Fathima F. An overview of human papilloma virus. WSN 2016; 53(3): 275-308.

[2] Palefsky JM, Rubin M. The epidemiology of anal human papillomavirus and related neoplasia. Obstet Gynecol Clin North Am 2009; 36(1): 187-200. [http://dx.doi.org/10.1016/j.ogc.2009.02.003] [PMID: 19344856]

[3] Bruni L. Human papillomavirus and related diseases report. L'Hospitalet de Llobregat: ICO Information Centre on HPV and Cancer 2014.

[4] Vinodhini K, Shanmughapriya S, Das BC, Natarajaseenivasan K. Prevalence and risk factors of HPV infection among women from various provinces of the world. Arch Gynecol Obstet 2012; 285(3): 771-7. [http://dx.doi.org/10.1007/s00404-011-2155-8] [PMID: 22159694]

[5] Wakeham K, Kavanagh K. The burden of HPV-associated anogenital cancers. Curr Oncol Rep 2014; 16(9): 402. [http://dx.doi.org/10.1007/s11912-014-0402-4] [PMID: 25118645]

[6] Comparison of risk factors for invasive squamous cell carcinoma and adenocarcinoma of the cervix: collaborative reanalysis of individual data on 8,097 women with squamous cell carcinoma and 1,374 women with adenocarcinoma from 12 epidemiological studies. Int J Cancer 2007; 120(4): 885-91. [http://dx.doi.org/10.1002/ijc.22357] [PMID: 17131323]

[7] Appleby P, Beral V, Berrington de González A, *et al.* Carcinoma of the cervix and tobacco smoking: collaborative reanalysis of individual data on 13,541 women with carcinoma of the cervix and 23,017 women without carcinoma of the cervix from 23 epidemiological studies. Int J Cancer 2006; 118(6): 1481-95. [http://dx.doi.org/10.1002/ijc.21493] [PMID: 16206285]

[8] Wallin KL, Wiklund F, Luostarinen T, *et al.* A population-based prospective study of *Chlamydia trachomatis* infection and cervical carcinoma. Int J Cancer 2002; 101(4): 371-4. [http://dx.doi.org/10.1002/ijc.10639] [PMID: 12209962]

[9] Palefsky JM. Cervical human papillomavirus infection and cervical intraepithelial neoplasia in women positive for human immunodeficiency virus in the era of highly active antiretroviral therapy. Curr Opin Oncol 2003; 15(5): 382-8. [http://dx.doi.org/10.1097/00001622-200309000-00007] [PMID: 12960521]

[10] Castellsagué X, Bosch FX, Muñoz N, *et al.* Male circumcision, penile human papillomavirus infection, and cervical cancer in female partners. N Engl J Med 2002; 346(15): 1105-12. [http://dx.doi.org/10.1056/NEJMoa011688] [PMID: 11948269]

[11] Kirti P. Human papillomavirus associated cervical cancer: A Review. Asian J Pharm Clin Res 2016; 9(3): 14-7.

[12] Melbye M, Sprøgel P. Aetiological parallel between anal cancer and cervical cancer. Lancet 1991; 338(8768): 657-9. [http://dx.doi.org/10.1016/0140-6736(91)91233-K] [PMID: 1679474]

[13] Frisch M, Glimelius B, van den Brule AJ, *et al.* Sexually transmitted infection as a cause of anal cancer. N Engl J Med 1997; 337(19): 1350-8. [http://dx.doi.org/10.1056/NEJM199711063371904] [PMID: 9358129]

[14] Daling JR, Weiss NS, Hislop TG, *et al.* Sexual practices, sexually transmitted diseases, and the incidence of anal cancer. N Engl J Med 1987; 317(16): 973-7. [http://dx.doi.org/10.1056/NEJM198710153171601] [PMID: 2821396]

[15] Moreno V, Bosch FX, Muñoz N, *et al.* Effect of oral contraceptives on risk of cervical cancer in women with human papillomavirus infection: the IARC multicentric case-control study. Lancet 2002; 359(9312): 1085-92. [http://dx.doi.org/10.1016/S0140-6736(02)08150-3] [PMID: 11943255]

[16] Palefsky J. Human papillomavirus and anal neoplasia. Curr HIV/AIDS Rep 2008; 5(2): 78-85. [http://dx.doi.org/10.1007/s11904-008-0013-5] [PMID: 18510893]

[17] Crum-Cianflone NF, Hullsiek KH, Marconi VC, *et al.* Anal cancers among HIV-infected persons: HAART is not slowing rising incidence. AIDS 2010; 24(4): 535-43. [http://dx.doi.org/10.1097/QAD.0b013e328331f6e2] [PMID: 19926961]

[18] Bower M, Powles T, Newsom-Davis T, *et al.* HIV-associated anal cancer: has highly active antiretroviral therapy reduced the incidence or improved the outcome? J Acquir Immune Defic Syndr 2004; 37(5): 1563-5. [http://dx.doi.org/10.1097/00126334-200412150-00004] [PMID: 15577408]

[19] Smith EM, Pawlita M, Rubenstein LM, Haugen TH, Hamsikova E, Turek LP. Risk factors and survival by HPV-16 E6 and E7 antibody status in human papillomavirus positive head and neck cancer. Int J Cancer 2010; 127(1): 111-7. [http://dx.doi.org/10.1002/ijc.25015] [PMID: 19876924]

[20] Diorio GJ, Leone AR, Spiess PE. Management of penile cancer. Urology 2016; 96: 15-21. [http://dx.doi.org/10.1016/j.urology.2015.12.041] [PMID: 26802797]

[21] Maden C, Sherman KJ, Beckmann AM, *et al.* History of circumcision, medical conditions, and sexual activity and risk of penile cancer. J Natl Cancer Inst 1993; 85(1): 19-24. [http://dx.doi.org/10.1093/jnci/85.1.19] [PMID: 8380060]

[22] Daling JR, Madeleine MM, Johnson LG, *et al.* Penile cancer: importance of circumcision, human papillomavirus and smoking in *in situ* and invasive disease. Int J Cancer 2005; 116(4): 606-16. [http://dx.doi.org/10.1002/ijc.21009] [PMID: 15825185]

[23] Lajous M, Mueller N, Cruz-Valdéz A, *et al.* Determinants of prevalence, acquisition, and persistence of human papillomavirus in healthy Mexican military men. Cancer Epidemiol Biomarkers Prev 2005; 14(7): 1710-6. [http://dx.doi.org/10.1158/1055-9965.EPI-04-0926] [PMID: 16030106]

[24] Bleeker MC, Hogewoning CJ, Van Den Brule AJ, *et al.* Penile lesions and human papillomavirus in male sexual partners of women with cervical intraepithelial neoplasia. J Am Acad Dermatol 2002; 47(3): 351-7.
[http://dx.doi.org/10.1067/mjd.2002.122198] [PMID: 12196743]

[25] Partridge JM, Hughes JP, Feng Q, *et al.* Genital human papillomavirus infection in men: incidence and risk factors in a cohort of university students. J Infect Dis 2007; 196(8): 1128-36.
[http://dx.doi.org/10.1086/521192] [PMID: 17955430]

[26] Ficarra V, Akduman B, Bouchot O, Palou J, Tobias-Machado M. Prognostic factors in penile cancer. Urology 2010; 76(2) (Suppl. 1): S66-73.
[http://dx.doi.org/10.1016/j.urology.2010.04.008] [PMID: 20691887]

[27] Strander B, Andersson-Ellström A, Milsom I, Sparén P. Long term risk of invasive cancer after treatment for cervical intraepithelial neoplasia grade 3: population based cohort study. BMJ 2007; 335(7629): 1077.
[http://dx.doi.org/10.1136/bmj.39363.471806.BE] [PMID: 17959735]

[28] Engels EA, Pfeiffer RM, Goedert JJ, *et al.* Trends in cancer risk among people with AIDS in the United States 1980-2002. AIDS 2006; 20(12): 1645-54.
[http://dx.doi.org/10.1097/01.aids.0000238411.75324.59] [PMID: 16868446]

[29] Engels EA, Pfeiffer RM, Fraumeni JF Jr, *et al.* Spectrum of cancer risk among US solid organ transplant recipients. JAMA 2011; 306(17): 1891-901.
[http://dx.doi.org/10.1001/jama.2011.1592] [PMID: 22045767]

[30] Madsen BS, Jensen HL, van den Brule AJ, Wohlfahrt J, Frisch M. Risk factors for invasive squamous cell carcinoma of the vulva and vagina--population-based case-control study in Denmark. Int J Cancer 2008; 122(12): 2827-34.
[http://dx.doi.org/10.1002/ijc.23446] [PMID: 18348142]

[31] Jones RW, Baranyai J, Stables S. Trends in squamous cell carcinoma of the vulva: the influence of vulvar intraepithelial neoplasia. Obstet Gynecol 1997; 90(3): 448-52.
[http://dx.doi.org/10.1016/S0029-7844(97)00298-6] [PMID: 9277660]

[32] Edgren G, Sparén P. Risk of anogenital cancer after diagnosis of cervical intraepithelial neoplasia: a prospective population-based study. Lancet Oncol 2007; 8(4): 311-6.
[http://dx.doi.org/10.1016/S1470-2045(07)70043-8] [PMID: 17395104]

[33] Palefsky J. Human papillomavirus-related disease in people with HIV. Curr Opin HIV AIDS 2009; 4(1): 52-6.
[http://dx.doi.org/10.1097/COH.0b013e32831a7246] [PMID: 19339939]

[34] van Seters M, van Beurden M, de Craen AJ. Is the assumed natural history of vulvar intraepithelial neoplasia III based on enough evidence? A systematic review of 3322 published patients. Gynecol Oncol 2005; 97(2): 645-51.
[http://dx.doi.org/10.1016/j.ygyno.2005.02.012] [PMID: 15863172]

[35] Joura EA, Lösch A, Haider-Angeler MG, Breitenecker G, Leodolter S. Trends in vulvar neoplasia. Increasing incidence of vulvar intraepithelial neoplasia and squamous cell carcinoma of the vulva in young women. J Reprod Med 2000; 45(8): 613-5.
[PMID: 10986677]

[36] Judson PL, Habermann EB, Baxter NN, Durham SB, Virnig BA. Trends in the incidence of invasive and *in situ* vulvar carcinoma. Obstet Gynecol 2006; 107(5): 1018-22.
[http://dx.doi.org/10.1097/01.AOG.0000210268.57527.a1] [PMID: 16648405]

[37] Srodon M, Stoler MH, Baber GB, Kurman RJ. The distribution of low and high-risk HPV types in vulvar and vaginal intraepithelial neoplasia (VIN and VaIN). Am J Surg Pathol 2006; 30(12): 1513-8.
[http://dx.doi.org/10.1097/01.pas.0000213291.96401.48] [PMID: 17122506]

[38] Conley LJ, Ellerbrock TV, Bush TJ, Chiasson MA, Sawo D, Wright TC. HIV-1 infection and risk of

vulvovaginal and perianal condylomata acuminata and intraepithelial neoplasia: a prospective cohort study. Lancet 2002; 359(9301): 108-13.
[http://dx.doi.org/10.1016/S0140-6736(02)07368-3] [PMID: 11809252]

[39] Burger MP, Hollema H, Emanuels AG, Krans M, Pras E, Bouma J. The importance of the groin node status for the survival of T1 and T2 vulval carcinoma patients. Gynecol Oncol 1995; 57(3): 327-34.
[http://dx.doi.org/10.1006/gyno.1995.1151] [PMID: 7774836]

[40] Gadducci A, Cionini L, Romanini A, Fanucchi A, Genazzani AR. Old and new perspectives in the management of high-risk, locally advanced or recurrent, and metastatic vulvar cancer. Crit Rev Oncol Hematol 2006; 60(3): 227-41.
[http://dx.doi.org/10.1016/j.critrevonc.2006.06.009] [PMID: 16945551]

[41] af Geijersstam V, Wang Z, Lewensohn-Fuchs I, *et al.* Trends in seroprevalence of human papillomavirus type 16 among pregnant women in Stockholm, Sweden, during 1969-1989. Int J Cancer 1998; 76(3): 341-4.
[http://dx.doi.org/10.1002/(SICI)1097-0215(19980504)76:3<341::AID-IJC10>3.0.CO;2-E] [PMID: 9579570]

[42] Laukkanen P, Koskela P, Pukkala E, *et al.* Time trends in incidence and prevalence of human papillomavirus type 6, 11 and 16 infections in Finland. J Gen Virol 2003; 84(Pt 8): 2105-9.
[http://dx.doi.org/10.1099/vir.0.18995-0] [PMID: 12867641]

[43] Mercer CH, Tanton C, Prah P, *et al.* Changes in sexual attitudes and lifestyles in Britain through the life course and over time: findings from the National Surveys of Sexual Attitudes and Lifestyles (Natsal). Lancet 2013; 382(9907): 1781-94.
[http://dx.doi.org/10.1016/S0140-6736(13)62035-8] [PMID: 24286784]

[44] Kangas I, Andersen B, McGarrigle CA, ØStergaard L. A comparison of sexual behaviour and attitudes of healthy adolescents in a Danish high school in 1982, 1996, and 2001. Popul Health Metr 2004; 2(1): 5.
[http://dx.doi.org/10.1186/1478-7954-2-5] [PMID: 15038827]

[45] Winer RL, Hughes JP, Feng Q, *et al.* Condom use and the risk of genital human papillomavirus infection in young women. N Engl J Med 2006; 354(25): 2645-54.
[http://dx.doi.org/10.1056/NEJMoa053284] [PMID: 16790697]

[46] Gray RH, Serwadda D, Kong X, *et al.* Male circumcision decreases acquisition and increases clearance of high-risk human papillomavirus in HIV-negative men: a randomized trial in Rakai, Uganda. J Infect Dis 2010; 201(10): 1455-62.
[http://dx.doi.org/10.1086/652184] [PMID: 20370483]

[47] Serwadda D, Wawer MJ, Makumbi F, *et al.* Circumcision of HIV-infected men: effects on high-risk human papillomavirus infections in a randomized trial in Rakai, Uganda. J Infect Dis 2010; 201(10): 1463-9.
[http://dx.doi.org/10.1086/652185] [PMID: 20370481]

[48] Xi LF, Koutsky LA, Castle PE, *et al.* Relationship between cigarette smoking and human papilloma virus types 16 and 18 DNA load. Cancer Epidemiol Biomarkers Prev 2009; 18(12): 3490-6.
[http://dx.doi.org/10.1158/1055-9965.EPI-09-0763] [PMID: 19959700]

[49] Cleveland JL, Junger ML, Saraiya M, Markowitz LE, Dunne EF, Epstein JB. The connection between human papillomavirus and oropharyngeal squamous cell carcinomas in the United States: implications for dentistry. J Am Dent Assoc 2011; 142(8): 915-24.
[http://dx.doi.org/10.14219/jada.archive.2011.0298] [PMID: 21804058]

[50] Calmon MF, Tasso Mota M, Vassallo J, Rahal P. Penile carcinoma: risk factors and molecular alterations. Sci World J 2011; 11: 269-82.
[http://dx.doi.org/10.1100/tsw.2011.24] [PMID: 21298218]

[51] Ferenczy A, Coutlée F, Franco E, Hankins C. Human papillomavirus and HIV coinfection and the risk of neoplasias of the lower genital tract: a review of recent developments. CMAJ 2003; 169(5): 431-4.

[PMID: 12952805]

[52] Uronis HE, Bendell JC. Anal cancer: an overview. Oncologist 2007; 12(5): 524-34. [http://dx.doi.org/10.1634/theoncologist.12-5-524] [PMID: 17522240]

CHAPTER 10

Diagnosis of HPV Infections, HPV Testing in Patients

Kimia Kardani, Elnaz Agi and **Azam Bolhassani***

Department of Pharmaceutical Biotechnology, School of Pharmacy, Shahid Beheshti University of Medical Sciences, Tehran, Iran

Department of Hepatitis and AIDS, Pasteur Institute of Iran, Tehran, Iran

Abstract: Human papillomaviruses are associated with various cutaneous or mucosal benign and malignant neoplasms. The majority of available data on routine HPV diagnostics has been focused on evaluating the cervix. There is limited data on the efficiency of HPV diagnostics in cutaneous lesions. The balance between analytical and clinical sensitivity is critical for the specificity of a routine HPV test. Furthermore, HPV16 and HPV18 confer a higher risk for the development of a cervical intraepithelial lesion 2+ compared to the other HPV high-risk types. Thus, it is suitable to detect these HPV types individually. Up till now, HPV diagnosis has been mainly based on DNA detection using available amplification methods. PCR techniques could be used as type-specific or consensus PCRs. Among the methods, the Hybrid Capture 2 test has become the gold standard in routine HPV testing due to its high clinical sensitivity and its relatively high specificity. Briefly, three tests have received FDA approval including CervistaTM, signal amplification; CobasTM HPV test, real-time PCR; APTIMATM HPV, RNA test. On the other hand, the broad cytology-based screening programs have reduced the incidence of cervical cancer by 70% in the developed world. However, more than 270,000 annual cervical cancer-related deaths occur in developing countries due to their inability to improve a high-quality cytology-based screening program. In this chapter, different diagnosis and screening methods of HPV infections are evaluated in women worldwide.

Keywords: Diagnosis, HPV infection, HPV test, Screening.

INTRODUCTION

Over the past two decades, the molecular methods were developed to quantify viral nucleic acid in clinical specimens and to use viral load assay in the diagnosis of patients suffering from viral infections [1, 2]. Cytological screening has been usually used as a clinical tool for the detection of precancerous and cancerous

* **Corresponding author Azam Bolhassani:** Department of Hepatitis and AIDS, Pasteur Institute of Iran, Tehran, Iran; Tel: 66953311-20; E-mails: A_bolhasani@pasteur.ac.ir, azam.bolhassani@yahoo.com

Azam Bolhassani (Ed.)

lesions. However, it is very difficult to detect an early HPV infection at a low-grade precancerous state [3 - 5]. Thus, it is important to detect the early cervical lesions by screening methods before cancer is developed [3]. In this line, other molecular techniques were developed to identify the presence of HR-HPV DNA/RNA and early diagnosis of precancerous cases [6 - 11]. According to the American Cancer Association guidelines, the Papanikolaou (Pap) test and the HPV DNA test are remarkable diagnostic tools in asymptomatic women and in the follow up of women after the treatment of pre-invasive cervical cancer [3, 12]. Molecular tests that detect HR-HPV infections constitute a combined approach more sensitive than cytology alone in cervical cancer screening, with a higher negative predictive value [1, 13, 14]. The Pap smear test detects the precancerous and cancerous cell lesions, and the HPV test detects infections caused by HPV types that could lead to cancer. Most of the HPV infections are self-curable and cannot cause precancerous cell changes; only chronic infection by specific HPV types could lead to cervical cell abnormalities. If these abnormalities (*i.e.,* precancerous or high grade lesions) are not treated, they may evolve into cervical cancer after many years [3]. However, the Pap smear test often produces a false negative or false positive result responsible for 10-50% of the incorrect diagnoses [15]. The limitations of cytological screening led to identify the type of DNA and to detect the copy number of DNA targets in biopsies or cytological smears using polymerase chain reaction (PCR) technique [4, 16]. Typical PCR tests use consensus primers based on highly conserved segments of the L1 gene for detection of novel HPV types. Distinction between known or novel types is achieved by sequencing the amplicon and comparing it against sequence databases [17 - 19]. However, the DNA-based detection methods are not enough for monitoring the progress state of cancer [15]. Moreover, HPV-based tests are used for management or follow-up of abnormal cervical cytology or histology. Numerous HPV-DNA assays are commercially available but only a few are clinically approved for screening or diagnosis. They rely on different molecular techniques of template and/or signal amplification and fluorescence detection [13] and widely differ in genotyping information [1]. Molecular detection of HPV DNA or RNA as a gold standard for detection of HPV infection in tissue samples include southern transfer hybridization (STH), dot blot hybridization (DB) and *in situ* hybridization (ISH), signal amplified hybridization assays and target amplification assays (*i.e.,* PCR and *in situ* PCR). The PCR-based detection of HPV is really sensitive and specific [3, 20], but other techniques showed low sensitivity and the need for large amounts of purified DNA [8, 21]. For the diagnosis of invasive cervical cancer, there are available imaging methods (colposcopy), biophysical methods (fluorescence spectroscopy, polar probe), molecular diagnostic methods (HPV DNA test), morphometric-cytometric methods (nuclear aneuploidy detection, DNA ploidy), new methods of cervical smear preparation (Thin prep, CytoRich) and methods of automated cervical smear examination (Papnet, Cytyc, Autocyte and Autopap 300) [3, 22]. Furthermore, detection of HPV E6/E7 mRNA in cervical specimens can be performed by reverse transcriptase (RT) PCR or by nucleic acid sequence-based amplification (NASBA) [3, 20]. Up to now, several companies have developed kits for detection of known HPV types in the clinical tests such as Roche Molecular Systems and Digene Diagnostics [17, 23 - 25]. This method allows for simultaneous genotyping of HPV-16 and -18 amplicon separately from other 12 HR types [3, 26]. According to the latest guidelines of the American Cancer Society, screening should be done at the age of 21 [3, 27]. Younger women should be screened neither with Pap test nor with HPV test. Women between 21-29 years should be screened with Pap test every 3 years [3]. The HPV test should be used in these ages only after abnormal Pap test findings. Women between 30-65 years should be screened with both Pap test and HPV test every 5 years. This type of screening is preferable, but the continuing of Pap test screening every 3 years is also acceptable. Data is inadequate to support longer interval time between tests in this age group after a number of negative tests [3, 28].

Pap Test

The Pap smear collection should not be done during menses, shower, and sexual intercourse. Use of tampon or local contraception or other vaginal products should be avoided 48 hrs before Pap test [3]. Pap test should not be offered every year because sometimes precancerous lesions are mentioned without really existing. These false positive results may lead to treatments that are not needed. The latest guidelines for mass population screening maintain the benefits of diagnostic tests but they reduce the risk of unnecessary treatment [3, 29, 30]. Women who have undergone total hysterectomy (including cervix) for benign diseases and do not have cervical cancer or severe precancerous lesions history should not be screened. Women who have been vaccinated against HPV infection should continue the screening according to the guidelines for their age group [3].

HPV DNA Test

Over the last years, several molecular methods were established to identify HPV integrated genomes in the cervical samples. HPV DNA and (to a lesser extent) RNA assays are currently used in clinical trial. The specificity of this method depends on some factors including the detection system, the cutoff values, and the age of the patient [31 - 36]. HPV DNA test has higher sensitivity than Pap smear in CIN detection. Moreover, HPV tests possess a predictive value which detects women more susceptible to develop cervical cancer in the future [37]. The molecular techniques for HPV DNA detection have been divided into three categories including nucleic acid-hybridization, signal amplification and target amplification methods [7, 38, 39]. The PCR techniques can be divided into type-specific and consensus PCRs. The products of consensus PCRs can also be used for genotyping by hybridizing them to multiple HPV types fixed on a membrane strip [31]. Target amplification methods use PCR techniques which require a low amount of target DNA initially. This is a sensitive and relatively fast method [40 - 47]. A complete genotyping is not required in primary screening and is used in epidemiological studies. As an unwanted result of a wider use of HPV-DNA based tests, over-treatment of HPV-positive early dysplastic lesions may have a negative impact on reproductive outcomes. Therefore, it is very important to use biomarkers able to identify HPV persistent infections with a high risk to develop cervical cancer [1]. Viral load in HPV infections has been an attractive candidate as a marker of cancer risk [1, 48 - 53]. Positive associations of HR-HPV DNA load with the risk of persistent infection and cervical pre-cancer lesions have been reported in some studies [1, 50] but not in others [1, 49 - 55]. The detection of HPV-DNA in cytological samples does not indicate an essential diagnosis of CIN or cancer, but elevated expression of HPV16/18 E6 is considered as a critical step for oncogenic transformation of cervical epithelial cells [41, 56]. Viral load has a limited use for screening or diagnostic purposes. Different possibilities in molecular diagnostics were opened by resolving the complex interactions between HR-HPVs and the infected host. Integration of HR-HPV into the host-cell genome is considered as a critical event in the pathogenesis of cervical neoplasia because of disruption of the HPV regulatory E2 gene leading to E6/E7 overexpression [1]. Considering that HPV-DNA testing has high sensitivity but low specificity in screening, triage of ASCUS (atypical squamous cells of undetermined significance) and in follow up after treatment, these processes can be monitored through biomarkers specific to each step in the progression toward neoplastic changes. In particular, detection of E6 and E7 mRNA levels, HPV genome integration status, and cellular protein detection could help in prediction of premalignant lesions evolution [1, 13, 57, 58]. The diagnosis of ASCUS is also important, because patients with this diagnosis will have approximately 10 percent risk of a coexisting high-grade squamous intraepithelial lesion and up to half the patients with an ASCUS diagnosis will have a low-grade CIN lesion [17, 59]. Testing for E6/E7 mRNA might be more specific than HPV-DNA testing alone; moreover, collection media for liquid-based cytology can preserve RNA sufficiently to allow transcript detection, after the first screening test [1]. Commercial tests have been approved for testing HR HPV E6/E7 mRNA, utilizing NASBA or TMA [60 - 62]. E2/E6 DNA copy number ratio is often considered as an alternative for HPV integration. If only the episomal form are present, the E2/E6 ratio would be close to 1, and if only the integrated form are present, the E2/E6 ratios would be close to zero; if the integrated form and episomal form are mixed, the E2/E6 ratios would be intermediate. Several studies considered E2/E6 ratio as a potential oncogenic biomarker for its correlation with lesion histological grade [1, 63, 64]. However, other study did not support HPV integration status to be considered as potential biomarkers of cervical disease [1, 65]. Therefore, before introducing HPV integration as a biomarker into clinical service, further studies is needed to determine how often E2 is disrupted during the natural history of HPV infection [1, 66]. In addition to viral genes, biomarkers of the cellular counterpart may be used as indicator for the presence of proliferative lesions. For example, over-expression of cyclin dependent kinases 4 and 6 (CDK4/CDK6) inhibitor p16 ($p16^{INK4a}$)-protein, and of the proliferation marker Ki-67 leads to HPV-induced deregulation of the cell cycle. Their immunohistochemical detection as a surrogate marker of oncogenic HPV process entered clinical use, but it is not as sensitive as most molecular-based methods [67, 68]. New technologies could be the next step in the search of better molecular markers. Methylation profiles in cell and viral genes [1, 69], genomic changes (losses and/or gains in specific chromosomal regions) [1, 70], miRNAs aberrant expression [1, 71], and telomerase activity deregulation are recently underway for determining lesion grade [1, 72]. Molecular markers either alone or in combination with more traditional techniques have the potential to further improve diagnostics, management, and treatment of cervical dysplasia and cervical cancer. A remarkable improvement would be HPV detection and genotyping tests applicable in POC settings, ultimately together with other Sexually Transmitted Infections [1, 73]. Accordingly, the detection of HPV-DNA associated with high levels of HPV16/18-E6 may be an interesting approach for CIN detection in cervical cancer prevention strategies [41]. In general, the molecular methods include hybridization assays (FISH), PCR-mediated methods (DIPS, RSPCR, APOT, qReal-time PCR) and whole genome sequence analysis [*i.e.*, next generation sequencing (NGS)] [7].

Fluorescent *In Situ* Hybridization (FISH)

The FISH assay is performed in cervical smears in order to detect chromosomal abnormalities in regions (3q26, 8q24, 5p15, 20q13, centromere 7) that are frequently detected in HPV-associated cancers as well as to identify the presence of HPV episomal or integrated HPV DNA [74 - 76]. The episomal form of HPV DNA is detected by a uniform signal in the nucleus of cell, while the integrated viral genomes are identified when a scatter signal is observed [7, 77]. It is possible that the episomal DNA can lose during FISH procedure, or the increased prevalence of integrated viral genomes might limit the detection of episomal DNA form [7, 78, 79]. In addition, the low copy number of viral genomes or loss of HPV DNA because of deregulated cell proliferation may prevent the detection of viral DNA [7, 80].

PCR-based Assays

The PCR-based techniques are highly sensitive and specific approaches [8]. The Detection of Integrated Papillomavirus Sequences (DIPS) method is an adaptor ligation-based PCR assay that has been designed specifically to identify integrated viral sequences of HPV DNA at the early stages of cervical lesions. A conventional PCR (*e.g.,* nested PCR) assay allows the amplification and identification of host DNA sequences flanking the integrated viral fragments [81 - 86]. Moreover, the restriction site PCR (RS-PCR) is a PCR-based assay that retrieves unknown sequences that are flanking a known sequence [83 - 86]. Although DIPS-PCR and RS-PCR assays facilitate the identification of the locus of viral insertion and the site of viral disruption with high specificity, they are not able to distinguish episomal or mixed HPV-DNA forms. An alternative method that can identify the episomal, mixed and integrated viral form with high sensitivity is the detection of HPV E6, E7 transcripts by RT-PCR (APOT) [7, 79, 87, 88].

Quantitative Real-Time PCR

The real-time PCR assay facilitates the rapid quantification of viral copy number and the physical state of HPV DNA (episomal, integrated or mixed) with high specificity and sensitivity. The studies showed that viral load assessment may not be clinically useful, except in the case of HPV16. Lowe *et al.* demonstrated differences in viral load between CIN I, CIN II and normal, but not between CIN II and CIN III [89 - 94]. The viral physical status (*i.e.,* episomal or integrated forms) is determined through analysis of E2/E6 ratio [7, 94]. This method may present false-negative rates in low-grade CINs which the E1 gene disruption is observed [7, 95, 96]. Recently, the simultaneous analysis of the E1/E6 and E2/E6 ratios was performed in each cervical sample determining the accuracy in the physical status of HPV16 DNA [7, 35]. However, the assay is not able to find the position of viral insertion into the host DNA [96, 97].

Next Generation Sequencing

The NGS technology as a whole genome sequencing method provides a wide range of data specific for each patient including the HPV genotype, the presence of multiple viral infections, the viral copy number, the physical status of viral DNA, the sites of viral disruption, the locus of viral insertion as well as the presence of chromosomal damages induced by HPV integrants, regardless the grade of cervical lesion [98 - 102]. However, data analysis and the increased cost of the assay remain the major issues for most clinical laboratories [103, 104]. Recently, the Illumina Hiseq NGS platform has been mainly used in clinical laboratories due to the highest throughput and lowest cost as compared to other

NGS platforms [105, 106].

HR-HPV Test

The US FDA recently approved HR-HPV testing as the primary screening tool for cervical cancer, alone or associated with the Pap test. Most of the HPV tests are DNA-based assays, which are more useful because of the stability of DNA in cervical samples. Recently, two lower cost molecular tests for HR-HPV have been developed: **a)** careHPV™ (QIAGEN, Gaithersburg, MD) detects the DNA for a pool of 14 HR-HPV genotypes [46, 107] and **b)** the OncoE6™ Cervical Test (Arbor Vita Corporation, Fremont, CA) detects hrHPV E6 oncoproteins from HPV16, 18 and 45 [107 - 120]. The studies showed that HPV DNA detection was more sensitive and less specific for cervical precancer and cancer than E6 detection [121 - 123].

Signal Amplification

Signal amplification methods use *in situ* hybridization techniques in liquid phase (*i.e.,* denatured target DNA (HPV) affixed to known labeled probes targeting mainly the L1 region of HPV genome). If the virus is present, a hybridization reaction occurs between denatured DNA and labeled specific and complementary probe. The reaction product is visualized by hybridization reaction immunoassays [40]. Two signal amplification technologies (Hybrid Capture 2TM, HC2, test, Qiagen, Gaithersburg, Md., USA; CervistaTM, Hologic, Bedford, Mass., USA) are commercially available [31, 124]. Nowadays, three DNA-based and one RNA-based assays have been approved by the US FDA for routine cervical cancer screening including the Digene Hybrid Capture 2 High-Risk HPV DNA test (HC2; Qiagen, Hilden, Germany), the Cervista HPV HR test (CER; Hologic, Madison, WI), the Cobas® HPV test (Roche, Pleasanton, USA) and the RNA-based Aptima® HPV assay (Hologic, San Diego, CA) [3].

Hybrid Capture 2 (HC2)

The Hybrid Capture 2 (HC2) method detects 13 high-risk HPV types (-16,-18,-31, -33,-35,-39,-45,-51,-52,-56,-58,-59 and -68), 5 low-risk types (-6, -11, -42, -43, and -44) [125 - 127] and also HR-HPV type 66 [128], in cervical scrapings and paraffin-embedded tissues (FFPE). This assay distinguishes between HR and LR groups, but was not designed for genotyping single HPV [129 - 131]. Moreover, the Hybrid Capture 2 (HC2) method can be used for semi-quantitative viral load. The assay presents high sensitivity (87-96%) for detecting high-grade CIN (*i.e.,* CIN3+), but relatively low specificity (20-85%) [132 - 138]. One disadvantage of the HC2 test is the lack of a control for the presence of human cellular material [139 - 143]. Another drawback is the potential for cross-reaction with certain low-risk HPV types, which occurs in 7.8% of all positive HC2 results [144]. Moreover, the clinical sensitivity of the HC2 test for CIN2⁺ is very high [145].

The Cervista™ HPV HR and Genfind™ DNA Extraction Kit, and the Cervista™ HPV16/18

The Cervista™ HPV HR and Genfind™ DNA Extraction Kit detects 14 HR HPV types (16/18/31/33/35/39/45/51/52/56/58/59/66 and 68) in cervical scrapings [146 - 149]. The clinical sensitivity and specificity of Cervista™ HPV HR for the detection of CIN2+ is 90 and 47%, respectively, and 95 and 87% for CINIII+ [150, 151]. In contrast to HC2, the Cervista™ HPV HR test contains an internal control that eliminates the false-negative results [152, 153]. On the other hand, this assay showed a lower false-positive rate, and high sensitivity and specificity to genotyping HPV16 / 18 [154].

Cobas HPV Test

In April 2014, the Cobas HPV (Roche Molecular) was approved by the FDA to be used for cervical cancer screening in women ≥ 25 years. After that, recent studies were published in 2015 indicating the value of co-testing, *e.g.,* cytology combined with HPV test [155, 156]. The CobasTM assay is a real-time consensus PCR which covers 14 HPV high-risk types as well as it differentiates HPV16 and HPV18 (Roche Molecular Diagnostics, Pleasanton, Calif., USA) [31]. The PCR amplification and detection occur in a single tube using HPV16, HPV18, 12 HR-HPV (-31, -33, -35, -39, -45, -51, -52, -56, -58, -59, -66, and -68) as a pool, and also β-globin as the control for extraction and amplification potential [8, 157 - 161]. Cobas HPV test has high clinical sensitivity for the detection of $CINII^+$ and $CINIII^+$ (> 93%), while the specificity of the assay is 59.3 and 56.8% for the detection of $CINII^+$ and $CINIII^+$, respectively [7, 162 - 168]. Finally, the Cobas HPV test achieves higher sensitivity and specificity in detecting HR-HPV genotypes and lower rate of cross-reactivity with LR-HPV genotypes than the HC2 [7, 167]. Cobas® 4800 is reliable in the detection of HR-HPV and has been clinically validated for ASCUS triage [8, 31, 168 - 172].

APTIMA HPV Test

The presence of E6 and E7 genes can be a specific marker for diagnosing precancerous lesions [173, 174]. In 2011, the FDA approved the APTIMA HPV test that is based on transcription-mediated amplification and probe hybridization for the simultaneous detection of E6/E7 mRNA of 14 HR genotypes (HPV16, 18, 31, 33, 35, 39, 45, 51, 52, 56, 58, 59, 66 and 68) in cervical scrapings. Aptima HPV test has similar sensitivity with HC2 (> 95%) for the detection of $CINII^+$ and $CINIII^+$, but the Aptima HPV test demonstrates significantly higher specificity

(42.2-94.5% for CINII$^+$ and CINIII$^+$) than the HC2. Moreover, the Aptima HPV test has higher specificity in detection of CIN II$^+$ and CINIII$^+$ than the Cobas HPV test [175 - 182].

Detection of p16 ^{INK4a} as a Biomarker

The increased expression of E7 gene results in the inactivation of the retinoblastoma gene product (pRB), and overexpression of the cyclin-dependent kinase inhibitor p16^{INK4a} retaining the cell proliferation. The p16^{INK4a} was determined as a specific marker for the neoplastic transformation of cervical squamous epithelial cells by HPVs in cytopathology specimens. Comparing to molecular HPV tests, the immunochemical detection of p16^{INK4a}-stained cells demonstrates a significantly improved specificity with good relative sensitivity [182 - 193].

Immunochromatography (IC)

The levels of serum anti-HPV antibodies (Abs) are important for determination of the efficiency of HPV vaccination. In the case of natural infection of HPVs, specific antibody responses are induced against the HPV antigens, and these antibodies are able to protect partially but not completely against the next infection [194, 195]. Vaccination by Cervarix was reported to sustain the high levels of serum anti-HPV Abs at 113 months post vaccination. Vaccination with Gardasil also showed that the anti-HPV antibodies were maintained at high levels 108 months post-vaccination. Herein, anti-HPV L1 antibody levels in serum have been measured by enzyme-linked immunosorbent assay (ELISA), competitive Luminex immunoassay (cLIA), and an *in vitro* neutralization assay called pseudovirion-based neutralization assay (PBNA). The titer of total anti-L1 Ab measured by ELISA highly correlates with that of HPV type-specific Abs by cLIA and that of neutralizing Ab by PBNA. These data suggest that the level of total anti-L1 Ab is a reliable marker for monitoring the efficacy of HPV vaccination. On the other hand, immunochromatography (IC) is widely used to detect target molecules in biological fluids. Recently, a low-cost immunochromatographic assay called the OncoE6 Cervical Test (Arbor Vita Corporation, Fremont, CA, USA) was developed to detect elevated expression of the HR-HPV 16/18 E6 oncoproteins (HPV16/18-E6). Furthermore, the relationship between the E7 concentration and the progress of cervical cancer has been studied by IC method [194 - 217].

PCR-based Methods for HPV Genotyping

Although several methods are available for HPV genotyping, clinical laboratories mainly use PCR-based assays to detect the HPV DNA [7, 8]. The comparative analyses between the HCII and conventional PCR revealed that HCII is more sensitive and specific than PCR for the detection of high-grade dysplasia, while PCR is more sensitive but less specific than HCII for the detection of low-grade dysplasia [218, 219]. On the other hand, the HPV-PCR protocols use consensus primers which allow amplification of a large number of HPV genotypes in a single reaction. Identification of specific HPV genotypes is performed through post-amplification analyses, including hybridization with type-specific probes, restriction fragment length polymorphism analysis (RFLP), direct sequence analysis, and nested PCR [220 - 232].

Hybridization

The hybridization with type-specific probes was performed through reverse methods for concurrent hybridization of a PCR product to multiple HPV type-specific oligonucleotide probes [7]. Briefly, after PCR, the biotinylated amplicons are denatured under alkaline conditions and are hybridized with the immobilized probes. Subsequently, streptavidine-peroxidase conjugate is added to bind to the biotinylated hybrids and color precipitates are formed in the presence of a chromogenic substrate. Several of these methods have been commercialized. For instance, the Linear Array® HPV Genotyping (Roche Molecular Diagnostics, Pleasanton, CA, USA) allows the discrimination of 36 HPV, including 15 HR (-16, -18, -31, -33, -35, -39, -45, -51, -52, -56, -58, -59, -68, -73 and -82), 3 probable HR (-26, -53 and -66), 10 LR (-6, -11, -40, -42, -54, -61, -70,-72, -81 and -CP6108) and 9 genotypes for which the risk is still undetermined (-55, -62, -64, -67, -69, -71, -83, -84 and -IS39). The test uses biotinylated PGMY09/11 primers to amplify a 450 bp fragment within the polymorphic L1 region of the HPV genome. The reports showed that linear array and HC2 are found to have similar sensitivity, but linear array is less specific than HC2 for the detection of high-grade dysplasia [233 - 254].

PCR-RFLP

The PCR-RFLP analysis is based on sequence-specific enzymatic digestion of PCR amplicons producing different size and number of DNA fragments. Genotyping by PCR-RFLP is easier and less expensive than sequencing. The pattern of generated bands is specific to each individual type-specific amplicon, enabling the discrimination of different HPV genotypes with significant sensitivity and specificity [255 - 259].

HPV Genome Sequencing

The dideoxy chain-termination technique (Sanger technique) is reliable as direct genome sequencing in cases with single HPV infection. In cases of multiple HPV infections, type-specific primers are used to perform HPVDNA-type-specific sequencing. Although sequencing is regarded as the 'gold standard' for HPV genotyping, it is time consuming, costly and not applicable for routine diagnosis. Similar to dideoxy sequencing methods, pyrosequencing is applicable to any source of DNA or RNA (blood, saliva, cell line, plasma, serum, tissue, paraffin-embedded samples, and whole genome-amplified DNA) that can be amplified by PCR. This method is based on the detection of the pyrophosphate released during DNA synthesis [260 - 264].

CONCLUDING REMARKS

In general, HPV diagnostic methods often involve PCR-based technologies with HPV DNA or RNA assays. The HPV genotyping can also identify women who have higher risk for development of CINII$^+$ and CINIII$^+$. However, the molecular assays that determine the physical state of HPV DNA (episomal or integrated forms) and the locus of viral insertion into the host genome should be involved in HPV diagnosis for the effective management of HPV infection.

CONFLICT OF INTEREST

The author (editor) declares no conflict of interest, financial or otherwise.

ACKNOWLEDGEMENT

Declare none.

REFERENCES

[1] Scagnolari C, Turriziani O, Monteleone K, Pierangeli A, Antonelli G. Consolidation of molecular testing in clinical virology. Expert Rev Anti Infect Ther 2017; 15(4): 387-400. [http://dx.doi.org/10.1080/14787210.2017.1271711] [PMID: 28002969]

[2] Chernesky MA. An evolutionary change in diagnostic virology. Yale J Biol Med 1989; 62(2): 89-92. [PMID: 2672623]

[3] Tsikouras P, Zervoudis S, Manav B, *et al.* Cervical cancer: screening, diagnosis and staging. J BUON 2016; 21(2): 320-5. [PMID: 27273940]

[4] Xiao Y, Sato S, Oguchi T, Kudo K, Yokoyama Y, Saito Y. High sensitivity of PCR *in situ* hybridization for the detection of human papillomavirus infection in uterine cervical neoplasias. Gynecol Oncol 2001; 82(2): 350-4. [http://dx.doi.org/10.1006/gyno.2001.6261] [PMID: 11531292]

[5] Willett GD, Kurman RJ, Reid R, Greenberg M, Jenson AB, Lorincz AT. Correlation of the histologic appearance of intraepithelial neoplasia of the cervix with human papillomavirus types. Emphasis on low grade lesions including so-called flat condyloma. Int J Gynecol Pathol 1989; 8(1): 18-25. [http://dx.doi.org/10.1097/00004347-198903000-00003] [PMID: 2540101]

[6] Crum CP, Mitao M, Levine RU, Silverstein S. Cervical papillomaviruses segregate within morphologically distinct precancerous lesions. J Virol 1985; 54(3): 675-81. [PMID: 2987521]

[7] Tsakogiannis D, Gartzonika C, Levidiotou-Stefanou S, Markoulatos P. Molecular approaches for HPV genotyping and HPV-DNA physical status. Expert Rev Mol Med 2017; 19: e1. [http://dx.doi.org/10.1017/erm.2017.2] [PMID: 28162121]

[8] Abreu AL, Souza RP, Gimenes F, Consolaro ME. A review of methods for detect human Papillomavirus infection. Virol J 2012; 9: 262. [http://dx.doi.org/10.1186/1743-422X-9-262] [PMID: 23131123]

[9] Castle PE, Stoler MH, Wright TC Jr, Sharma A, Wright TL, Behrens CM. Performance of carcinogenic human papillomavirus (HPV) testing and HPV16 or HPV18 genotyping for cervical cancer screening of women aged 25 years and older: a subanalysis of the ATHENA study. Lancet Oncol 2011; 12(9): 880-90. [http://dx.doi.org/10.1016/S1470-2045(11)70188-7] [PMID: 21865084]

[10] Cox JT, Castle PE, Behrens CM, Sharma A, Wright TC Jr, Cuzick J. Comparison of cervical cancer screening strategies incorporating different combinations of cytology, HPV testing, and genotyping for HPV 16/18: results from the ATHENA HPV study. Am J Obstet Gynecol 2013; 208(3): 184.e1-184.e11. [http://dx.doi.org/10.1016/j.ajog.2012.11.020] [PMID: 23174289]

[11] Schiffman M, Wentzensen N. A suggested approach to simplify and improve cervical screening in the United States. J Low Genit Tract Dis 2016; 20(1): 1-7. [http://dx.doi.org/10.1097/LGT.0000000000000170] [PMID: 26704326]

[12] Bergeron C, von Knebel Doeberitz M. The role of cytology in the 21st century: The integration of cells and molecules. Acta Cytol 2016; 60(6): 540-2. [http://dx.doi.org/10.1159/000449402] [PMID: 27788516]

[13] Luhn P, Wentzensen N. HPV-based Tests for Cervical Cancer Screening and Management of Cervical Disease. Curr Obstet Gynecol Rep 2013; 2(2): 76-85. [http://dx.doi.org/10.1007/s13669-013-0040-0] [PMID: 23705102]

[14] Ronco G, Dillner J, Elfström KM, *et al.* Efficacy of HPV-based screening for prevention of invasive cervical cancer: follow-up of four European randomised controlled trials. Lancet 2014; 383(9916): 524-32. [http://dx.doi.org/10.1016/S0140-6736(13)62218-7] [PMID: 24192252]

[15] Kim JH, Cho HI, Seo SM, *et al.* Immuno-chromatographic analysis for HPV-16 and 18 E7 proteins as a biomarker of cervical cancer caused by human papillomavirus. Bull Korean Chem Soc 2009; 30(12): 2999-3005. [http://dx.doi.org/10.5012/bkcs.2009.30.12.2999]

[16] Tyring S. Perspectives on human papillomavirus infection. Am J Med 1997; 102(5A): 1-2. [http://dx.doi.org/10.1016/S0002-9343(97)00176-9] [PMID: 9217655]

[17] Garcea RL, Dimaio D. The papillomaviruses. Springer Science & Business Media 2007. [http://dx.doi.org/10.1007/978-0-387-36523-7]

[18] Jacobs MV, de Roda Husman AM, van den Brule AJ, Snijders PJ, Meijer CJ, Walboomers JM. Group-specific differentiation between high- and low-risk human papillomavirus genotypes by general primer-mediated PCR and two cocktails of oligonucleotide probes. J Clin Microbiol 1995; 33(4): 901-5. [PMID: 7790457]

[19] Antonsson A, Forslund O, Ekberg H, Sterner G, Hansson BG. The ubiquity and impressive genomic diversity of human skin papillomaviruses suggest a commensalic nature of these viruses. J Virol 2000; 74(24): 11636-41. [http://dx.doi.org/10.1128/JVI.74.24.11636-11641.2000] [PMID: 11090162]

[20] Lie AK, Kristensen G. Human papillomavirus E6/E7 mRNA testing as a predictive marker for cervical carcinoma. Expert Rev Mol Diagn 2008; 8(4): 405-15.

[http://dx.doi.org/10.1586/14737159.8.4.405] [PMID: 18598223]

[21] Villa LL, Denny L. Methods for detection of HPV infection and its clinical utility. Int J Gynaecol Obstet 2006; 94: 71-80.
[http://dx.doi.org/10.1016/S0020-7292(07)60013-7]

[22] Fontaine PL, Saslow D, King VJ. ACS/ASCCP/ASCP guidelines for the early detection of cervical cancer. Am Fam Physician 2012; 86(6): 501-, 506-507.
[PMID: 23062041]

[23] Gravitt PE, Peyton CL, Apple RJ, Wheeler CM. Genotyping of 27 human papillomavirus types by using L1 consensus PCR products by a single-hybridization, reverse line blot detection method. J Clin Microbiol 1998; 36(10): 3020-7.
[PMID: 9738060]

[24] Ferris DG, Wright TC Jr, Litaker MS, *et al.* Comparison of two tests for detecting carcinogenic HPV in women with Papanicolaou smear reports of ASCUS and LSIL. J Fam Pract 1998; 46(2): 136-41.
[PMID: 9487319]

[25] Smits HL, van Gemen B, Schukkink R, *et al.* Application of the NASBA nucleic acid amplification method for the detection of human papillomavirus type 16 E6-E7 transcripts. J Virol Methods 1995; 54(1): 75-81.
[http://dx.doi.org/10.1016/0166-0934(95)00032-P] [PMID: 7559859]

[26] Agorastos T, Chatzistamatiou K, Katsamagkas T, *et al.* Primary screening for cervical cancer based on high-risk human papillomavirus (HPV) detection and HPV 16 and HPV 18 genotyping, in comparison to cytology. PLoS One 2015; 10(3): e0119755.
[http://dx.doi.org/10.1371/journal.pone.0119755] [PMID: 25793281]

[27] Koss LG. Chapter Part I: Inflammatory processes; Part II: Other benign disorders of the cervix and vagina.Diagnostic Cytology. 4th ed. Philadelphia: JB Lippincott Co 1992; pp. 314-70.

[28] Saslow D, Solomon D, Lawson HW, *et al.* American Cancer Society, American Society for Colposcopy and Cervical Pathology, and American Society for Clinical Pathology screening guidelines for the prevention and early detection of cervical cancer. Am J Clin Pathol 2012; 137(4): 516-42.
[http://dx.doi.org/10.1309/AJCPTGD94EVRSJCG] [PMID: 22431528]

[29] Saslow D, Solomon D, Lawson HW, *et al.* American Cancer Society, American Society for Colposcopy and Cervical Pathology, and American Society for Clinical Pathology screening guidelines for the prevention and early detection of cervical cancer. CA Cancer J Clin 2012; 62(3): 147-72.
[http://dx.doi.org/10.3322/caac.21139] [PMID: 22422631]

[30] Saslow D, Solomon D, Lawson HW, *et al.* American Cancer Society, American Society for Colposcopy and Cervical Pathology, and American Society for Clinical Pathology screening guidelines for the prevention and early detection of cervical cancer. J Low Genit Tract Dis 2012; 16(3): 175-204.
[http://dx.doi.org/10.1097/LGT.0b013e31824ca9d5] [PMID: 22418039]

[31] Ikenberg H. Laboratory diagnosis of human papillomavirus infection. Curr Probl Dermatol 2014; 45: 166-74.
[http://dx.doi.org/10.1159/000356515] [PMID: 24643185]

[32] Hesselink AT, van den Brule AJ, Brink AA, *et al.* Comparison of hybrid capture 2 with *in situ* hybridization for the detection of high-risk human papillomavirus in liquid-based cervical samples. Cancer 2004; 102(1): 11-8.
[http://dx.doi.org/10.1002/cncr.11904] [PMID: 14968413]

[33] Wang SS, Schiffman M, Shields TS, *et al.* Seroprevalence of human papillomavirus-16, -18, -31, and -45 in a population-based cohort of 10000 women in Costa Rica. Br J Cancer 2003; 89(7): 1248-54.
[http://dx.doi.org/10.1038/sj.bjc.6601272] [PMID: 14520455]

[34] Belinson JL, Wu R, Belinson SE, *et al.* A population-based clinical trial comparing endocervical high-risk HPV testing using hybrid capture 2 and Cervista from the SHENCCAST II Study. Am J Clin Pathol 2011; 135(5): 790-5.
[http://dx.doi.org/10.1309/AJCPKA6ATAPBZ6JQ] [PMID: 21502436]

[35] Tsakogiannis D, Kyriakopoulou Z, Ruether IG, *et al.* Determination of human papillomavirus 16 physical status through E1/E6 and E2/E6 ratio analysis. J Med Microbiol 2014; 63(Pt 12): 1716-23.
[http://dx.doi.org/10.1099/jmm.0.076810-0] [PMID: 25212758]

[36] Li H, Yang Y, Zhang R, *et al.* Preferential sites for the integration and disruption of human papillomavirus 16 in cervical lesions. J Clin Virol 2013; 56(4): 342-7.
[http://dx.doi.org/10.1016/j.jcv.2012.12.014] [PMID: 23290390]

[37] Nowak-Markwitz E, Spaczyński M. [Is the PAP smear era coming to an end?]. Ginekol Pol 2015; 86(12): 947-50.
[http://dx.doi.org/10.17772/gp/60709] [PMID: 26995946]

[38] Castle PE, de Sanjosé S, Qiao YL, Belinson JL, Lazcano-Ponce E, Kinney W. Introduction of human papillomavirus DNA screening in the world: 15 years of experience. Vaccine 2012; 30(5) (Suppl. 5): F117-22.
[http://dx.doi.org/10.1016/j.vaccine.2012.05.071] [PMID: 23199954]

[39] Cuzick J, Szarewski A, Mesher D, *et al.* Long-term follow-up of cervical abnormalities among women screened by HPV testing and cytology-Results from the Hammersmith study. Int J Cancer 2008; 122(10): 2294-300.
[http://dx.doi.org/10.1002/ijc.23339] [PMID: 18240149]

[40] Eide ML, Debaque H. HPV detection methods and genotyping techniques in screening for cervical cancer. Ann Pathol 2012; 32(6): e15-e23, 401-409.
[http://dx.doi.org/10.1016/j.annpat.2012.09.231] [PMID: 23244480]

[41] Mariano VS, Lorenzi AT, Scapulatempo-Neto C, *et al.* A low-cost HPV immunochromatographic assay to detect high-grade cervical intraepithelial neoplasia. PLoS One 2016; 11(10): e0164892.
[http://dx.doi.org/10.1371/journal.pone.0164892] [PMID: 27764154]

[42] Sankaranarayanan R, Budukh AM, Rajkumar R. Effective screening programmes for cervical cancer in low- and middle-income developing countries. Bull World Health Organ 2001; 79(10): 954-62.
[PMID: 11693978]

[43] Kitchener HC, Castle PE, Cox JT. Chapter 7: Achievements and limitations of cervical cytology screening. Vaccine 2006; 24(3): S3/63-70.

[44] Blumenthal PD, Gaffikin L, Deganus S, Lewis R, Emerson M, Adadevoh S. Cervical cancer prevention: safety, acceptability, and feasibility of a single-visit approach in Accra, Ghana. Am J Obstet Gynecol 2007; 196(4): 407.e1-8.
[http://dx.doi.org/10.1016/j.ajog.2006.12.031] [PMID: 17403438]

[45] Longatto-Filho A, Schmitt FC. Gynecological cytology: too old to be a pop star but too young to die. Diagn Cytopathol 2007; 35(10): 672-3.
[http://dx.doi.org/10.1002/dc.20700] [PMID: 17854085]

[46] Qiao YL, Sellors JW, Eder PS, *et al.* A new HPV-DNA test for cervical-cancer screening in developing regions: a cross-sectional study of clinical accuracy in rural China. Lancet Oncol 2008; 9(10): 929-36.
[http://dx.doi.org/10.1016/S1470-2045(08)70210-9] [PMID: 18805733]

[47] Zhao FH, Lewkowitz AK, Chen F, *et al.* Pooled analysis of a self-sampling HPV DNA Test as a cervical cancer primary screening method. J Natl Cancer Inst 2012; 104(3): 178-88.
[http://dx.doi.org/10.1093/jnci/djr532] [PMID: 22271765]

[48] Swan DC, Tucker RA, Tortolero-Luna G, *et al.* Human papillomavirus (HPV) DNA copy number is dependent on grade of cervical disease and HPV type. J Clin Microbiol 1999; 37(4): 1030-4.

[PMID: 10074522]

[49] Cheung JL, Lo KW, Cheung TH, Tang JW, Chan PK. Viral load, E2 gene disruption status, and lineage of human papillomavirus type 16 infection in cervical neoplasia. J Infect Dis 2006; 194(12): 1706-12.
[http://dx.doi.org/10.1086/509622] [PMID: 17109343]

[50] Moberg M, Gustavsson I, Gyllensten U. Type-specific associations of human papillomavirus load with risk of developing cervical carcinoma in situ. Int J Cancer 2004; 112(5): 854-9.
[http://dx.doi.org/10.1002/ijc.20480] [PMID: 15386375]

[51] Andersson S, Safari H, Mints M, Lewensohn-Fuchs I, Gyllensten U, Johansson B. Type distribution, viral load and integration status of high-risk human papillomaviruses in pre-stages of cervical cancer (CIN). Br J Cancer 2005; 92(12): 2195-200.
[http://dx.doi.org/10.1038/sj.bjc.6602648] [PMID: 15942630]

[52] Molano M, Van den Brule A, Plummer M, *et al.* Determinants of clearance of human papillomavirus infections in Colombian women with normal cytology: a population-based, 5-year follow-up study. Am J Epidemiol 2003; 158(5): 486-94.
[http://dx.doi.org/10.1093/aje/kwg171] [PMID: 12936904]

[53] Kulmala SM, Shabalova IP, Petrovitchev N, *et al.* Type-specific persistence of high-risk human papillomavirus infections in the New Independent States of the former Soviet Union Cohort Study. Cancer Epidemiol Biomarkers Prev 2007; 16(1): 17-22.
[http://dx.doi.org/10.1158/1055-9965.EPI-06-0649] [PMID: 17220327]

[54] Constandinou-Williams C, Collins SI, Roberts S, Young LS, Woodman CB, Murray PG. Is human papillomavirus viral load a clinically useful predictive marker? A longitudinal study. Cancer Epidemiol Biomarkers Prev 2010; 19(3): 832-7.
[http://dx.doi.org/10.1158/1055-9965.EPI-09-0838] [PMID: 20200441]

[55] Depuydt CE, Criel AM, Benoy IH, Arbyn M, Vereecken AJ, Bogers JJ. Changes in type-specific human papillomavirus load predict progression to cervical cancer. J Cell Mol Med 2012; 16(12): 3096-104.
[http://dx.doi.org/10.1111/j.1582-4934.2012.01631.x] [PMID: 22978795]

[56] Isaacson Wechsler E, Wang Q, Roberts I, *et al.* Reconstruction of human papillomavirus type 16-mediated early-stage neoplasia implicates E6/E7 deregulation and the loss of contact inhibition in neoplastic progression. J Virol 2012; 86(11): 6358-64.
[http://dx.doi.org/10.1128/JVI.07069-11] [PMID: 22457518]

[57] Schiffman M, Castle PE, Jeronimo J, Rodriguez AC, Wacholder S. Human papillomavirus and cervical cancer. Lancet 2007; 370(9590): 890-907.
[http://dx.doi.org/10.1016/S0140-6736(07)61416-0] [PMID: 17826171]

[58] Snijders PJ, Steenbergen RD, Heideman DA, Meijer CJ. HPV-mediated cervical carcinogenesis: concepts and clinical implications. J Pathol 2006; 208(2): 152-64.
[http://dx.doi.org/10.1002/path.1866] [PMID: 16362994]

[59] Wright TC Jr, Schiffman M, Solomon D, *et al.* Interim guidance for the use of human papillomavirus DNA testing as an adjunct to cervical cytology for screening. Obstet Gynecol 2004; 103(2): 304-9.
[http://dx.doi.org/10.1097/01.AOG.0000109426.82624.f8] [PMID: 14754700]

[60] Burger EA, Kornør H, Klemp M, Lauvrak V, Kristiansen IS. HPV mRNA tests for the detection of cervical intraepithelial neoplasia: a systematic review. Gynecol Oncol 2011; 120(3): 430-8.
[http://dx.doi.org/10.1016/j.ygyno.2010.11.013] [PMID: 21130490]

[61] Coquillard G, Palao B, Patterson BK. Quantification of intracellular HPV E6/E7 mRNA expression increases the specificity and positive predictive value of cervical cancer screening compared to HPV DNA. Gynecol Oncol 2011; 120(1): 89-93.
[http://dx.doi.org/10.1016/j.ygyno.2010.09.013] [PMID: 20950847]

[62] Verdoodt F, Szarewski A, Halfon P, Cuschieri K, Arbyn M. Triage of women with minor abnormal cervical cytology: meta-analysis of the accuracy of an assay targeting messenger ribonucleic acid of 5 high-risk human papillomavirus types. Cancer Cytopathol 2013; 121(12): 675-87. [http://dx.doi.org/10.1002/cncy.21325] [PMID: 23881840]

[63] Hudelist G, Manavi M, Pischinger KI, *et al.* Physical state and expression of HPV DNA in benign and dysplastic cervical tissue: different levels of viral integration are correlated with lesion grade. Gynecol Oncol 2004; 92(3): 873-80. [http://dx.doi.org/10.1016/j.ygyno.2003.11.035] [PMID: 14984955]

[64] Manawapat A, Stubenrauch F, Russ R, Munk C, Kjaer SK, Iftner T. Physical state and viral load as predictive biomarkersfor persistence and progression of HPV16-positive cervical lesions: results from a population based long-term prospective cohort study. Am J Cancer Res 2012; 2(2): 192-203. [PMID: 22432058]

[65] Marongiu L, Godi A, Parry JV, Beddows S. Human Papillomavirus 16, 18, 31 and 45 viral load, integration and methylation status stratified by cervical disease stage. BMC Cancer 2014; 14: 384. [http://dx.doi.org/10.1186/1471-2407-14-384] [PMID: 24885011]

[66] Leonard SM, Pereira M, Roberts S, *et al.* Evidence of disrupted high-risk human papillomavirus DNA in morphologically normal cervices of older women. Sci Rep 2016; 6: 20847. [http://dx.doi.org/10.1038/srep20847] [PMID: 26875676]

[67] Mulvany NJ, Allen DG, Wilson SM. Diagnostic utility of p16INK4a: a reappraisal of its use in cervical biopsies. Pathology 2008; 40(4): 335-44. [http://dx.doi.org/10.1080/00313020802035907] [PMID: 18446622]

[68] Uijterwaal MH, Polman NJ, Witte BI, *et al.* Triaging HPV-positive women with normal cytology by p16/Ki-67 dual-stained cytology testing: baseline and longitudinal data. Int J Cancer 2015; 136(10): 2361-8. [http://dx.doi.org/10.1002/ijc.29290] [PMID: 25345358]

[69] Leonard SM, Wei W, Collins SI, *et al.* Oncogenic human papillomavirus imposes an instructive pattern of DNA methylation changes which parallel the natural history of cervical HPV infection in young women. Carcinogenesis 2012; 33(7): 1286-93. [http://dx.doi.org/10.1093/carcin/bgs157] [PMID: 22552403]

[70] Pett MR, Alazawi WO, Roberts I, *et al.* Acquisition of high-level chromosomal instability is associated with integration of human papillomavirus type 16 in cervical keratinocytes. Cancer Res 2004; 64(4): 1359-68. [http://dx.doi.org/10.1158/0008-5472.CAN-03-3214] [PMID: 14973079]

[71] Deftereos G, Corrie SR, Feng Q, *et al.* Expression of mir-21 and mir-143 in cervical specimens ranging from histologically normal through to invasive cervical cancer. PLoS One 2011; 6(12): e28423. [http://dx.doi.org/10.1371/journal.pone.0028423] [PMID: 22194833]

[72] Kudela E, Holubekova V, Farkasova A, Danko J. Determination of malignant potential of cervical intraepithelial neoplasia. Tumour Biol 2016; 37(2): 1521-5. [http://dx.doi.org/10.1007/s13277-015-4677-3] [PMID: 26695139]

[73] Song K, Nimse SB, An H, Kim T. HPV genotyping 9G membrane test: a point-of-care diagnostic platform. Sensors (Basel) 2014; 14(10): 19162-75. [http://dx.doi.org/10.3390/s141019162] [PMID: 25320905]

[74] Houldsworth J. FHACT: the FISH-based HPV-associated cancer test that detects nonrandom gain at four genomic loci as biomarkers of disease progression. Expert Rev Mol Diagn 2014; 14(8): 921-34. [http://dx.doi.org/10.1586/14737159.2014.965685] [PMID: 25308338]

[75] Olthof NC, Huebbers CU, Kolligs J, *et al.* Viral load, gene expression and mapping of viral integration sites in HPV16-associated HNSCC cell lines. Int J Cancer 2015; 136(5): E207-18.

[http://dx.doi.org/10.1002/ijc.29112] [PMID: 25082736]

[76] Gimenes F, Souza RP, de Abreu AL, Pereira MW, Consolaro ME, da Silva VR. Simultaneous detection of human papillomavirus integration and c-MYC gene amplification in cervical lesions: an emerging marker for the risk to progression. Arch Gynecol Obstet 2016; 293(4): 857-63. [http://dx.doi.org/10.1007/s00404-015-3870-3] [PMID: 26315473]

[77] De Marchi Triglia R, Metze K, Zeferino LC, Lucci De Angelo Andrade LA. HPV *in situ* hybridization signal patterns as a marker for cervical intraepithelial neoplasia progression. Gynecol Oncol 2009; 112(1): 114-8. [http://dx.doi.org/10.1016/j.ygyno.2008.09.047] [PMID: 19007972]

[78] Hopman AH, Kamps MA, Smedts F, Speel EJ, Herrington CS, Ramaekers FC. HPV in situ hybridization: impact of different protocols on the detection of integrated HPV. Int J Cancer 2005; 115(3): 419-28. [http://dx.doi.org/10.1002/ijc.20862] [PMID: 15688369]

[79] Theelen W, Litjens RJ, Vinokurova S, *et al.* Human papillomavirus multiplex ligation-dependent probe amplification assay for the assessment of viral load, integration, and gain of telomerase-related genes in cervical malignancies. Hum Pathol 2013; 44(11): 2410-8. [http://dx.doi.org/10.1016/j.humpath.2013.04.026] [PMID: 23968641]

[80] Sokolova I, Algeciras-Schimnich A, Song M, *et al.* Chromosomal biomarkers for detection of human papillomavirus associated genomic instability in epithelial cells of cervical cytology specimens. J Mol Diagn 2007; 9(5): 604-11. [http://dx.doi.org/10.2353/jmoldx.2007.070007] [PMID: 17975027]

[81] Luft F, Klaes R, Nees M, *et al.* Detection of integrated papillomavirus sequences by ligation-mediated PCR (DIPS-PCR) and molecular characterization in cervical cancer cells. Int J Cancer 2001; 92(1): 9-17. [http://dx.doi.org/10.1002/1097-0215(200102)9999:9999<::AID-IJC1144>3.0.CO;2-L] [PMID: 11279600]

[82] Zaravinos A, Mammas IN, Sourvinos G, Spandidos DA. Molecular detection methods of human papillomavirus (HPV). Int J Biol Markers 2009; 24(4): 215-22. [http://dx.doi.org/10.5301/JBM.2010.754] [PMID: 20108214]

[83] Sarkar G, Turner RT, Bolander ME. Restriction-site PCR: a direct method of unknown sequence retrieval adjacent to a known locus by using universal primers. PCR Methods Appl 1993; 2(4): 318-22. [http://dx.doi.org/10.1101/gr.2.4.318] [PMID: 8391890]

[84] Thorland EC, Myers SL, Gostout BS, Smith DI. Common fragile sites are preferential targets for HPV16 integrations in cervical tumors. Oncogene 2003; 22(8): 1225-37. [http://dx.doi.org/10.1038/sj.onc.1206170] [PMID: 12606949]

[85] Thorland EC, Myers SL, Persing DH, *et al.* Human papillomavirus type 16 integrations in cervical tumors frequently occur in common fragile sites. Cancer Res 2000; 60(21): 5916-21. [PMID: 11085503]

[86] Tsakogiannis D, Bletsa M, Kyriakopoulou Z, *et al.* Identification of rearranged sequences of HPV16 DNA in precancerous and cervical cancer cases. Mol Cell Probes 2016; 30(1): 6-12. [http://dx.doi.org/10.1016/j.mcp.2015.11.004] [PMID: 26627739]

[87] Lu X, Lin Q, Lin M, *et al.* Multiple-integrations of HPV16 genome and altered transcription of viral oncogenes and cellular genes are associated with the development of cervical cancer. PLoS One 2014; 9(7): e97588. [http://dx.doi.org/10.1371/journal.pone.0097588] [PMID: 24992025]

[88] Klaes R, Woerner SM, Ridder R, *et al.* Detection of high-risk cervical intraepithelial neoplasia and cervical cancer by amplification of transcripts derived from integrated papillomavirus oncogenes. Cancer Res 1999; 59(24): 6132-6.

[PMID: 10626803]

[89] Monnier-Benoit S, Dalstein V, Riethmuller D, Lalaoui N, Mougin C, Prétet JL. Dynamics of HPV16 DNA load reflect the natural history of cervical HPV-associated lesions. J Clin Virol 2006; 35(3): 270-7.
[http://dx.doi.org/10.1016/j.jcv.2005.09.001] [PMID: 16214397]

[90] Hesselink AT, van Ham MA, Heideman DA, *et al.* Comparison of GP5+/6+-PCR and SPF10-line blot assays for detection of high-risk human papillomavirus in samples from women with normal cytology results who develop grade 3 cervical intraepithelial neoplasia. J Clin Microbiol 2008; 46(10): 3215-21.
[http://dx.doi.org/10.1128/JCM.00476-08] [PMID: 18685007]

[91] Xi LF, Koutsky LA, Castle PE, *et al.* Human papillomavirus type 18 DNA load and 2-year cumulative diagnoses of cervical intraepithelial neoplasia grades 2-3. J Natl Cancer Inst 2009; 101(3): 153-61.
[http://dx.doi.org/10.1093/jnci/djn461] [PMID: 19176451]

[92] Lowe B, O'Neil D, Loeffert D, Nazarenko I. Distribution of Human papillomavirus load in clinical specimens. J Virol Methods 2011; 173(1): 150-2.
[http://dx.doi.org/10.1016/j.jviromet.2011.01.018] [PMID: 21295613]

[93] Gravitt PE, Kovacic MB, Herrero R, *et al.* High load for most high risk human papillomavirus genotypes is associated with prevalent cervical cancer precursors but only HPV16 load predicts the development of incident disease. Int J Cancer 2007; 121(12): 2787-93.
[http://dx.doi.org/10.1002/ijc.23012] [PMID: 17722112]

[94] Peitsaro P, Johansson B, Syrjänen S. Integrated human papillomavirus type 16 is frequently found in cervical cancer precursors as demonstrated by a novel quantitative real-time PCR technique. J Clin Microbiol 2002; 40(3): 886-91.
[http://dx.doi.org/10.1128/JCM.40.3.886-891.2002] [PMID: 11880410]

[95] Cricca M, Venturoli S, Leo E, Costa S, Musiani M, Zerbini M. Disruption of HPV 16 E1 and E2 genes in precancerous cervical lesions. J Virol Methods 2009; 158(1-2): 180-3.
[http://dx.doi.org/10.1016/j.jviromet.2009.01.005] [PMID: 19187786]

[96] Tsakogiannis D, Gortsilas P, Kyriakopoulou Z, *et al.* Sites of disruption within E1 and E2 genes of HPV16 and association with cervical dysplasia. J Med Virol 2015; 87(11): 1973-80.
[http://dx.doi.org/10.1002/jmv.24256] [PMID: 25959607]

[97] Yoshida T, Sano T, Kanuma T, *et al.* Quantitative real-time polymerase chain reaction analysis of the type distribution, viral load, and physical status of human papillomavirus in liquid-based cytology samples from cervical lesions. Int J Gynecol Cancer 2008; 18(1): 121-7.
[http://dx.doi.org/10.1111/j.1525-1438.2007.00979.x] [PMID: 17506843]

[98] Chen CY. DNA polymerases drive DNA sequencing-by-synthesis technologies: both past and present. Front Microbiol 2014; 5: 305.
[http://dx.doi.org/10.3389/fmicb.2014.00305] [PMID: 25009536]

[99] Soper SA, Williams DC, Xu Y, *et al.* Sanger DNA-sequencing reactions performed in a solid-phase nanoreactor directly coupled to capillary gel electrophoresis. Anal Chem 1998; 70(19): 4036-43.
[http://dx.doi.org/10.1021/ac980288z] [PMID: 9784746]

[100] Datta S, Budhauliya R, Das B, Chatterjee S, Vanlalhmuaka , Veer V. Next-generation sequencing in clinical virology: Discovery of new viruses. World J Virol 2015; 4(3): 265-76.
[http://dx.doi.org/10.5501/wjv.v4.i3.265] [PMID: 26279987]

[101] Akagi K, Li J, Broutian TR, *et al.* Genome-wide analysis of HPV integration in human cancers reveals recurrent, focal genomic instability. Genome Res 2014; 24(2): 185-99.
[http://dx.doi.org/10.1101/gr.164806.113] [PMID: 24201445]

[102] Wang L, Dai SZ, Chu HJ, Cui HF, Xu XY. Integration sites and genotype distributions of human papillomavirus in cervical intraepithelial neoplasia. Asian Pac J Cancer Prev 2013; 14(6): 3837-41.
[http://dx.doi.org/10.7314/APJCP.2013.14.6.3837] [PMID: 23886192]

[103] Liu L, Li Y, Li S, *et al.* Comparison of next-generation sequencing systems. J Biomed Biotechnol 2012; 2012: 251364.

[104] Buermans HP, den Dunnen JT. Next generation sequencing technology: Advances and applications. Biochim Biophys Acta 2014; 1842(10): 1932-41. [http://dx.doi.org/10.1016/j.bbadis.2014.06.015] [PMID: 24995601]

[105] Mardis ER. The impact of next-generation sequencing technology on genetics. Trends Genet 2008; 24(3): 133-41. [http://dx.doi.org/10.1016/j.tig.2007.12.007] [PMID: 18262675]

[106] Goodwin S, McPherson JD, McCombie WR. Coming of age: ten years of next-generation sequencing technologies. Nat Rev Genet 2016; 17(6): 333-51. [http://dx.doi.org/10.1038/nrg.2016.49] [PMID: 27184599]

[107] Valdez M, Jeronimo J, Bansil P, *et al.* Effectiveness of novel, lower cost molecular human papillomavirus-based tests for cervical cancer screening in rural china. Int J Cancer 2016; 138(6): 1453-61. [http://dx.doi.org/10.1002/ijc.29877] [PMID: 26421807]

[108] Naucler P, Ryd W, Törnberg S, *et al.* Human papillomavirus and Papanicolaou tests to screen for cervical cancer. N Engl J Med 2007; 357(16): 1589-97. [http://dx.doi.org/10.1056/NEJMoa073204] [PMID: 17942872]

[109] Sankaranarayanan R, Nene BM, Shastri SS, *et al.* HPV screening for cervical cancer in rural India. N Engl J Med 2009; 360(14): 1385-94. [http://dx.doi.org/10.1056/NEJMoa0808516] [PMID: 19339719]

[110] Dillner J, Rebolj M, Birembaut P, *et al.* Long term predictive values of cytology and human papillomavirus testing in cervical cancer screening: joint European cohort study. BMJ 2008; 337: a1754. [http://dx.doi.org/10.1136/bmj.a1754] [PMID: 18852164]

[111] Castle PE, Glass AG, Rush BB, *et al.* Clinical human papillomavirus detection forecasts cervical cancer risk in women over 18 years of follow-up. J Clin Oncol 2012; 30(25): 3044-50. [http://dx.doi.org/10.1200/JCO.2011.38.8389] [PMID: 22851570]

[112] Kjær SK, Frederiksen K, Munk C, Iftner T. Long-term absolute risk of cervical intraepithelial neoplasia grade 3 or worse following human papillomavirus infection: role of persistence. J Natl Cancer Inst 2010; 102(19): 1478-88. [http://dx.doi.org/10.1093/jnci/djq356] [PMID: 20841605]

[113] Cuzick J, Bergeron C, von Knebel Doeberitz M, *et al.* New technologies and procedures for cervical cancer screening. Vaccine 2012; 30(5) (Suppl. 5): F107-16. [http://dx.doi.org/10.1016/j.vaccine.2012.05.088] [PMID: 23199953]

[114] Cuzick J, Cadman L, Mesher D, *et al.* Comparing the performance of six human papillomavirus tests in a screening population. Br J Cancer 2013; 108(4): 908-13. [http://dx.doi.org/10.1038/bjc.2013.22] [PMID: 23370211]

[115] Cuzick J, Myers O, Hunt WC, *et al.* Human papillomavirus testing 2007-2012: co-testing and triage utilization and impact on subsequent clinical management. Int J Cancer 2015; 136(12): 2854-63. [http://dx.doi.org/10.1002/ijc.29337] [PMID: 25447979]

[116] Giorgi Rossi P, Carozzi F, Collina G, *et al.* HPV testing is an efficient management choice for women with inadequate liquid-based cytology in cervical cancer screening. Am J Clin Pathol 2012; 138(1): 65-71. [http://dx.doi.org/10.1309/AJCP6J2OEFOYTRFD] [PMID: 22706859]

[117] Schiffman M, Wentzensen N, Wacholder S, Kinney W, Gage JC, Castle PE. Human papillomavirus testing in the prevention of cervical cancer. J Natl Cancer Inst 2011; 103(5): 368-83. [http://dx.doi.org/10.1093/jnci/djq562] [PMID: 21282563]

[118] Cubie HA, Cuschieri K. Understanding HPV tests and their appropriate applications. Cytopathology 2013; 24(5): 289-308.
[PMID: 23998275]

[119] Litjens RJ, Hopman AH, van de Vijver KK, Ramaekers FC, Kruitwagen RF, Kruse AJ. Molecular biomarkers in cervical cancer diagnosis: a critical appraisal. Expert Opin Med Diagn 2013; 7(4): 365-77.
[http://dx.doi.org/10.1517/17530059.2013.808621] [PMID: 23777477]

[120] Schweizer J, Lu PS, Mahoney CW, *et al.* Feasibility study of a human papillomavirus E6 oncoprotein test for diagnosis of cervical precancer and cancer. J Clin Microbiol 2010; 48(12): 4646-8.
[http://dx.doi.org/10.1128/JCM.01315-10] [PMID: 20926711]

[121] Zhao FH, Jeronimo J, Qiao YL, *et al.* An evaluation of novel, lower-cost molecular screening tests for human papillomavirus in rural China. Cancer Prev Res (Phila) 2013; 6(9): 938-48.
[http://dx.doi.org/10.1158/1940-6207.CAPR-13-0091] [PMID: 23878179]

[122] Sherman ME, Lorincz AT, Scott DR, *et al.* Baseline cytology, human papillomavirus testing, and risk for cervical neoplasia: a 10-year cohort analysis. J Natl Cancer Inst 2003; 95(1): 46-52.
[http://dx.doi.org/10.1093/jnci/95.1.46] [PMID: 12509400]

[123] Wentzensen N, Wacholder S. From differences in means between cases and controls to risk stratification: a business plan for biomarker development. Cancer Discov 2013; 3(2): 148-57.
[http://dx.doi.org/10.1158/2159-8290.CD-12-0196] [PMID: 23299199]

[124] Hwang SJ, Shroyer KR. Biomarkers of cervical dysplasia and carcinoma. J Oncol 2012; 2012: 507286.

[125] Bozzetti M, Nonnenmacher B, Mielzinska I, *et al.* Comparison between hybrid capture II and polymerase chain reaction results among women at low risk for cervical cancer. Ann Epidemiol 2000; 10(7): 466.
[http://dx.doi.org/10.1016/S1047-2797(00)00147-2] [PMID: 11018389]

[126] Origoni M, Carminati G, Rolla S, *et al.* Human papillomavirus viral load expressed as relative light units (RLU) correlates with the presence and grade of preneoplastic lesions of the uterine cervix in atypical squamous cells of undetermined significance (ASCUS) cytology. Eur J Clin Microbiol Infect Dis 2012; 31(9): 2401-6.
[http://dx.doi.org/10.1007/s10096-012-1582-1] [PMID: 22382821]

[127] Iftner T, Villa LL. Chapter 12: Human papillomavirus technologies. J Natl Cancer Inst Monogr 2003; 31(31): 80-8.
[http://dx.doi.org/10.1093/oxfordjournals.jncimonographs.a003487] [PMID: 12807950]

[128] Halec G, Alemany L, Lloveras B, *et al.* Pathogenic role of the eight probably/possibly carcinogenic HPV types 26, 53, 66, 67, 68, 70, 73 and 82 in cervical cancer. J Pathol 2014; 234(4): 441-51.
[http://dx.doi.org/10.1002/path.4405] [PMID: 25043390]

[129] Wright TC Jr, Schiffman M. Adding a test for human papillomavirus DNA to cervical-cancer screening. N Engl J Med 2003; 348(6): 489-90.
[http://dx.doi.org/10.1056/NEJMp020178] [PMID: 12571255]

[130] Frazer IH, Leggatt GR, Mattarollo SR. Prevention and treatment of papillomavirus-related cancers through immunization. Annu Rev Immunol 2011; 29: 111-38.
[http://dx.doi.org/10.1146/annurev-immunol-031210-101308] [PMID: 21166538]

[131] Otero-Motta AP, Ordóñez JL, González-Celador R, *et al.* Prevalence of human papillomavirus genotypes in cytologic abnormalities from unvaccinated women living in north-western Spain. APMIS 2011; 119(3): 204-15.
[http://dx.doi.org/10.1111/j.1600-0463.2010.02711.x] [PMID: 21284738]

[132] Lorincz AT. Sexually transmissible viral pathogens: human papillomaviruses and herpes simplex viruses.Nucleic Acid Testing for Human Disease. Boca Raton: Taylor Francis CRC Press 2006; pp. 244-73.

[http://dx.doi.org/10.1201/9781420016888]

[133] Ratnam S, Coutlee F, Fontaine D, *et al.* Aptima HPV E6/E7 mRNA test is as sensitive as Hybrid Capture 2 Assay but more specific at detecting cervical precancer and cancer. J Clin Microbiol 2011; 49(2): 557-64.
[http://dx.doi.org/10.1128/JCM.02147-10] [PMID: 21147950]

[134] Luu HN, Dahlstrom KR, Mullen PD, VonVille HM, Scheurer ME. Comparison of the accuracy of Hybrid Capture II and polymerase chain reaction in detecting clinically important cervical dysplasia: a systematic review and meta-analysis. Cancer Med 2013; 2(3): 367-90.
[http://dx.doi.org/10.1002/cam4.83] [PMID: 23930214]

[135] Meijer CJ, Berkhof J, Castle PE, *et al.* Guidelines for human papillomavirus DNA test requirements for primary cervical cancer screening in women 30 years and older. Int J Cancer 2009; 124(3): 516-20.
[http://dx.doi.org/10.1002/ijc.24010] [PMID: 18973271]

[136] Castle PE, Schiffman M, Wheeler CM. Hybrid capture 2 viral load and the 2-year cumulative risk of cervical intraepithelial neoplasia grade 3 or cancer. Am J Obstet Gynecol 2004; 191(5): 1590-7.
[http://dx.doi.org/10.1016/j.ajog.2004.05.018] [PMID: 15547529]

[137] Gravitt PE, Belinson JL, Salmeron J, Shah KV. Looking ahead: a case for human papillomavirus testing of self-sampled vaginal specimens as a cervical cancer screening strategy. Int J Cancer 2011; 129(3): 517-27.
[http://dx.doi.org/10.1002/ijc.25974] [PMID: 21384341]

[138] Fotiadis DI. HPV Detection Methods, Handbook of Research on Trends in the Diagnosis and Treatment of Chronic Conditions. Hershey, Pennsylvania, USA: IGI Global 2016; pp. 99-132.
[http://dx.doi.org/10.4018/978-1-4666-8828-5]

[139] Castle PE, Wheeler CM, Solomon D, Schiffman M, Peyton CL. Interlaboratory reliability of Hybrid Capture 2. Am J Clin Pathol 2004; 122(2): 238-45.
[http://dx.doi.org/10.1309/BA43HMCAJ26VWQH3] [PMID: 15323141]

[140] Quint WG, Pagliusi SR, Lelie N, de Villiers EM, Wheeler CM. Results of the first World Health Organization international collaborative study of detection of human papillomavirus DNA. J Clin Microbiol 2006; 44(2): 571-9.
[http://dx.doi.org/10.1128/JCM.44.2.571-579.2006] [PMID: 16455914]

[141] Castle PE, Cox JT, Jeronimo J, *et al.* An analysis of high-risk human papillomavirus DNA-negative cervical precancers in the ASCUS-LSIL Triage Study (ALTS). Obstet Gynecol 2008; 111(4): 847-56.
[http://dx.doi.org/10.1097/AOG.0b013e318168460b] [PMID: 18378743]

[142] Castle PE, Gutierrez EC, Leitch SV, *et al.* Evaluation of a new DNA test for detection of carcinogenic human papillomavirus. J Clin Microbiol 2011; 49(8): 3029-32.
[http://dx.doi.org/10.1128/JCM.00422-11] [PMID: 21632892]

[143] Youens KE, Hosler GA, Washington PJ, Jenevein EP, Murphy KM. Clinical experience with the Cervista HPV HR assay: correlation of cytology and HPV status from 56,501 specimens. J Mol Diagn 2011; 13(2): 160-6.
[http://dx.doi.org/10.1016/j.jmoldx.2010.11.016] [PMID: 21354050]

[144] Castle PE, Solomon D, Wheeler CM, Gravitt PE, Wacholder S, Schiffman M. Human papillomavirus genotype specificity of hybrid capture 2. J Clin Microbiol 2008; 46(8): 2595-604.
[http://dx.doi.org/10.1128/JCM.00824-08] [PMID: 18579716]

[145] Goldstone SE, Lowe B, Rothmann T, Nazarenko I. Evaluation of the hybrid capture 2 assay for detecting anal high-grade dysplasia. Int J Cancer 2012; 131(7): 1641-8.
[http://dx.doi.org/10.1002/ijc.27431] [PMID: 22234750]

[146] Thai H, Rangwala S, Gay T, *et al.* An HPV 16, 18, and 45 genotyping test based on Hybrid Capture technology. J Clin Virol 2009; 45(1) (Suppl. 1): S93-7.
[http://dx.doi.org/10.1016/S1386-6532(09)70014-9] [PMID: 19651375]

[147] Day SP, Hudson A, Mast A, *et al.* Analytical performance of the Investigational Use Only Cervista HPV HR test as determined by a multi-center study. J Clin Virol 2009; 45(1) (Suppl. 1): S63-72. [http://dx.doi.org/10.1016/S1386-6532(09)70010-1] [PMID: 19651371]

[148] Einstein MH, Martens MG, Garcia FA, *et al.* Clinical validation of the Cervista HPV HR and 16/18 genotyping tests for use in women with ASC-US cytology. Gynecol Oncol 2010; 118(2): 116-22. [http://dx.doi.org/10.1016/j.ygyno.2010.04.013] [PMID: 20488510]

[149] Kinney W, Stoler MH, Castle PE. Special commentary: patient safety and the next generation of HPV DNA tests. Am J Clin Pathol 2010; 134(2): 193-9. [http://dx.doi.org/10.1309/AJCPRI8XPQUEAA3K] [PMID: 20660320]

[150] Tao K, Yang J, Yang H, *et al.* Comparative study of the cervista and hybrid capture 2 methods in detecting high-risk human papillomavirus in cervical lesions. Diagn Cytopathol 2014; 42(3): 213-7. [http://dx.doi.org/10.1002/dc.23025] [PMID: 23904341]

[151] Johnson LR, Starkey CR, Palmer J, *et al.* A comparison of two methods to determine the presence of high-risk HPV cervical infections. Am J Clin Pathol 2008; 130(3): 401-8. [http://dx.doi.org/10.1309/4DXEAFG2JXYF34N3] [PMID: 18701413]

[152] Boehmer G, Wang L, Iftner A, *et al.* A population-based observational study comparing Cervista and Hybrid Capture 2 methods: improved relative specificity of the Cervista assay by increasing its cut-off. BMC Infect Dis 2014; 14: 674. [http://dx.doi.org/10.1186/s12879-014-0674-1] [PMID: 25487281]

[153] Quigley NB, Potter NT, Chivukula M, Knight MZ, Welch JR, Olson MC. Rate of detection of high-risk HPV with two assays in women ≥ 30 years of age. J Clin Virol 2011; 52(1): 23-7. [http://dx.doi.org/10.1016/j.jcv.2011.05.014] [PMID: 21724457]

[154] Bartholomew DA, Luff RD, Quigley NB, Curtis M, Olson MC. Analytical performance of Cervista HPV 16/18 genotyping test for cervical cytology samples. J Clin Virol 2011; 51(1): 38-43. [http://dx.doi.org/10.1016/j.jcv.2011.01.016] [PMID: 21376660]

[155] Valentine K, Vanden Broeck D, Benoy I, Truyens M, Bogers J. Cytology at the time of HPV: Some things to think about when discussing HPV. Acta Cytol 2016; 60(6): 527-33. [http://dx.doi.org/10.1159/000450821] [PMID: 27816982]

[156] Blatt AJ, Kennedy R, Luff R, Austin RM, Rabin D. Blatt AJ, Kennedy R, Luff R, Austin RM, Rabin DS. Comparison of cervical cancer screening results among 256,648 women in multiple clinical practices. Cancer Cytopathology 2015. doi:10.1002/cncy.21544. Cancer Cytopathol 2016; 124(5): 362-3. [http://dx.doi.org/10.1002/cncy.21616] [PMID: 27176737]

[157] Heideman DA, Hesselink AT, Berkhof J, *et al.* Clinical validation of the cobas 4800 HPV test for cervical screening purposes. J Clin Microbiol 2011; 49(11): 3983-5. [http://dx.doi.org/10.1128/JCM.05552-11] [PMID: 21880968]

[158] Zheng B, Li Z, Griffith CC, *et al.* Prior high-risk HPV testing and Pap test results for 427 invasive cervical cancers in China's largest CAP-certified laboratory. Cancer Cytopathol 2015; 123(7): 428-34. [http://dx.doi.org/10.1002/cncy.21557] [PMID: 25954852]

[159] Tao X, Griffith CC, Zhou X, *et al.* History of high-risk HPV and Pap test results in a large cohort of patients with invasive cervical carcinoma: experience from the largest women's hospital in China. Cancer Cytopathol 2015; 123(7): 421-7. [http://dx.doi.org/10.1002/cncy.21545] [PMID: 25955972]

[160] Bekker JB, John TS, Leiman G. Confirming suboptimal adherence to HPV cotesting guidelines in an academic center in Vermont. Am J Clin Pathol 2013; 139(2): 259-60. [http://dx.doi.org/10.1309/AJCP41LLYKYUGXVD] [PMID: 23355212]

[161] Tatsas AD, Phelan DF, Gravitt PE, Boitnott JK, Clark DP. Practice patterns in cervical cancer screening and human papillomavirus testing. Am J Clin Pathol 2012; 138(2): 223-9.

[http://dx.doi.org/10.1309/AJCPPVX91HQMNYZZ] [PMID: 22904133]

[162] Rao A, Young S, Erlich H, *et al.* Development and characterization of the cobas human papillomavirus test. J Clin Microbiol 2013; 51(5): 1478-84. [http://dx.doi.org/10.1128/JCM.03386-12] [PMID: 23447640]

[163] Kleter B, van Doorn LJ, Schrauwen L, *et al.* Development and clinical evaluation of a highly sensitive PCR-reverse hybridization line probe assay for detection and identification of anogenital human papillomavirus. J Clin Microbiol 1999; 37(8): 2508-17. [PMID: 10405393]

[164] Jacobs MV, Snijders PJ, van den Brule AJ, Helmerhorst TJ, Meijer CJ, Walboomers JM. A general primer $GP5^{+}/GP6(^{+})$-mediated PCR-enzyme immunoassay method for rapid detection of 14 high-risk and 6 low-risk human papillomavirus genotypes in cervical scrapings. J Clin Microbiol 1997; 35(3): 791-5. [PMID: 9041439]

[165] Gravitt PE, Peyton CL, Alessi TQ, *et al.* Improved amplification of genital human papillomaviruses. J Clin Microbiol 2000; 38(1): 357-61. [PMID: 10618116]

[166] Snijders PJ, van den Brule AJ, Meijer CJ. The clinical relevance of human papillomavirus testing: relationship between analytical and clinical sensitivity. J Pathol 2003; 201(1): 1-6. [http://dx.doi.org/10.1002/path.1433] [PMID: 12950011]

[167] Cui M, Chan N, Liu M, *et al.* Clinical performance of Roche Cobas 4800 HPV Test. J Clin Microbiol 2014; 52(6): 2210-1. [http://dx.doi.org/10.1128/JCM.00883-14] [PMID: 24719443]

[168] Castle PE, Eaton B, Reid J, Getman D, Dockter J. Comparison of human papillomavirus detection by Aptima HPV and cobas HPV tests in a population of women referred for colposcopy following detection of atypical squamous cells of undetermined significance by Pap cytology. J Clin Microbiol 2015; 53(4): 1277-81. [http://dx.doi.org/10.1128/JCM.03558-14] [PMID: 25653409]

[169] Karlsen F, Kalantari M, Jenkins A, *et al.* Use of multiple PCR primer sets for optimal detection of human papillomavirus. J Clin Microbiol 1996; 34(9): 2095-100. [PMID: 8862564]

[170] Qu W, Jiang G, Cruz Y, *et al.* PCR detection of human papillomavirus: comparison between MY09/MY11 and GP5+/GP6+ primer systems. J Clin Microbiol 1997; 35(6): 1304-10. [PMID: 9163434]

[171] Mateos ML, Chacón de Antonio J, Rodríguez-Domínguez M, Sanz I, Rubio MD. [Evaluation of a prototype real-time PCR assay for the separate detection of human papilloma virus genotypes 16 and 18 and other high risk human papillomavirus in cervical cancer screening]. Enferm Infecc Microbiol Clin 2011; 29(6): 411-4. [http://dx.doi.org/10.1016/j.eimc.2011.01.007] [PMID: 21435749]

[172] Martínez SB, Palomares JC, Artura A, *et al.* Comparison of the Cobas 4800 Human Papillomavirus test against a combination of the Amplicor Human Papillomavirus and the Linear Array tests for detection of HPV types 16 and 18 in cervical samples. J Virol Methods 2012; 180(1-2): 7-10. [http://dx.doi.org/10.1016/j.jviromet.2011.12.002] [PMID: 22197189]

[173] Rosenblatt C, Lucon AM, Pereyra EA. HPV in Clinical Practice. São Paulo: Atheneu 2005; pp. 25-37.

[174] Wentzensen N, von Knebel Doeberitz M. Biomarkers in cervical cancer screening. Dis Markers 2007; 23(4): 315-30. [http://dx.doi.org/10.1155/2007/678793] [PMID: 17627065]

[175] Dockter J, Schroder A, Eaton B, *et al.* Analytical characterization of the APTIMA HPV Assay. J Clin Virol 2009; 45(1) (Suppl. 1): S39-47.

[http://dx.doi.org/10.1016/S1386-6532(09)70007-1] [PMID: 19651368]

[176] Molden T, Kraus I, Karlsen F, Skomedal H, Nygård JF, Hagmar B. Comparison of human papillomavirus messenger RNA and DNA detection: a cross-sectional study of 4,136 women >30 years of age with a 2-year follow-up of high-grade squamous intraepithelial lesion. Cancer Epidemiol Biomarkers Prev 2005; 14(2): 367-72. [http://dx.doi.org/10.1158/1055-9965.EPI-04-0410] [PMID: 15734959]

[177] Cuschieri K, Wentzensen N. Human papillomavirus mRNA and p16 detection as biomarkers for the improved diagnosis of cervical neoplasia. Cancer Epidemiol Biomarkers Prev 2008; 17(10): 2536-45. [http://dx.doi.org/10.1158/1055-9965.EPI-08-0306] [PMID: 18842994]

[178] Castle PE, Dockter J, Giachetti C, *et al.* A cross-sectional study of a prototype carcinogenic human papillomavirus E6/E7 messenger RNA assay for detection of cervical precancer and cancer. Clin Cancer Res 2007; 13(9): 2599-605. [http://dx.doi.org/10.1158/1078-0432.CCR-06-2881] [PMID: 17473189]

[179] Szarewski A, Mesher D, Cadman L, *et al.* Comparison of predictors for high grade cervical intraepithelial neoplasia in women with abnormal smears. J Clin Microbiol 2012; 50(6): 1867-73. [http://dx.doi.org/10.1128/JCM.00181-12] [PMID: 22422852]

[180] Castle PE, Reid J, Dockter J, Getman D. The reliability of high-risk human papillomavirus detection by Aptima HPV assay in women with ASC-US cytology. J Clin Virol 2015; 69: 52-5. [http://dx.doi.org/10.1016/j.jcv.2015.05.006] [PMID: 26209379]

[181] Schmitt M, Dalstein V, Waterboer T, Clavel C, Gissmann L, Pawlita M. Diagnosing cervical cancer and high-grade precursors by HPV16 transcription patterns. Cancer Res 2010; 70(1): 249-56. [http://dx.doi.org/10.1158/0008-5472.CAN-09-2514] [PMID: 20028865]

[182] Haedicke J, Iftner T. A review of the clinical performance of the Aptima HPV assay. J Clin Virol 2016; 76(1) (Suppl. 1): S40-8. [http://dx.doi.org/10.1016/j.jcv.2015.10.027] [PMID: 26614686]

[183] Darragh TM, Colgan TJ, Thomas Cox J, *et al.* The lower anogenital squamous terminology standardization project for HPV-associated lesions: background and consensus recommendations from the College of American Pathologists and the American Society for Colposcopy and Cervical Pathology. Int J Gynecol Pathol 2013; 32(1): 76-115. [http://dx.doi.org/10.1097/PGP.0b013e31826916c7] [PMID: 23202792]

[184] Stoler M, Colgan TJ, Ferenczy A, *et al.* Squamous cell tumors and precursors.WHO Classification of Tumours of Female Reproductive Organs. Lyon: IARC 2014; pp. 1-12.

[185] Bergeron C, Ronco G, Reuschenbach M, *et al.* The clinical impact of using p16(INK4a) immunochemistry in cervical histopathology and cytology: an update of recent developments. Int J Cancer 2015; 136(12): 2741-51. [http://dx.doi.org/10.1002/ijc.28900] [PMID: 24740700]

[186] Reuschenbach M, Seiz M, von Knebel Doeberitz C, *et al.* Evaluation of cervical cone biopsies for coexpression of p16INK4a and Ki-67 in epithelial cells. Int J Cancer 2012; 130(2): 388-94. [http://dx.doi.org/10.1002/ijc.26017] [PMID: 21387293]

[187] Schmidt D, Bergeron C, Denton KJ, Ridder R. p16/ki-67 dual-stain cytology in the triage of ASCUS and LSIL papanicolaou cytology: results from the European equivocal or mildly abnormal Papanicolaou cytology study. Cancer Cytopathol 2011; 119(3): 158-66. [http://dx.doi.org/10.1002/cncy.20140] [PMID: 21442767]

[188] Waldstrøm M, Christensen RK, Ørnskov D. Evaluation of p16(INK4a)/Ki-67 dual stain in comparison with an mRNA human papillomavirus test on liquid-based cytology samples with low-grade squamous intraepithelial lesion. Cancer Cytopathol 2013; 121(3): 136-45. [http://dx.doi.org/10.1002/cncy.21233] [PMID: 22987560]

[189] Ziemke P, Marquardt K, Griesser H. Predictive value of the combined p16 and Ki-67

immunocytochemistry in low-grade squamous intraepithelial lesions. Acta Cytol 2014; 58(5): 489-94. [http://dx.doi.org/10.1159/000367838] [PMID: 25342512]

[190] Bergeron C, Ikenberg H, Sideri M, *et al.* Prospective evaluation of p16/Ki-67 dual-stained cytology for managing women with abnormal Papanicolaou cytology: PALMS study results. Cancer Cytopathol 2015; 123(6): 373-81.
[http://dx.doi.org/10.1002/cncy.21542] [PMID: 25891096]

[191] Ronco G, Meijer CJ, Snijders PJ, Cuzick J. screening for cervical cancer with primary testing for human papillomavirus; in Anttila A, Arbyn M, de Vuyst H, Dillner J, Dillner L, Franceschi S, Patnick J, Ronco G, Segnan N, Suonio E, Tornberg S, von Karsa L (eds): Supplements to European Guidelines for Quality Assurance in Cervical Cancer Screening, ed 2-Supplements. Luxembourg, European Commission 2015.

[192] Bergeron C, Giorgi-Rossi P, Cas F, *et al.* Informed cytology for triaging HPV-positive women: substudy nested in the NTCC randomized controlled trial. J Natl Cancer Inst 2015; 107(2): dju423.
[http://dx.doi.org/10.1093/jnci/dju423] [PMID: 25568167]

[193] Carozzi F, Gillio-Tos A, Confortini M, *et al.* Risk of high-grade cervical intraepithelial neoplasia during follow-up in HPV-positive women according to baseline p16-INK4A results: a prospective analysis of a nested substudy of the NTCC randomised controlled trial. Lancet Oncol 2013; 14(2): 168-76.
[http://dx.doi.org/10.1016/S1470-2045(12)70529-6] [PMID: 23261355]

[194] Endo F, Tabata T, Sadato D, *et al.* Development of a simple and quick immunochromatography method for detection of anti-HPV-16/-18 antibodies. PLoS One 2017; 12(2): e0171314.
[http://dx.doi.org/10.1371/journal.pone.0171314] [PMID: 28158224]

[195] Wentzensen N, Rodriguez AC, Viscidi R, *et al.* A competitive serological assay shows naturally acquired immunity to human papillomavirus infections in the Guanacaste Natural History Study. J Infect Dis 2011; 204(1): 94-102.
[http://dx.doi.org/10.1093/infdis/jir209] [PMID: 21628663]

[196] Dobson SR, McNeil S, Dionne M, *et al.* Immunogenicity of 2 doses of HPV vaccine in younger adolescents vs 3 doses in young women: a randomized clinical trial. JAMA 2013; 309(17): 1793-802.
[http://dx.doi.org/10.1001/jama.2013.1625] [PMID: 23632723]

[197] Schiller JT, Lowy DR. Immunogenicity testing in human papillomavirus virus-like-particle vaccine trials. J Infect Dis 2009; 200(2): 166-71.
[http://dx.doi.org/10.1086/599988] [PMID: 19519255]

[198] Kollmann TR, Marchant A. Towards predicting protective vaccine responses in the very young. Trends Immunol 2016; 37(8): 523-34.
[http://dx.doi.org/10.1016/j.it.2016.05.005] [PMID: 27344245]

[199] Naud PS, Roteli-Martins CM, De Carvalho NS, *et al.* Sustained efficacy, immunogenicity, and safety of the HPV-16/18 AS04-adjuvanted vaccine: final analysis of a long-term follow-up study up to 9.4 years post-vaccination. Hum Vaccin Immunother 2014; 10(8): 2147-62.
[http://dx.doi.org/10.4161/hv.29532] [PMID: 25424918]

[200] Nygård M, Saah A, Munk C, *et al.* Evaluation of the long-term anti-human papillomavirus 6 (HPV6), 11, 16, and 18 immune responses generated by the Quadrivalent HPV vaccine. Clin Vaccine Immunol 2015; 22(8): 943-8.
[http://dx.doi.org/10.1128/CVI.00133-15] [PMID: 26084514]

[201] Lehtinen M, Paavonen J, Wheeler CM, *et al.* Overall efficacy of HPV-16/18 AS04-adjuvanted vaccine against grade 3 or greater cervical intraepithelial neoplasia: 4-year end-of-study analysis of the randomised, double-blind PATRICIA trial. Lancet Oncol 2012; 13(1): 89-99.
[http://dx.doi.org/10.1016/S1470-2045(11)70286-8] [PMID: 22075171]

[202] Kreimer AR, González P, Katki HA, *et al.* Efficacy of a bivalent HPV 16/18 vaccine against anal HPV 16/18 infection among young women: a nested analysis within the Costa Rica Vaccine Trial. Lancet

Oncol 2011; 12(9): 862-70.
[http://dx.doi.org/10.1016/S1470-2045(11)70213-3] [PMID: 21865087]

[203] Naud PS, Roteli-Martins CM, De Carvalho NS, *et al.* Sustained efficacy, immunogenicity, and safety of the HPV-16/18 AS04-adjuvanted vaccine: final analysis of a long-term follow-up study up to 9.4 years post-vaccination. Hum Vaccin Immunother 2014; 10(8): 2147-62.
[http://dx.doi.org/10.4161/hv.29532] [PMID: 25424918]

[204] Garland SM, Hernandez-Avila M, Wheeler CM, *et al.* Quadrivalent vaccine against human papillomavirus to prevent high-grade cervical lesions. N Engl J Med 2007; 356(19): 1915-27.
[http://dx.doi.org/10.1056/NEJMoa061760] [PMID: 17494925]

[205] Garland SM, Hernandez-Avila M, Wheeler CM, *et al.* Quadrivalent vaccine against human papillomavirus to prevent anogenital diseases. N Engl J Med 2007; 356(19): 1928-43.
[http://dx.doi.org/10.1056/NEJMoa061760] [PMID: 17494926]

[206] Garland SM, Kjaer SK, Muñoz N, *et al.* Impact and effectiveness of the quadrivalent human papillomavirus vaccine: A systematic review of ten years of real-world experience. Clin Infect Dis 2016; 63(4): 519-27.
[http://dx.doi.org/10.1093/cid/ciw354] [PMID: 27230391]

[207] Zhou J, Sun XY, Stenzel DJ, Frazer IH. Expression of vaccinia recombinant HPV 16 L1 and L2 ORF proteins in epithelial cells is sufficient for assembly of HPV virion-like particles. Virology 1991; 185(1): 251-7.
[http://dx.doi.org/10.1016/0042-6822(91)90772-4] [PMID: 1656586]

[208] Kirnbauer R, Booy F, Cheng N, Lowy DR, Schiller JT. Papillomavirus L1 major capsid protein self-assembles into virus-like particles that are highly immunogenic. Proc Natl Acad Sci USA 1992; 89(24): 12180-4.
[http://dx.doi.org/10.1073/pnas.89.24.12180] [PMID: 1334560]

[209] Ruiz W, McClements WL, Jansen KU, Esser MT. Kinetics and isotype profile of antibody responses in rhesus macaques induced following vaccination with HPV 6, 11, 16 and 18 L1-virus-like particles formulated with or without Merck aluminum adjuvant. J Immune Based Ther Vaccines 2005; 3(1): 2.
[http://dx.doi.org/10.1186/1476-8518-3-2] [PMID: 15842730]

[210] Pagliusi SR, Garland SM. International standard reagents for HPV detection. Dis Markers 2007; 23(4): 283-96.
[http://dx.doi.org/10.1155/2007/591826] [PMID: 17627063]

[211] Schiller JT, Castellsagué X, Garland SM. A review of clinical trials of human papillomavirus prophylactic vaccines. Vaccine 2012; 30(5) (Suppl. 5): F123-38.
[http://dx.doi.org/10.1016/j.vaccine.2012.04.108] [PMID: 23199956]

[212] Brown DR, Garland SM, Ferris DG, *et al.* The humoral response to Gardasil over four years as defined by total IgG and competitive Luminex immunoassay. Hum Vaccin 2011; 7(2): 230-8.
[http://dx.doi.org/10.4161/hv.7.2.13948] [PMID: 21307649]

[213] Dessy FJ, Giannini SL, Bougelet CA, *et al.* Correlation between direct ELISA, single epitope-based inhibition ELISA and pseudovirion-based neutralization assay for measuring anti-HPV-16 and anti-HPV-18 antibody response after vaccination with the AS04-adjuvanted HPV-16/18 cervical cancer vaccine. Hum Vaccin 2008; 4(6): 425-34.
[http://dx.doi.org/10.4161/hv.4.6.6912] [PMID: 18948732]

[214] Kemp TJ, García-Piñeres A, Falk RT, *et al.* Evaluation of systemic and mucosal anti-HPV16 and anti-HPV18 antibody responses from vaccinated women. Vaccine 2008; 26(29-30): 3608-16.
[http://dx.doi.org/10.1016/j.vaccine.2008.04.074] [PMID: 18541349]

[215] Paek SH, Lee SH, Cho JH, Kim YS. Development of rapid one-step immunochromatographic assay. Methods 2000; 22(1): 53-60.
[http://dx.doi.org/10.1006/meth.2000.1036] [PMID: 11020318]

[216] Ganguly N, Parihar SP. Human papillomavirus E6 and E7 oncoproteins as risk factors for tumorigenesis. J Biosci 2009; 34(1): 113-23.
[http://dx.doi.org/10.1007/s12038-009-0013-7] [PMID: 19430123]

[217] Yim EK, Park JS. The role of HPV E6 and E7 oncoproteins in HPV-associated cervical carcinogenesis. Cancer Res Treat 2005; 37(6): 319-24.
[http://dx.doi.org/10.4143/crt.2005.37.6.319] [PMID: 19956366]

[218] Sotlar K, Diemer D, Dethleffs A, *et al.* Detection and typing of human papillomavirus by e6 nested multiplex PCR. J Clin Microbiol 2004; 42(7): 3176-84.
[http://dx.doi.org/10.1128/JCM.42.7.3176-3184.2004] [PMID: 15243079]

[219] Tsakogiannis D, Diamantidou V, Toska E, *et al.* Multiplex PCR assay for the rapid identification of human papillomavirus genotypes 16, 18, 45, 35, 66, 33, 51, 58, and 31 in clinical samples. Arch Virol 2015; 160(1): 207-14.
[http://dx.doi.org/10.1007/s00705-014-2261-6] [PMID: 25344303]

[220] de Roda Husman AM, Walboomers JM, van den Brule AJ, Meijer CJ, Snijders PJ. The use of general primers GP5 and GP6 elongated at their 3′ ends with adjacent highly conserved sequences improves human papillomavirus detection by PCR. J Gen Virol 1995; 76(Pt 4): 1057-62.
[http://dx.doi.org/10.1099/0022-1317-76-4-1057] [PMID: 9049358]

[221] Kleter B, van Doorn LJ, Schrauwen L, *et al.* Development and clinical evaluation of a highly sensitive PCR-reverse hybridization line probe assay for detection and identification of anogenital human papillomavirus. J Clin Microbiol 1999; 37(8): 2508-17.
[PMID: 10405393]

[222] Sasagawa T, Minemoto Y, Basha W, *et al.* A new PCR-based assay amplifies the E6-E7 genes of most mucosal human papillomaviruses (HPV). Virus Res 2000; 67(2): 127-39.
[http://dx.doi.org/10.1016/S0168-1702(00)00137-4] [PMID: 10867192]

[223] Lin H, Moh JS, Ou YC, *et al.* A simple method for the detection and genotyping of high-risk human papillomavirus using seminested polymerase chain reaction and reverse hybridization. Gynecol Oncol 2005; 96(1): 84-91.
[http://dx.doi.org/10.1016/j.ygyno.2004.09.043] [PMID: 15589585]

[224] Camargo M, Soto-De Leon S, Sanchez R, *et al.* Detection by PCR of human papillomavirus in Colombia: Comparison of GP5+/6+ and MY09/11 primer sets. J Virol Methods 2011; 178(1-2): 68-74.
[http://dx.doi.org/10.1016/j.jviromet.2011.08.014] [PMID: 21884728]

[225] Depuydt CE, Boulet GA, Horvath CA, Benoy IH, Vereecken AJ, Bogers JJ. Comparison of MY09/11 consensus PCR and type-specific PCRs in the detection of oncogenic HPV types. J Cell Mol Med 2007; 11(4): 881-91.
[http://dx.doi.org/10.1111/j.1582-4934.2007.00073.x] [PMID: 17760847]

[226] Coser J, Boeira TdaR, Fonseca AS, Ikuta N, Lunge VR. Human papillomavirus detection and typing using a nested-PCR-RFLP assay. Braz J Infect Dis 2011; 15(5): 467-72.
[http://dx.doi.org/10.1590/S1413-86702011000500009] [PMID: 22230854]

[227] Carvalho NdeO, del Castillo DM, Perone C, Januário JN, Melo VH, Brasileiro Filho G. Comparison of HPV genotyping by type-specific PCR and sequencing. Mem Inst Oswaldo Cruz 2010; 105(1): 73-8.
[http://dx.doi.org/10.1590/S0074-02762010000100011] [PMID: 20209333]

[228] Shen-Gunther J, Rebeles J. Genotyping human papillomaviruses: development and evaluation of a comprehensive DNA microarray. Gynecol Oncol 2013; 128(3): 433-41.
[http://dx.doi.org/10.1016/j.ygyno.2012.11.028] [PMID: 23200917]

[229] Maver PJ, Poljak M, Seme K, Kocjan BJ. Detection and typing of low-risk human papillomavirus genotypes HPV 6, HPV 11, HPV 42, HPV 43 and HPV 44 by polymerase chain reaction and restriction fragment length polymorphism. J Virol Methods 2010; 169(1): 215-8.
[http://dx.doi.org/10.1016/j.jviromet.2010.07.007] [PMID: 20637805]

[230] Naqvi SH, Wajid S, Mitra AB. Restriction fragment length polymorphism of L1 amplicon using Rsa 1 detects five different human papillomavirus types and their co-infections among women attending a gynaecological outpatient department. J Virol Methods 2004; 117(1): 91-5. [http://dx.doi.org/10.1016/j.jviromet.2003.12.002] [PMID: 15019264]

[231] Militello V, Lavezzo E, Costanzi G, *et al.* Accurate human papillomavirus genotyping by 454 pyrosequencing. Clin Microbiol Infect 2013; 19(10): E428-34. [http://dx.doi.org/10.1111/1469-0691.12219] [PMID: 23573945]

[232] Brandstetter T, Böhmer S, Prucker O, *et al.* A polymer-based DNA biochip platform for human papilloma virus genotyping. J Virol Methods 2010; 163(1): 40-8. [http://dx.doi.org/10.1016/j.jviromet.2009.07.027] [PMID: 19664659]

[233] Ngou J, Gilham C, Omar T, *et al.* Comparison of analytical and clinical performances of the digene HC2 HPV DNA assay and the INNO-LiPA HPV genotyping assay for detecting high-risk HPV infection and cervical neoplasia among HIV-positive African women. J Acquir Immune Defic Syndr 2015; 68(2): 162-8. [http://dx.doi.org/10.1097/QAI.0000000000000428] [PMID: 25394189]

[234] Pista A, Verdasca N, Oliveira A. Clinical performance of the CLART human papillomavirus 2 assay compared with the hybrid capture 2 test. J Med Virol 2011; 83(2): 272-6. [http://dx.doi.org/10.1002/jmv.21952] [PMID: 21181922]

[235] Alberizzi P, Spinillo A, Gardella B, Cesari S, Silini EM. Evaluation of the HPV typing INNO-LiPA EXTRA assay on formalin-fixed paraffin-embedded cervical biopsy samples. J Clin Virol 2014; 61(4): 535-9. [http://dx.doi.org/10.1016/j.jcv.2014.10.016] [PMID: 25464970]

[236] van Hamont D, van Ham MA, Bakkers JM, Massuger LF, Melchers WJ. Evaluation of the SPF10-INNO LiPA human papillomavirus (HPV) genotyping test and the roche linear array HPV genotyping test. J Clin Microbiol 2006; 44(9): 3122-9. [http://dx.doi.org/10.1128/JCM.00517-06] [PMID: 16954236]

[237] Gravitt PE, Schiffman M, Solomon D, Wheeler CM, Castle PE. A comparison of linear array and hybrid capture 2 for detection of carcinogenic human papillomavirus and cervical precancer in ASCUS-LSIL triage study. Cancer Epidemiol Biomarkers Prev 2008; 17(5): 1248-54. [http://dx.doi.org/10.1158/1055-9965.EPI-07-2904] [PMID: 18483347]

[238] Kocjan BJ, Seme K, Poljak M. Comparison of the Abbott RealTime High Risk HPV test and INNO-LiPA HPV Genotyping Extra test for the detection of human papillomaviruses in formalin-fixed, paraffin-embedded cervical cancer specimens. J Virol Methods 2011; 175(1): 117-9. [http://dx.doi.org/10.1016/j.jviromet.2011.04.006] [PMID: 21513740]

[239] Sukasem C, Pairoj W, Saekang N, *et al.* Molecular epidemiology of human papillomavirus genotype in women with high-grade squamous intraepithelial lesion and cervical cancer: will a quadrivalent vaccine be necessary in Thailand? J Med Virol 2011; 83(1): 119-26. [http://dx.doi.org/10.1002/jmv.21948] [PMID: 21108348]

[240] Schopp B, Holz B, Zago M, *et al.* Evaluation of the performance of the novel PapilloCheck HPV genotyping test by comparison with two other genotyping systems and the HC2 test. J Med Virol 2010; 82(4): 605-15. [http://dx.doi.org/10.1002/jmv.21719] [PMID: 20166179]

[241] Lenselink CH, de Bie RP, van Hamont D, *et al.* Detection and genotyping of human papillomavirus in self-obtained cervicovaginal samples by using the FTA cartridge: new possibilities for cervical cancer screening. J Clin Microbiol 2009; 47(8): 2564-70. [http://dx.doi.org/10.1128/JCM.00285-09] [PMID: 19553570]

[242] Schmeink CE, Bekkers RL, Massuger LF, Melchers WJ. The potential role of self-sampling for high-risk human papillomavirus detection in cervical cancer screening. Rev Med Virol 2011; 21(3): 139-53. [http://dx.doi.org/10.1002/rmv.686] [PMID: 21538664]

[243] Dobec M, Bannwart F, Kilgus S, Kaeppeli F, Cassinotti P. Human papillomavirus infection among women with cytological abnormalities in Switzerland investigated by an automated linear array genotyping test. J Med Virol 2011; 83(8): 1370-6.
[http://dx.doi.org/10.1002/jmv.22126] [PMID: 21678440]

[244] Dalstein V, Merlin S, Bali C, Saunier M, Dachez R, Ronsin C. Analytical evaluation of the PapilloCheck test, a new commercial DNA chip for detection and genotyping of papillomavirus in cervical and anal scraps. J Virol Methods 2011; 156(1-2): 77-83.
[http://dx.doi.org/10.1016/j.jviromet.2008.11.002] [PMID: 19041893]

[245] Weaver B, Shew M, Qadadri B, *et al.* Low-level persistence of human papillomavirus 16 DNA in a cohort of closely followed adolescent women. J Med Virol 2011; 83(8): 1362-9.
[http://dx.doi.org/10.1002/jmv.22116] [PMID: 21678439]

[246] Ejegod DM, Rebolj M, Bonde J. Comparison of analytical and clinical performance of CLART HPV2 genotyping assay to Linear Array and Hybrid Capture 2: a split-sample study. BMC Cancer 2015; 15: 216.
[http://dx.doi.org/10.1186/s12885-015-1223-z] [PMID: 25886410]

[247] Crosbie EJ, Bailey A, Sargent A, Gilham C, Peto J, Kitchener HC. The PapilloCheck assay for detection of high-grade cervical intraepithelial neoplasia. J Clin Microbiol 2015; 53(11): 3553-9.
[http://dx.doi.org/10.1128/JCM.01578-15] [PMID: 26338859]

[248] Bryant D, Rai N, Rowlands G, *et al.* Human papillomavirus type distribution in vulval intraepithelial neoplasia determined using PapilloCheck DNA Microarray. J Med Virol 2011; 83(8): 1358-61.
[http://dx.doi.org/10.1002/jmv.22107] [PMID: 21618551]

[249] Didelot MN, Boulle N, Damay A, Costes V, Segondy M. Comparison of the PapilloCheck® assay with the digene HC2 HPV DNA assay for the detection of 13 high-risk human papillomaviruses in cervical and anal scrapes. J Med Virol 2011; 83(8): 1377-82.
[http://dx.doi.org/10.1002/jmv.22148] [PMID: 21678441]

[250] Barcellos RB, Almeida SE, Sperhacke RD, *et al.* Evaluation of a novel microplate colorimetric hybridization genotyping assay for human papillomavirus. J Virol Methods 2011; 177(1): 38-43.
[http://dx.doi.org/10.1016/j.jviromet.2011.06.010] [PMID: 21807028]

[251] Zubach V, Smart G, Ratnam S, Severini A. Novel microsphere-based method for detection and typing of 46 mucosal human papillomavirus types. J Clin Microbiol 2012; 50(2): 460-4.
[http://dx.doi.org/10.1128/JCM.06090-11] [PMID: 22116162]

[252] Oh Y, Bae SM, Kim YW, *et al.* Polymerase chain reaction-based fluorescent Luminex assay to detect the presence of human papillomavirus types. Cancer Sci 2007; 98(4): 549-54.
[http://dx.doi.org/10.1111/j.1349-7006.2007.00427.x] [PMID: 17425592]

[253] Jiang HL, Zhu HH, Zhou LF, Chen F, Chen Z. Genotyping of human papillomavirus in cervical lesions by L1 consensus PCR and the Luminex xMAP system. J Med Microbiol 2006; 55(Pt 6): 715-20.
[http://dx.doi.org/10.1099/jmm.0.46493-0] [PMID: 16687589]

[254] Seme K, Lepej SZ, Lunar MM, *et al.* Digene HPV Genotyping RH Test RUO: comparative evaluation with INNO-LiPA HPV Genotyping Extra Test for detection of 18 high-risk and probable high-risk human papillomavirus genotypes. J Clin Virol 2009; 46(2): 176-9.
[http://dx.doi.org/10.1016/j.jcv.2009.07.017] [PMID: 19683958]

[255] Nogara PR, Gimenes F, Consolaro ME. Distribution of HPV genotypes and HPV-16 and HPV-18 E2 gene disruption in South Brazilian women with cervical abnormalities. Int J Gynaecol Obstet 2012; 117(3): 289-90.
[http://dx.doi.org/10.1016/j.ijgo.2012.01.003] [PMID: 22425011]

[256] Chen L, Watanabe K, Haruyama T, Kobayashi N. Simple and rapid human papillomavirus genotyping method by restriction fragment length polymorphism analysis with two restriction enzymes. J Med

Virol 2013; 85(7): 1229-34.
[http://dx.doi.org/10.1002/jmv.23582] [PMID: 23918541]

[257] Santiago E, Camacho L, Junquera ML, Vázquez F. Full HPV typing by a single restriction enzyme. J Clin Virol 2006; 37(1): 38-46.
[http://dx.doi.org/10.1016/j.jcv.2006.06.001] [PMID: 16861031]

[258] Gimenes F, Medina FS, Abreu AL, *et al.* Sensitive simultaneous detection of seven sexually transmitted agents in semen by multiplex-PCR and of HPV by single PCR. PLoS One 2014; 9(6): e98862.
[http://dx.doi.org/10.1371/journal.pone.0098862] [PMID: 24921247]

[259] Milutin Gasperov N, Sabol I, Matovina M, Spaventi S, Grce M. Detection and typing of human papillomaviruses combining different methods: polymerase chain reaction, restriction fragment length polymorphism, line probe assay and sequencing. Pathol Oncol Res 2008; 14(4): 355-63.
[http://dx.doi.org/10.1007/s12253-008-9084-2] [PMID: 18752054]

[260] Sanger F, Nicklen S, Coulson AR. DNA sequencing with chain-terminating inhibitors. 1977. Biotechnology 1992; 24: 104-8.
[PMID: 1422003]

[261] Wang L, Wang P, Ren Y, *et al.* Prevalence of high-risk human papillomavirus (HR-HPV) genotypes and multiple infections in cervical abnormalities from Northern Xinjiang, China. PLoS One 2016; 11(8): e0160698.
[http://dx.doi.org/10.1371/journal.pone.0160698] [PMID: 27494179]

[262] Smith LM, Sanders JZ, Kaiser RJ, *et al.* Fluorescence detection in automated DNA sequence analysis. Nature 1986; 321(6071): 674-9.
[http://dx.doi.org/10.1038/321674a0] [PMID: 3713851]

[263] Lee LG, Connell CR, Woo SL, *et al.* DNA sequencing with dye-labeled terminators and T7 DNA polymerase: effect of dyes and dNTPs on incorporation of dye-terminators and probability analysis of termination fragments. Nucleic Acids Res 1992; 20(10): 2471-83.
[http://dx.doi.org/10.1093/nar/20.10.2471] [PMID: 1598205]

[264] Novais RC, Thorstenson YR. The evolution of Pyrosequencing® for microbiology: From genes to genomes. J Microbiol Methods 2011; 86(1): 1-7.
[http://dx.doi.org/10.1016/j.mimet.2011.04.006] [PMID: 21514329]

CHAPTER 11

Prevention of HPV-Associated Diseases

Azam Bolhassani* and **Elnaz Agi**

Department of Hepatitis and AIDS, Pasteur Institute of Iran, Tehran, Iran

Abstract: HPV infection as the etiologic agent of cervical cancer and also other epithelial cancers, has led to the development of three FDA-approved prophylactic HPV vaccines composed of virus-like particles (VLPs). Development of prophylactic HPV vaccines could decrease HPV-associated diseases especially HPV-16 and -18 in the world. Recently, in order to enhance protection against other HPV genotypes, second-generation vaccines are underway. For example, A novel safe HPV L1-based nonavalent vaccine was designed to prevent precancerous lesions related to high-risk HPV types 16/18/31/33/45/52/58, as well as anogenital warts associated with HPV types 6/11. This vaccine is in the advanced stage of phase III clinical trials. Other second-generation vaccines were based on L1-pentameric subunits and also the minor capsid protein L2 that have shown to be effective in preclinical studies. In this chapter, some major methods about the prevention of HPV-associated diseases will be discussed.

Keywords: Cancer, HPV, Preventive study.

INTRODUCTION

Widespread use of HPV vaccine has the potential to reduce incidence of HPV-associated cancers. The National Comprehensive Cancer Control Program (NCCCP) can play a role in increasing HPV vaccination coverage through cancer prevention and access to partners in the healthcare community [1]. In recent years, increasing knowledge about HPVs and their interactions with host cells, tissues and the immune system, led to design safe and effective prophylactic vaccination against HPV infections as well as development of sensitive and specific molecular diagnostic tools for HPV detection in women, men and children. However, these achievements demonstrated new challenges in health care systems which play a main role for control of HPV infections [2]. The impact of Prophylactic HPV vaccination has been observed especially among girls vaccinated before HPV exposure in countries with high vaccine uptake. Maximal reductions for HPV

* **Corresponding author Azam Bolhassani:** Department of Hepatitis and AIDS, Pasteur Institute of Iran, Tehran, Iran; Tel: 66953311-20; E-mails: A_bolhasani@pasteur.ac.ir, azam.bolhassani@yahoo.com

6/11/16/18 infection, genital wart, low-grade cervical cancer, and high-grade cervical cancer were reported approximately 90%, 90%, 45%, and 85%, respectively [3]. At present, second-generation prophylactic HPV vaccines are suggested in clinical trials due to some benefits compared to the current vaccines such as protection against further oncogenic HPV serotypes, effective oral and mucosal routes of injection, and less dependence on cold chain storage [4, 5]. The second-generation prophylactic HPV vaccine developed in phase III clinical trial is a nonavalent vaccine targeting five oncogenic HPV types (*i.e.*, 31, 33, 45, 52, and 58) which offers an additional 15-30% reduction in incidence of cervical cancer. However, the actual impact of this vaccine depends on the prevalence of co-infections with various HPV types and vaccine cross-protective effects against other oncogenic types not covered by the vaccine [6, 7].

Prophylactic Vaccines

The FDA-approved quadrivalent (Gardasil) and bivalent (Cervarix) HPV vaccines were shown to be safe, with a long-term durability of protection against high-risk HPV-16 and -18 infections and a moderate degree of cross-protection against some non-vaccine HPV types. Next-generation vaccines targeting additional oncogenic genotypes are underway in clinical trials. Childhood vaccination programs are important worldwide, because stronger immune responses to the HPV vaccines along with the durability of protection against infection are generated at younger ages compared to adolescents [2].

Protection Against More HPV Types

The first-generation vaccines specifically target about 70% of infections that may lead to cervical cancer. In 2014, Merck developed a second-generation nonavalent vaccine containing VLPs of nine HPV types (HPV-16, -18, -31, -33, -45, -52, -58, -6 and -11) found commonly in cervical cancer [8]. Indeed, the nonavalent vaccine showed more than 95% efficiency against novel persistent infections and CIN2 [9]. Recently, a cross-reactive prophylactic L2-based vaccine is also underway [10]. Up to now, several prokaryotic and eukaryotic systems such as insect, yeast, plant, and *E. coli* were used to express the recombinant proteins especially for VLP production [11]. One main challenge is VLP purification in insect and yeast leading to high cost of these vaccines. Our group developed a novel strategy to generate HPVL1 VLP using stably transfected *leishmania* cells that could induce effective immune responses similar to HPVL1 VLP produced in *baculovirus*-infected insect cells [12]. On the other hand, among different vaccination strategies, live vector-based vaccines have attracted a special attention. Our data indicated that subcutaneous immunization of mice with the recombinant *leishmania tarentolae* expressing HPV16 L1 (*L.tar*-L1) was able to induce humoral immunity in mice without need of any adjuvant [13]. In this line, immunological and protective efficacy of whole recombinant killed *Pichia pastoris* and *Leishmania tarentolae* expressing HPV16 L1 capsid protein (*Pichia*-L1 and *L.tar*-L1) was evaluated in tumor mice model. The data showed that the group receiving killed *Pichia*-L1 generated significantly the anti-tumor protective effects in vaccinated mice as compared to killed *L.tar*-L1 and control groups [14]. Another study showed that vaccination with the full-length or a polypeptide containing residues 11-200 of BPV4 L2 induced complete protection in cattle against papillomas after BPV4 challenge similar to vaccination with BPV4 L1 VLP. However, the levels of neutralizing antibodies induced by L2 vaccination were lower than those generated by L1 VLP vaccination. This result was confirmed in the rabbit model indicating that antibodies generated by HPV L2 polypeptide can cross-neutralize a broad range of HPV genotypes [15]. Moreover, one possible approach to extend protection to more genotypes might be to vaccinate with L1/L2 VLP rather than with L1-only VLPs, as L2 co-assembles with L1 into VLPs. Unfortunately, L2 is immunologically subdominant to L1 in an L1/L2 VLP and even virion, thus, no more cross-protection is observed in animals vaccinated with L1/L2 VLPs as compared to L1-only VLPs because they generate only L1-specific neutralizing antibodies. Indeed, the neutralizing epitopes on L2 may be partially buried and revealed only during infection. These data led to optimize L2 vaccine through multimerization, epitope display and/or the use of adjuvants [15].

Diagnostic Methods

Diagnostic screening for HPV lesions is generally performed in the developed countries. Indeed, novel tests for molecular biomarkers of infection can determine the degree of present and future risk [2].

Therapeutic Methods for Persistent Infections

At present, new therapies are required to be minimally toxic on normal tissues and organs along with high efficiency. The therapeutic resources include therapeutic vaccines and specific immune stimulants to augment natural immunity and stop the growth of tumors [2]. Several therapeutic vaccines based on induction of effective immune responses against HPV E6/ E7 proteins are underway in patients with cervical cancer [10].

CONCLUDING REMARKS

HPV-related diseases remain a significant source of morbidity and mortality in developing and developed countries indicating the need for HPV vaccination programs with high population coverage. Second-generation HPV vaccines that protect against additional oncogenic HPV types have the potential to improve cervical cancer prevention. Co-infection with multiple HPV infections and unidentifiable HPV types can influence vaccine potency, but its importance may be moderated by vaccine cross-protective effects. However, the cost of these vaccines should be evaluated to use in developing or low-income countries.

CONFLICT OF INTEREST

The author (editor) declares no conflict of interest, financial or otherwise.

ACKNOWLEDGEMENT

Declare none.

REFERENCES

[1] Townsend JS, Steele CB, Hayes N, Bhatt A, Moore AR. Human papillomavirus vaccine as an anticancer vaccine: Collaborative efforts to promote human papillomavirus vaccine in the National Comprehensive Cancer Control Program. J Womens Health (Larchmt) 2017; 26(3): 200-6. [http://dx.doi.org/10.1089/jwh.2017.6351] [PMID: 28263672]

[2] Bosch FX, Broker TR, Forman D, *et al.* Comprehensive control of human papillomavirus infections and related diseases. Vaccine 2013; 31 (Suppl. 5): F1-F31. [http://dx.doi.org/10.1016/j.vaccine.2013.10.001] [PMID: 24331745]

[3] Garland SM, Kjaer SK, Muñoz N, *et al.* Impact and effectiveness of the quadrivalent human papillomavirus vaccine: A systematic review of 10 years of real-world experience. Clin Infect Dis 2016; 63(4): 519-27. [http://dx.doi.org/10.1093/cid/ciw354] [PMID: 27230391]

[4] Schiller JT, Nardelli-Haefliger D. Chapter 17: Second generation HPV vaccines to prevent cervical cancer. Vaccine 2006; 24 (3): S3/147-53.

[5] Stanley M. Prospects for new human papillomavirus vaccines. Curr Opin Infect Dis 2010; 23(1): 70-5. [http://dx.doi.org/10.1097/QCO.0b013e328334c0e1] [PMID: 19926987]

[6] http:// clinicaltrials.gov/ct2/show/NCT00543543

[7] Kiatpongsan S, Campos NG, Kim JJ. Potential benefits of second-generation human papillomavirus vaccines. PLoS One 2012; 7(11): e48426. [http://dx.doi.org/10.1371/journal.pone.0048426] [PMID: 23144879]

[8] Joura EA, Giuliano AR, Iversen OE, *et al.* A 9-valent HPV vaccine against infection and intraepithelial neoplasia in women. N Engl J Med 2015; 372(8): 711-23. [http://dx.doi.org/10.1056/NEJMoa1405044] [PMID: 25693011]

[9] Lowy DR. HPV vaccination to prevent cervical cancer and other HPV-associated disease: from basic science to effective interventions. J Clin Invest 2016; 126(1): 5-11. [http://dx.doi.org/10.1172/JCI85446] [PMID: 26727228]

[10] Jin L, Xu ZX. Recent advances in the study of HPV-associated carcinogenesis. Virol Sin 2015; 30(2): 101-6. [http://dx.doi.org/10.1007/s12250-015-3586-3] [PMID: 25910482]

[11] Shirbaghaee Z, Bolhassani A. Different applications of virus-like particles in biology and medicine: Vaccination and delivery systems. Biopolymers 2016; 105(3): 113-32. [http://dx.doi.org/10.1002/bip.22759] [PMID: 26509554]

[12] Bolhassani A, Shirbaghaee Z, Agi E, Davoudi N. VLP production in *Leishmania tarentolae*: A novel expression system for purification and assembly of HPV16 L1. Protein Expr Purif 2015; 116: 7-11. [http://dx.doi.org/10.1016/j.pep.2015.08.024] [PMID: 26304732]

[13] Shirbaghaee Z, Bolhassani A, Mirshafiey A, Motevalli F, Zohrei N. A live vector expressing HPV16 L1 generates an adjuvant-induced antibody response *in vivo*. Iran J Cancer Prev 2015; 8(6): e3991. [http://dx.doi.org/10.17795/ijcp-3991] [PMID: 26855722]

[14] Bolhassani A, Muller M, Roohvand F, *et al.* Whole recombinant *Pichia pastoris* expressing HPV16 L1 antigen is superior in inducing protection against tumor growth as compared to killed transgenic *Leishmania.* Hum Vaccin Immunother 2014; 10(12): 3499-508. [http://dx.doi.org/10.4161/21645515.2014.979606] [PMID: 25668661]

[15] Karanam B, Jagu S, Huh WK, Roden RB. Developing vaccines against minor capsid antigen L2 to prevent papillomavirus infection. Immunol Cell Biol 2009; 87(4): 287-99. [http://dx.doi.org/10.1038/icb.2009.13] [PMID: 19421199]

CHAPTER 12

Treatment and Follow up of HPV Infection-Related Cancers

Azam Bolhassani* and **Niloofar Naderi**

Department of Hepatitis and AIDS, Pasteur Institute of Iran, Tehran, Iran

Abstract: In spite of the use of prophylactic vaccines to prevent some HPV infections, HPV-associated diseases have remained as a significant public health problem for decades especially in the developing world. There is an urgent need for the treatment of existing HPV-related lesions. The current treatment of neoplastic HPV-associated conditions includes HPV vaccines, targeted therapy of cervical cancer, drug therapy, and stem cell therapy. Herein, some recent findings on therapy of HPV-induced intraepithelial neoplasias will be summarized.

Keywords: Drug therapy, HPV infection-related cancers, Stem cell therapy, Treatment, Vaccine.

INTRODUCTION

Human papillomavirus (HPV) as a necessary agent for many gynecologic malignancies has shown the opportunity to control HPV-related cancers through vaccination. While prophylactic HPV vaccines are efficient in prevention of infection, they are not effective at clearing pre-existing HPV infections. Thus, there is an urgent need for therapeutic vaccines to treat existing HPV-associated lesions. Unlike prophylactic vaccines which generate neutralizing antibodies, therapeutic vaccines enhance cell-mediated immunity against HPV antigens [1]. On the other hand, the use of drug, and target therapy are other important pathways against HPV infection. In Europe, surgery, home therapies such as podophyllotoxin, imiquimod, or sinecatechins, laser therapy and cryotherapy have been successful for the treatment of anogenital warts [2].

Current Treatment of HPV-Related Disease

One of the most common therapeutic methods for HPV-related cancer is a loop electrosurgical excision procedure. Cryotherapy is also a treatment widely used in

* **Corresponding author Azam Bolhassani:** Department of Hepatitis and AIDS, Pasteur Institute of Iran, Tehran, Iran; Tel: 66953311-20; E-mails: A_bolhasani@pasteur.ac.ir, azam.bolhassani@yahoo.com

Azam Bolhassani (Ed.)

many countries due to its ease of use [3, 4]. The advanced cervical cancer is treated with chemoradiotherapy using cisplatin-based regimens (~ 66-79%). Moreover, the topical agent imiquimod (*i.e.,* an immune response modifier), and also photodynamic therapy (*i.e.,* direct damage of tumor and augmentation of anti-tumor immunity) have shown useful efficiency (~ 50-60%) in treatment of high-grade vulvar intraepithelial neoplasia (VIN) [3, 4]. On the other hand, there are promising results from clinical trials using topical therapies for the treatment of high-grade anogenital intraepithelial neoplasias (AIN) such as 5-fluoruracil (5-FU), imiquimod, and topical cidofovir. Also, surgical treatment and topical chemotherapy agents (5-FU, imiquimod) are the best options for penile intraepithelial neoplasias (PeIN) and penile cancer. The fractionated radiotherapy combined with cisplatin is used to treat oropharyngeal squamous cell carcinomas. The surgical treatment and adjuvant therapy are recommended for recurrent respiratory papillomatosis (RRP) [3, 4].

Development of Novel Treatments

The immune system plays an important role in controlling the development of HPV-associated cancer through specific immunity to the E6 and E7 oncogenes. Thus, therapeutic E6/E7 vaccines have attracted a special interest for treatment of high-risk HPV- associated cancers, *e.g.*, high-grade VIN patients using development of HPV-specific T-cell responses and modulation of key local immune factors in tumor microenvironment. Recently, treatments that can locally shift the balance of immune effectors (*e.g.,* imiquimod) in combination with vaccination have been tested in HPV-induced tumors [3, 4]. Moreover, combination of immunotherapy with new drugs targeting molecular pathways mediated by HPV, are being tested as an effective treatment in HPV-associated cancer. For instance, small molecule inhibitors targeting the DNA-binding activities of HPV E1/E2 or the anti-apoptotic properties of E6/E7 oncogenes have been used in preclinical studies. On the other hand, proteosome and histone deacetylase inhibitors enhancing apoptosis in HPV-positive tumor cells are being tested in early clinical trials [3, 4]. However, lesion infiltration of effectors and the use of effective adjuvants in vaccines are required to develop successfully immunotherapeutic regimens in the future.

Follow-up After Treatment of High-grade CIN

After treatment of cervical pre-cancer lesions, HPV testing accelerates follow-up recurrent high-grade CIN compared to cytology with higher sensitivity and without any decrease in specificity [3, 5].

Drug Treatment for HPV-related Neoplasias

Standard treatment of HPV-related Neoplasias includes cryotherapy and laser treatment. Researchers showed that CIN can be treated with pharmaceutical agents, *e.g.,* treatment of CIN2 and CIN3 patients with oral administration of diindolylmethane (DIM) derived from indole-3-carbinol (I3C) found in Brassica vegetables and /or topical chemotherapy of CIN2 patients using cidofovir drug [6, 7]. Moreover, an immune response modifier, topical imiquimod cream was also used effectively for treatment of skin diseases, genital warts and CIN2 and CIN3 patients, alone and/ or in combination with HPV therapeutic vaccination in patients with AIN and VIN [8 - 10]. The increased local infiltration of CD8 and CD4 T cells, and also HPV clearance rates were significantly observed in AIN and VIN patients [11].

Target Therapy

Based on international guidelines, treatment of cervical cancer (CC) includes surgery in early stages and chemoradiation in advanced stages. Recent clinical trials focus on using the anti-angiogenesis agents in advanced or recurrent cervical cancer. For instance, Bevacizumab, a humanized anti- vascular endothelial growth factor (VEGF) monoclonal antibody, in combination with chemotherapies increased the survival in patients with recurrent or metastatic cervical cancer compared to chemotherapy alone [11 - 14].

Stem Cells in Therapy of HPV-Associated Cancers

As known, cancer stem cells (CSCs) maintain the ability of normal tissue stem cells such as unlimited self-regeneration and differentiation into different cell types, and express the specific surface markers. For instance, the markers for cervical cancer stem cells including p63, cytokeratin 17 (CK17), Nanog, Musashi-1 (Msi1), Nucleostemin (NS), CD49f, ALDH1, and CD44. Nanog, NS, and Msi1 are highly expressed in cervical carcinomas compared to normal cervix [15]. Also, the markers of embryonic stem cells (*e.g.,* Sox2, Oct4) are highly expressed in cervical cell carcinomas [16]. Indeed, HPVs infect stem cells for the initiation of cervical epithelial cancers through modulation of several cellular pathways by HPV E6 and E7 oncoproteins in the carcinogenic process [17, 18]. The effects of HPV16 E6/E7 on stem cells within hair follicles showed that the number of quiescent cells as well as stem cell markers is reduced [19]. Moreover, the studies indicated that CSCs of head and neck squamous cell carcinoma (HNSCC) do not correlate with HPV infections. These CSCs were more resistant to cisplatin than non-CSCs and HPVs do not affect the response of CSCs to the treatment of cisplatin [20]. However, the role of HPV oncogenic E6/E7 in the formation of cervix CSCs and the potential therapeutic significance of CSCs in

HPV-positive cancers are still unknown [11].

Therapeutic Vaccines

The HPV E6 and E7 antigens represent ideal targets for development of therapeutic vaccines. Several therapeutic vaccines targeting E6 and E7 proteins were generated to control HPV infection through cell-mediated immunity in preclinical and clinical studies [21, 22]. However, the use of novel adjuvants, and further understanding of tumor biology will develop the combinational therapies along with HPV vaccines in the future.

CONCLUDING REMARKS

Among all treatment methods of HPV infections, therapeutic vaccines have attracted a special interest among all researchers. Moreover, the combinational therapies along with HPV vaccines are known as a promising approach against HPV-associated neoplasia. However, further understanding of the tumor microenvironment and molecular mechanisms inhibiting immune system will lead to find novel targets for treatment of HPV infections in the future.

CONFLICT OF INTEREST

The author (editor) declares no conflict of interest, financial or otherwise.

ACKNOWLEDGEMENT

Declare none.

REFERENCES

[1] Yang A, Farmer E, Lin J, Wu TC, Hung CF. The current state of therapeutic and T cell-based vaccines against human papillomaviruses. Virus Res 2017; 231: 148-65. [http://dx.doi.org/10.1016/j.virusres.2016.12.002] [PMID: 27932207]

[2] Mosa C, Trizzino A, Trizzino A, Di Marco F, D'Angelo P, Farruggia P. Treatment of human papillomavirus infection with interferon alpha and ribavirin in a patient with acquired aplastic anemia. Int J Infect Dis 2014; 23: 25-7. [http://dx.doi.org/10.1016/j.ijid.2013.11.021] [PMID: 24661930]

[3] Bosch FX, Broker TR, Forman D, *et al.* Comprehensive control of human papillomavirus infections and related diseases. Vaccine 2013; 31 (Suppl. 5): F1-F31. [http://dx.doi.org/10.1016/j.vaccine.2013.10.001] [PMID: 24331745]

[4] Stern PL, van der Burg SH, Hampson IN, *et al.* Therapy of human papillomavirus-related disease. Vaccine 2012; 30(S5) (Suppl. 5): F71-82. [http://dx.doi.org/10.1016/j.vaccine.2012.05.091] [PMID: 23199967]

[5] Arbyn M, Ronco G, Anttila A, *et al.* Evidence regarding human papillomavirus testing in secondary prevention of cervical cancer. Vaccine 2012; 30(S5) (Suppl. 5): F88-99. [http://dx.doi.org/10.1016/j.vaccine.2012.06.095] [PMID: 23199969]

[6] Del Priore G, Gudipudi DK, Montemarano N, Restivo AM, Malanowska-Stega J, Arslan AA. Oral diindolylmethane (DIM): pilot evaluation of a nonsurgical treatment for cervical dysplasia. Gynecol Oncol 2010; 116(3): 464-7.
[http://dx.doi.org/10.1016/j.ygyno.2009.10.060] [PMID: 19939441]

[7] Van Pachterbeke C, Bucella D, Rozenberg S, *et al.* Topical treatment of CIN 2+ by cidofovir: results of a phase II, double-blind, prospective, placebo-controlled study. Gynecol Oncol 2009; 115(1): 69-74.
[http://dx.doi.org/10.1016/j.ygyno.2009.06.042] [PMID: 19647859]

[8] Grimm C, Polterauer S, Natter C, *et al.* Treatment of cervical intraepithelial neoplasia with topical imiquimod: a randomized controlled trial. Obstet Gynecol 2012; 120(1): 152-9.
[http://dx.doi.org/10.1097/AOG.0b013e31825bc6e8] [PMID: 22914404]

[9] Hibbitts S. TA-CIN, a vaccine incorporating a recombinant HPV fusion protein (HPV16 L2E6E7) for the potential treatment of HPV16-associated genital diseases. Curr Opin Mol Ther 2010; 12(5): 598-606.
[PMID: 20886392]

[10] Daayana S, Elkord E, Winters U, *et al.* Phase II trial of imiquimod and HPV therapeutic vaccination in patients with vulval intraepithelial neoplasia. Br J Cancer 2010; 102(7): 1129-36.
[http://dx.doi.org/10.1038/sj.bjc.6605611] [PMID: 20234368]

[11] Jin L, Xu ZX. Recent advances in the study of HPV-associated carcinogenesis. Virol Sin 2015; 30(2): 101-6.
[http://dx.doi.org/10.1007/s12250-015-3586-3] [PMID: 25910482]

[12] Wright JD, Viviano D, Powell MA, *et al.* Bevacizumab combination therapy in heavily pretreated, recurrent cervical cancer. Gynecol Oncol 2006; 103(2): 489-93.
[http://dx.doi.org/10.1016/j.ygyno.2006.03.023] [PMID: 16647106]

[13] Tewari KS, Sill MW, Long HJ III, *et al.* Improved survival with bevacizumab in advanced cervical cancer. N Engl J Med 2014; 370(8): 734-43.
[http://dx.doi.org/10.1056/NEJMoa1309748] [PMID: 24552320]

[14] Monk BJ, Mas Lopez L, Zarba JJ, *et al.* Phase II, open-label study of pazopanib or lapatinib monotherapy compared with pazopanib plus lapatinib combination therapy in patients with advanced and recurrent cervical cancer. J Clin Oncol 2010; 28(22): 3562-9.
[http://dx.doi.org/10.1200/JCO.2009.26.9571] [PMID: 20606083]

[15] Ye F, Zhou C, Cheng Q, Shen J, Chen H. Stem-cell-abundant proteins Nanog, Nucleostemin and Musashi1 are highly expressed in malignant cervical epithelial cells. BMC Cancer 2008; 8: 108-12.
[http://dx.doi.org/10.1186/1471-2407-8-108] [PMID: 18419830]

[16] Ji J, Wei X, Wang Y. Embryonic stem cell markers Sox-2 and OCT4 expression and their correlation with WNT signal pathway in cervical squamous cell carcinoma. Int J Clin Exp Pathol 2014; 7(5): 2470-6.
[PMID: 24966958]

[17] López J, Poitevin A, Mendoza-Martínez V, Pérez-Plasencia C, García-Carrancá A. Cancer-initiating cells derived from established cervical cell lines exhibit stem-cell markers and increased radioresistance. BMC Cancer 2012; 12: 48.
[http://dx.doi.org/10.1186/1471-2407-12-48] [PMID: 22284662]

[18] Gu W, Yeo E, McMillan N, Yu C. Silencing oncogene expression in cervical cancer stem-like cells inhibits their cell growth and self-renewal ability. Cancer Gene Ther 2011; 18(12): 897-905.
[http://dx.doi.org/10.1038/cgt.2011.58] [PMID: 21904396]

[19] Michael S, Lambert PF, Strati K. The HPV16 oncogenes cause aberrant stem cell mobilization. Virology 2013; 443(2): 218-25.
[http://dx.doi.org/10.1016/j.virol.2013.04.008] [PMID: 23664148]

[20] Tang AL, Owen JH, Hauff SJ, *et al.* Head and neck cancer stem cells: the effect of HPV--an *in vitro*

and mouse study. Otolaryngol Head Neck Surg 2013; 149(2): 252-60. [http://dx.doi.org/10.1177/0194599813486599] [PMID: 23585151]

[21] http://clinicaltrials.gov/ct2/show/NCT00943722

[22] Lin K, Doolan K, Hung CF, Wu TC. Perspectives for preventive and therapeutic HPV vaccines. J Formos Med Assoc 2010; 109(1): 4-24. [http://dx.doi.org/10.1016/S0929-6646(10)60017-4] [PMID: 20123582]

CHAPTER 13

Preventive Human Papillomavirus (HPV) Vaccines: Immunogenicity, Efficacy and Safety

Amitis Ramezani and **Arezoo Aghakhani***

Clinical Research Department, Pasteur Institute of Iran, Tehran, Iran

Abstract: Human papillomaviruses (HPV) infection can cause cervical, vaginal and vulvar cancers in women and penile cancer in men. HPV can also cause oropharyngeal and anal cancers and genital warts in both women and men. HPV types 16 and 18 are the most carcinogenic types and are responsible for about 70% of the cervical cancers. HPV types 31, 33, 35, 45, 52 and 58 account for an additional 20% of the cervical malignancies worldwide. Currently, three vaccines are available on the market that prevent HPV infection including bivalent Cervarix targeting HPV types 16 and 18, quadrivalent Gardasil targeting HPV 16, 18, 6 and 11, and 9-valent Gardasil-9 targeting HPV 31, 33, 45, 52 and 58 in addition to HPV 16, 18, 6 and 11. The present chapter discusses the HPV vaccines and their immunogenicity, efficacy, safety and side effects.

Keywords: Efficacy, Human papillomavirus (HPV), Immunogenicity, Safety, Side effects, Vaccine.

INTRODUCTION

Human papillomavirus (HPV) is a small, non-enveloped, double-stranded DNA virus belonging to the family *Papillomaviridae* [1]. HPV is the most common sexually transmitted viral infection and 80% of sexually active women and men will be infected with HPV at some points in their lives [2]. There are more than 100 types of HPV and more than 40 types are transmitted through sexual contact and infect the anogenital region [3].

HPVs are divided in to "high-risk" and "low-risk" groups based on the degree that they put a person at risk of malignancy. HPV 16 and 18 are the most carcinogenic types and are responsible for about 70% of the cervical cancers. HPV types 31, 33, 35, 45, 52 and 58 account for an additional 20% of the cervical cancers, the third most common cancer in women throughout the world [4 - 7]. HPV infection

* **Corresponding author Arezoo Aghakhani:** Clinical Research Dept., Pasteur Institute of Iran, Tehran, Iran; Tel: 66953311-20; E-mail: araghakhani@hotmail.com

can also cause vaginal and vulvar cancers in women and penile cancer in men. HPV also linked to oropharyngeal and anal cancers in both women and men [8 - 11]. Low-risk HPV types (especially types 6 and 11) can cause genital warts and respiratory papillomatosis. These HPV types are causative agents of about 90% of genital warts in women and men [12].

Currently, three HPV vaccines are available that can prevent the most common types of HPV infection including bivalent Cervarix, targeting HPV types 16 and 18, quadrivalent Gardasil, targeting HPV 16, 18, 6 and 11, and 9-valent Gardasil-9, targeting HPV 31, 33, 45, 52 and 58, in addition to HPV 16, 18, 6 and 11 [13 - 18].

Quadrivalent HPV vaccine (Gardasil, Merck, USA) targeting HPV 16, 18, 6 and 11 was approved by the FDA in June 2006. The vaccine is approved for females and males 9 to 26 years of age. Each 0.5 mL dose of Gardasil contains 20 μg of each HPV 6 and 18 L1 proteins and 40 μg of each HPV 11 and 16 L1 proteins. The vaccine antigen is adsorbed on amorphous aluminium hydroxyphosphate sulfate adjuvant. The vaccine also includes L-histidine, sodium chloride, sodium borate, polysorbate 80 and water. Gardasil does not include any preservative or antibiotic. The vaccine is supplied either in a single-dose vial or in a prefilled syringe [13, 14].

Bivalent vaccine (Cervarix, GSK Biologicals, Belgium) contains the recombinant HPV L1 capsid proteins from HPV types 16 and 18 and was approved by the FDA in October 2009. The vaccine was approved for females 9 to 25 years of age. Cervarix uses the proprietary adjuvant, aluminum hydroxide with 3-deacylated monophosphoryl lipid A (ASO4). Each 0.5 mL dose contains 20 μg of each HPV 16 and 18 L1 protein. Cervarix also does not contain any preservative or antibiotic. This vaccine is available in two forms of prefilled syringes [14, 15].

On December 2014, the FDA announced approval of a third HPV vaccine, a 9-valent vaccine (Gardasil-9, Merck, USA). Gardasil-9 protects against infection with the HPV types covered by Gardasil (HPV 16, 18, 6 and 11) and also protects against five other HPV types (HPV 31, 33, 45, 52 and 58). This vaccine was approved for women and men aged 9 to 26 years old [16, 17]. Gardasil-9 prevents infections with additional cancer causing HPV types 31, 33, 45, 52 and 58 with 98% effectiveness which adds protection against an additional 20% of cervical cancers not previously prevented by Gardasil and Cervarix [16 - 18].

In all HPV vaccines, the L1 surface proteins of the targeted HPV types are used as the antigen. The L1 protein undergoes conformal changes to self-assemble into virus-like particles (VLPs) in artificial production systems. VLPs lack the infectious viral genome, so they are non-infective and non-pathogenic. Adjuvants used to ensure robust and long-term immunogenicity include aluminium phosphate and ASO4 in the Cervarix and aluminium hydroxyl-phosphate sulphate in the Gardasil and Gardasil-9 [19, 20].

Vaccination Schedule and Use

For most effectiveness of HPV vaccines, they should be administrated before exposure of cases to HPV through sexual contact; however subjects with prior exposure to HPV should also be vaccinated. HPV vaccines are highly effective and can provide full protection against HPV types they target when given before exposure to the virus. Vaccination will be less effective in persons who have already been exposed with one or more of the HPV vaccine types. Pre-vaccination examinations such as Pap testing or screening for high-risk HPV-DNA or HPV antibody are not recommended before HPV vaccination at any age [18, 19, 21].

The CDC Advisory Committee on Immunization Practices (ACIP) recommends routine administration of Gardasil or Gardasil-9 for males and Gardasil, Gardasil-9 or Cervarix for females aged 11-12 years. Female vaccination with HPV vaccines prevents cervical cancers and precancerous lesions. Gardasil and Gardasil-9 are also preventing genital warts. HPV vaccination can be started at age 9 years. Early HPV vaccination is recommended because HPV vaccines are effective in preventing, but not treating HPV infections, which are transmitted through sexual contact. HPV vaccination at ages 11-12 years provides protection before the adolescence and initiation of sexual contact and thus before the chance of HPV exposure [22 - 24].

In October 2016, CDC recommended that healthy adolescents who initiated HPV vaccination before age 15 years should receive two doses of any HPV vaccine. The second dose of HPV vaccine should be given 6-12 months after the first dose (0, 6-12 month schedule). Cases that start the HPV vaccine series at ages 15-26 years, need three doses of HPV vaccine to protect against cancer-causing HPV infections [25]. Three dose series are still recommended for cases with immunocompromising conditions aged 9-26 years [25].

The recommendations for adult immunization schedule are as follows:

-Adult females through age 26 years and adult males through age 21 years who have not received any HPV vaccine should receive a 3-dose series of HPV vaccine at 0, 1–2 and 6 months. Males aged 22-26 years old can be received 3-dose HPV vaccine schedule at 0, 1-2 and 6 months.

-Adult females through age 26 years and adult males through age 21 years (and also 22-26 years males who may receive HPV vaccine) who initiated the HPV vaccination series before age 15 years and received 2 doses at least 5 months apart are considered adequately vaccinated and do not need an additional dose of HPV vaccine.

-Adult females through age 26 years and adult males through age 21 years (and also 22-26 years males who may receive HPV vaccine) who initiated the HPV vaccination series before age 15 years and received only 1 dose or 2 doses less than 5 months apart, are not considered adequately vaccinated and should receive 1 additional dose of HPV vaccine [25 - 27].

ACIP recommends 3-dose series HPV vaccination with Gardasil or Gardasil-9 for immunocompromised males and men who have sex with men (MSM). Cervarix is not licensed for males. Adult females and males through age 26 years with immunocompromising conditions such as HIV infection, malignant neoplasm, transplantation, autoimmune disease and immunosuppressive therapy should receive a 3-dose series of HPV vaccine at 0, 1-2, and 6 months. Because HPV vaccines are subunit vaccines, they can be administered to immunosuppressed subjects. However, the immune response and vaccine efficacy might be less than immunocompetent persons. Women who are breastfeeding may receive HPV vaccine. Females and males who are victims of sexual abuse or assault should receive HPV vaccine through the recommended ages if they have not already been vaccinated [28].

Contraindications and Precautions to Vaccination

A severe allergic reaction to a vaccine component or following a previous dose of HPV vaccine is a contraindication of HPV vaccine receipt. Anaphylactic allergy to latex is a contraindication to bivalent HPV vaccine because prefilled syringe of Cervarix contains natural rubber latex [29].

A moderate or severe acute illness is a precaution to HPV vaccination and vaccination should be postponed until the acute illness symptoms improve. A minor acute illness (like mild upper respiratory tract infection or diarrhea) is not a contraindication of HPV vaccination [29].

HPV vaccine is not recommended during pregnancy. Data regarding HPV vaccination during pregnancy are scant. Although HPV vaccine has not been associated with adverse pregnancy outcomes or adverse effects on the fetus, but it is better to not use HPV vaccine during pregnancy. Pregnancy testing before vaccination is not needed. If a woman is found to be pregnant after initiation of the vaccination series, no intervention is indicated but the remainder of the series should be deferred until after delivery [29].

Immunogenicity and Vaccine Efficacy

The immunogenic particle of the available HPV vaccines is a DNA-free VLP. The L1 VLP is highly immunogenic. However, because the L1 protein is type-specific, effective vaccines must be polyvalent, containing multiple VLPs from different HPV types. VLPs have now been developed for types 6, 11, 16, 18, 31, 33, 45, 52, and 58 [30].

HPV vaccines are highly immunogenic. More than 99% of vaccine recipients develop antibody response to HPV vaccine types one month after completion the vaccine series. However, at the present time, there is no correlation between immune response and HPV protection. Moreover there is no data about antibody titer which correlates with HPV protection. After HPV vaccination, L1 proteins are recognized by the immune system in the regional lymph nodes to create strong antibody response (IgG). L1 VLP vaccines are highly immunogenic and generating antibody titers higher than the antibody levels induced by the natural HPV infections. The IgG is exuded at the possible sites of infection such as mucosa of genital tract and neutralizes the HPV, and prevents its entry into the cells. HPV vaccination generates both components of the antibody memory response (serological and reactive memory) and with reactivation of memory B-cells and plasma cells allows generation and exudation of protecting IgG each time that body is exposed to HPV infection [20].

Both Gardasil and Cervarix are effective against their respective HPV types. In addition to protection against the HPV types included in these vaccines, the vaccines provide cross-protection against additional HPV types that can cause cancer. Cervarix also has more cross-protection against oncogenic HPV types in addition to types 16 and 18 than Gardasil [31 - 35]. Cervarix uses a novel aluminum salt (AS04) adjuvant, which is responsible for eliciting a strong immunologic response [35, 36]. So after vaccination with Cervarix, higher anti-HPV 16 and 18 antibodies and neutralization titers are observed in comparison to Gardasil, although whether that correlates with clinical endpoints is unknown [27]. Avidity of antibodies is similar between the two vaccines [37].

In subjects who was not infected with HPV types 16 and 18, both Cervarix and Gardasil prevent 96-100% of cervical intraepithelial neoplasia (CIN) 1 to CIN3 cases caused by HPV16 and 18 [38, 39]. Both vaccines protect against 70% of cervical cancer cases [37]. In addition to protection against HPV16 and 18, Gardasil also prevents HPV 6 and 11, which are associated with 90-99% of genital warts [40]. It was reported that clinical efficacy of Gardasil and Cervarix against HPV 16 or 18 related cervical adenocarcinoma in situ (AIS) was 97% and 93%, respectively [30].

It has been showed that both Cervarix and Gardasil are safe and highly immunogenic in male and female HIV positive cases regardless of CD4 counts and seroconversion to HPV can be demonstrated in 75-100% of HPV-vaccinated HIV patients [41 - 43]. Both vaccines will reduce incidences of penile cancers in HIV-positive men, cervical cancers in HIV-positive women and anogenital cancers in both men and women [3].

The CDC mentions that both Cervarix and Gardasil vaccines maintain their efficacy for at least 10 years based on ongoing research. The ACIP states that no booster dose is recommended for Cervarix and Gardasil [44].

Although high efficacy of HPV vaccines is demonstrated among cases without evidence of prior HPV infection with vaccine HPV types, there is no evidence of efficacy of HPV vaccines against disease caused by vaccine HPV types which subjects were infected with them at the time of vaccination. It means that HPV vaccines have no therapeutic effect on existing HPV infection or disease. Cases that infected with one or more vaccine HPV types prior to vaccination were protected against disease caused by the other HPV vaccine types. Prior infection with one HPV type did not reduce efficacy of the vaccine against other vaccine HPV types [44].

The newly FDA approved Gardasil-9 has the highest number of L1 VLPs among three HPV vaccines. Despite the concern that adding the more HPV types to Gardasil might compromise the immunogenicity of HPV 6, 11, 16 and 18; but the geometric mean antibody titers to HPV 6, 11, 16 and 18 in Gardasil-9 are not lower than Gardasil. Besides, Gardasil-9 targets HPV types 31, 33, 45, 52 and 58 in addition to HPV types 16, 18, 6, 11 and therefore reduces persistent HPV infections and incidence of VIN, CIN2 and 3, and AIS better than Gardasil [45]. It is reported that Gardasil-9 provides protection against 90% of HPV types related to cervical cancers and genital warts in women and 80-95% of other HPV associated anogenital cancers in both men and women [46]. However, in respect to the variation of the prevalence and distribution of HPV types in different geographical areas, Gardasil-9 will protect against 92% of HPV associated cervical cancers in North America, 91.7% in Africa, 90.9% in Europe, 89.5% in Latin America and the Caribbean, 87.7% in Asia and 86.5% in Australia [47 - 52].

Other Efficacy Considerations

Although most clinical trials have focused on the efficacy of HPV vaccines in cervical and vulvo-vaginal cancers and precancerous lesions, some reports are also published on vaccine efficacy in the prevention of other HPV related genital and oropharyngeal diseases. In an investigation, in women of Costa Rica who vaccinated with Cervarix, the efficacy of vaccine against anal infection with HPV

16 and 18 was reported to be about 83.6% [53]. In another survey, an estimated HPV vaccine efficacy was 93.3% in oropharyngeal HPV related cancers [54]. In another study, Gardasil had 90% efficacy in preventing HPV 6, 11, 16 and 18 related external genital lesions in men aged 16-26 years [55].

It is expected that Gardasil-9 prevents 80-85% of HPV related vaginal cancers, 85-90% of HPV associated vulvar cancers, 90-95% of HPV related anal cancers [46] and 86% of HPV associated penile cancers [56]. It is also demonstrated that Gardasil-9 may protect 90% of HPV associated recurrent respiratory papillomatosis and 93% of HPV related head and neck malignancies [57].

Adverse Reactions Following Vaccination

All Randomized controlled trials (RCTs) of the Cervarix, Gardasil and Gardasil-9 reported a favorable safety profile. In addition, post-marketing surveillance and longitudinal studies have showed the safety of the HPV vaccines [58, 59]. Safety reports from the Vaccine Adverse Event Reporting System (VAERS) indicate thatless than 1% of HPV vaccine recipients showed adverse effects and 92% of them were non-serious including pain, redness or swelling at the site of vaccine injection in 20% of cases and headache or fainting immediately following vaccination. Recipients should always be seated during vaccine administration. Clinicians should consider observing recipient for 15 minutes after vaccination. Guillain-Barre Syndrome, seizures, stroke, venous thromboembolism and appendicitis were not more common after HPV vaccination than other adolescent vaccinations [59 - 61]. A variety of systemic adverse reactions were reported by vaccine recipients including fever, nausea, dizziness, myalgia and malaise. However, these symptoms occurred with equal frequency among both vaccine and placebo recipients. Severe adverse effects such as persistent headache, gastroenteritis, hypertension and bronchospasm were reported in no more than 0.5% of cases [58]. No increased risk of autoimmune, venous thromboembolic or neurologic disease has been shown among HPV vaccine recipients in long-term studies [60, 61].

CONCLUDING REMARKS

Given the studies, both commercial preventive vaccines including Gardasil and Cervarix demonstrated remarkably high and similar efficacy for a range of cervical endpoints from persistent infection to CIN3 in women. However, there are some limitations (*e.g.,* duration of protection, cross-protection, tolerability and side effects) for using these vaccines. Recently, several second-generation prophylactic vaccines are underway, aimed at resolving some of these limitations including nonavalent vaccine and/or L2-based vaccine.

CONFLICT OF INTEREST

The author (editor) declares no conflict of interest, financial or otherwise.

ACKNOWLEDGEMENT

Declare none.

REFERENCES

[1] Muñoz N, Bosch FX, de Sanjosé S, *et al.* Epidemiologic classification of human papillomavirus types associated with cervical cancer. N Engl J Med 2003; 348(6): 518-27. [http://dx.doi.org/10.1056/NEJMoa021641] [PMID: 12571259]

[2] Einstein MH, Schiller JT, Viscidi RP, *et al.* Clinician's guide to human papillomavirus immunology: knowns and unknowns. Lancet Infect 2009; Dis 9:347-56.. [http://dx.doi.org/10.1016/S1473-3099(09)70108-2]

[3] Parkin DM, Bray F. Chapter 2: The burden of HPV-related cancers. Vaccine 2006; 24: S3/11-25.

[4] Balanda M, Quiero A, Vergara N, *et al.* Prevalence of human papillomavirus infection among women presenting for cervical cancer screening in Chile, 2014-2015. Med Microbiol Immunol (Berl) 2016; 205(6): 585-94. [http://dx.doi.org/10.1007/s00430-016-0473-y] [PMID: 27539577]

[5] Centers for Disease Control and Prevention Genital HPV Infection – CDC Fact Sheet. 2009.http://www.cdc.gov/std/HPV/STDFact-HPV.htm

[6] Bruni L, Barrionuevo-Rosas L, Albero G, *et al.* Information Centre on HPV and Cancer (HPV Information Centre). Human Papillomavirus and Related Diseases in the World. Summary Report 7 October 2016.

[7] Aghakhani A, Mamishi S, Sabeti S, *et al.* Gender and age-specific seroprevalence of human papillomavirus 16 and 18 in general population in Tehran, Iran. Med Microbiol Immunol (Berl) 2017; 206(2): 105-10. [http://dx.doi.org/10.1007/s00430-016-0487-5] [PMID: 27858157]

[8] Bodelon C, Untereiner ME, Machiela MJ, Vinokurova S, Wentzensen N. Genomic characterization of viral integration sites in HPV-related cancers. Int J Cancer 2016; 139(9): 2001-11. [http://dx.doi.org/10.1002/ijc.30243] [PMID: 27343048]

[9] Di Giuseppe G, Abbate R, Liguori G, Albano L, Angelillo IF. Human papillomavirus and vaccination: knowledge, attitudes, and behavioural intention in adolescents and young women in Italy. Br J Cancer 2008; 99(2): 225-9. [http://dx.doi.org/10.1038/sj.bjc.6604454] [PMID: 18628763]

[10] Far AE, Aghakhani A, Hamkar R, *et al.* Frequency of human papillomavirus infection in oesophageal squamous cell carcinoma in Iranian patients. Scand J Infect Dis 2007; 39(1): 58-62. [http://dx.doi.org/10.1080/00365540600740496] [PMID: 17366014]

[11] Aghakhani A, Hamkar R, Parvin M, *et al.* The role of human papillomavirus infection in prostate carcinoma. Scand J Infect Dis 2011; 43(1): 64-9. [http://dx.doi.org/10.3109/00365548.2010.502904] [PMID: 20662618]

[12] Poljak M, Seme K, Maver PJ, *et al.* Human papillomavirus prevalence and type-distribution, cervical cancer screening practices and current status of vaccination implementation in Central and Eastern Europe. Vaccine 2013; 31 (Suppl. 7): H59-70. [http://dx.doi.org/10.1016/j.vaccine.2013.03.029] [PMID: 24332298]

[13] Markowitz LE, Dunne EF, Saraiya M, Lawson HW, Chesson H, Unger ER. Quadrivalent human

papillomavirus vaccine. Recommendations of the Advisory Committee on Immunization Practices (ACIP). MMWR Recomm Rep 2007; 56(RR-2): 1-24.
[PMID: 17380109]

[14] Schiller JT, Lowy DR, Markowitz LE. Human papillomavirus vaccines.Vaccines. 6th ed. China: Saunders 2012; pp. 235-56.

[15] FDA licensure of bivalent human papillomavirus vaccine (HPV2, Cervarix) for use in females and updated HPV vaccination recommendations from the Advisory Committee on Immunization Practices (ACIP). MMWR Morb Mortal Wkly Rep 2010; 59(20): 626-9.
[PMID: 20508593]

[16] http://www.fda.gov/NewsEvents/Newsroom/PressAnnouncements/ucm426485.htm2014.

[17] Saraiya M, Unger ER, Thompson TD, *et al.* US assessment of HPV types in cancers: implications for current and 9-valent HPV vaccines. J Natl Cancer Inst 2015; 107(6): djv086.
[http://dx.doi.org/10.1093/jnci/djv086] [PMID: 25925419]

[18] Markowitz LE, Dunne EF, Saraiya M, *et al.* Human papillomavirus vaccination: recommendations of the Advisory Committee on Immunization Practices (ACIP). MMWR Recomm Rep 2014; 63(RR-05): 1-30.
[PMID: 25167164]

[19] 2016.http://www.who.int/immunization/diseases/hpv/en

[20] Sankaranarayanan R, Bhatla N, Basu P. Current global status & impact of human papillomavirus vaccination: Implications for India. Indian J Med Res 2016; 144(2): 169-80.
[http://dx.doi.org/10.4103/0971-5916.195023] [PMID: 27934795]

[21] Isidean SD, Tota JE, Gagnon JA, Franco EL. Human papillomavirus vaccines: key factors in planning cost-effective vaccination programs. Expert Rev Vaccines 2015; 14(1): 119-33.
[http://dx.doi.org/10.1586/14760584.2015.964213] [PMID: 25266065]

[22] Petrosky E, Bocchini JA Jr, Hariri S, *et al.* Use of 9-valent human papillomavirus (HPV) vaccine: updated HPV vaccination recommendations of the advisory committee on immunization practices. MMWR Morb Mortal Wkly Rep 2015; 64(11): 300-4.
[PMID: 25811679]

[23] Saraiya M, Sawaya G, Garcia F. 2014.http://emergency.cdc.gov/coca/calls/2014/callinfo_112014.asp

[24] Hendry M, Lewis R, Clements A, Damery S, Wilkinson C. "HPV? Never heard of it!": a systematic review of girls' and parents' information needs, views and preferences about human papillomavirus vaccination. Vaccine 2013; 31(45): 5152-67.
[http://dx.doi.org/10.1016/j.vaccine.2013.08.091] [PMID: 24029117]

[25] CDC recommends only two HPV shots for younger adolescents. MMWR 2016; 65(49): 1405-8.
[PMID: 27977643]

[26] Kim DK, Riley LE, Harriman KH, Hunter P, Bridges CB. Advisory Committee on Immunization Practices Recommended Immunization Schedule for Adults Aged 19 Years or Older - United States, 2017. MMWR Morb Mortal Wkly Rep 2017; 66(5): 136-8.
[http://dx.doi.org/10.15585/mmwr.mm6605e2] [PMID: 28182599]

[27] MMWR Morb Mortal Wkly Rep 2017; 66www.cdc.gov/mmwr/volumes/66/wr/mm6605e2.htm

[28] Human Papillomavirus Vaccination: Recommendations of the Advisory Committee on Immunization Practices (ACIP). (MMWR) 2014; 63(RR05):1-30.

[29] CDC. Who Should NOT Get Vaccinated with these Vaccines 2016.https://www.cdc.gov/vaccines/vpd/should-not-vacc.html

[30] Jorge S, Wright JD. Update: HPV prevention. Contemp Ob Gyn 2016; 25(February)
http://contemporaryobgyn.modernmedicine.com/contemporary-obgyn/news/update-hpv-prevention

[31] Demarteau N, Tang CH, Chen HC, Chen CJ, Van Kriekinge G. Cost-effectiveness analysis of the bivalent compared with the quadrivalent human papillomavirus vaccines in Taiwan. Value Health 2012; 15(5): 622-31.
[http://dx.doi.org/10.1016/j.jval.2012.02.012] [PMID: 22867770]

[32] Paavonen J, Naud P, Salmerón J, *et al.* Efficacy of human papillomavirus (HPV)-16/18 AS04-adjuvanted vaccine against cervical infection and precancer caused by oncogenic HPV types (PATRICIA): final analysis of a double-blind, randomised study in young women. Lancet 2009; 374(9686): 301-14.
[http://dx.doi.org/10.1016/S0140-6736(09)61248-4] [PMID: 19586656]

[33] Quadrivalent vaccine against human papillomavirus to prevent high-grade cervical lesions. N Engl J Med 2007; 356(19): 1915-27.
[http://dx.doi.org/10.1056/NEJMoa061741] [PMID: 17494925]

[34] Harper DM, Franco EL, Wheeler CM, *et al.* Sustained efficacy up to 4.5 years of a bivalent L1 virus-like particle vaccine against human papillomavirus types 16 and 18: follow-up from a randomised control trial. Lancet 2006; 367(9518): 1247-55.
[http://dx.doi.org/10.1016/S0140-6736(06)68439-0] [PMID: 16631880]

[35] Wheeler CM, Castellsagué X, Garland SM, *et al.* Cross-protective efficacy of HPV-16/18 AS04-adjuvanted vaccine against cervical infection and precancer caused by non-vaccine oncogenic HPV types: 4-year end-of-study analysis of the randomised, double-blind PATRICIA trial. Lancet Oncol 2012; 13(1): 100-10.
[http://dx.doi.org/10.1016/S1470-2045(11)70287-X] [PMID: 22075170]

[36] Szarewski A. HPV vaccine: Cervarix. Expert Opin Biol Ther 2010; 10(3): 477-87.
[http://dx.doi.org/10.1517/14712591003601944] [PMID: 20132062]

[37] Herrin DM, Coates EE, Costner PJ, *et al.* Comparison of adaptive and innate immune responses induced by licensed vaccines for Human Papillomavirus. Hum Vaccin Immunother 2014; 10(12): 3446-54.
[http://dx.doi.org/10.4161/hv.34408] [PMID: 25483691]

[38] Apter D, Wheeler CM, Paavonen J, *et al.* Efficacy of human papillomavirus 16 and 18 (HPV-16/18) AS04-adjuvanted vaccine against cervical infection and precancer in young women: final event-driven analysis of the randomized, double-blind PATRICIA trial. Clin Vaccine Immunol 2015; 22 (4), 361e373.

[39] Dillner J, Kjaer SK, Wheeler CM, *et al.* Four year efficacy of prophylactic human papillomavirus quadrivalent vaccine against low grade cervical, vulvar, and vaginal intraepithelial neoplasia and anogenital warts: randomised controlled trial. BMJ 2010; 341: c3493.
[http://dx.doi.org/10.1136/bmj.c3493] [PMID: 20647284]

[40] Ljubojevic S, Skerlev M. HPV-associated diseases. Clin Dermatol 2014; 32(2): 227-34.
[http://dx.doi.org/10.1016/j.clindermatol.2013.08.007] [PMID: 24559558]

[41] Levin MJ, Moscicki AB, Song LY, *et al.* Safety and immunogenicity of a quadrivalent human papillomavirus (types 6, 11, 16, and 18) vaccine in HIV infected children 7 to 12 years old. J Acquir Immune Defic Syndr 2010; 55 (2): 197e204.

[42] Kojic EM, Kang M, Cespedes MS, *et al.* Immunogenicity and safety of the quadrivalent human papillomavirus vaccine in HIV-1-infected women. Clin Infect Dis 2014; 59 (1): 127e135.

[43] Toft L, Storgaard M, Muller M, *et al.* Comparison of the immunogenicity and reactogenicity of Cervarix and Gardasil human papillomavirus vaccines in HIV-infected adults: a randomized, double-blind clinical trial. J Infect Dis 2014; 209(8): 1165e1173.

[44] 2014.http://www.cdc.gov/vaccines/vpd-vac/hpv/vac-faqs.htm

[45] Joura EA, Giuliano AR, Iversen OE, *et al.* 2015.http://www.mercknewsroom.com/news-release/prescriptionmedicine-news/fda-approves-mercks-hpv-vaccine-gardasil9-prevent-cancersan

[46] Yang DY, Bracken K. Update on the new 9-valent vaccine for human papillomavirus prevention. Can Fam Physician 2016; 62(5): 399-402.
[PMID: 27255620]

[47] Muñoz N, Bosch FX, Castellsagué X, *et al.* Against which human papillomavirus types shall we vaccinate and screen? The international perspective. Int J Cancer 2004; 111(2): 278-85.
[http://dx.doi.org/10.1002/ijc.20244] [PMID: 15197783]

[48] Ogembo RK, Gona PN, Seymour AJ, *et al.* Prevalence of human papillomavirus genotypes among African women with normal cervical cytology and neoplasia: a systematic review and meta-analysis. PLoS One 2015; 10(4): e0122488.
[http://dx.doi.org/10.1371/journal.pone.0122488] [PMID: 25875167]

[49] Bao YP, Li N, Smith JS, Qiao YL. Human papillomavirus type distribution in women from Asia: a meta-analysis. Int J Gynecol Cancer 2008; 18(1): 71-9.
[http://dx.doi.org/10.1111/j.1525-1438.2007.00959.x] [PMID: 17466054]

[50] Bosch FX, Burchell AN, Schiffman M, *et al.* Epidemiology and natural history of human papillomavirus infections and type-specific implications in cervical neoplasia. Vaccine 2008; 26 (Suppl. 10): K1-K16.
[http://dx.doi.org/10.1016/j.vaccine.2008.05.064] [PMID: 18847553]

[51] Ciapponi A, Bardach A, Glujovsky D, Gibbons L, Picconi MA. Type-specific HPV prevalence in cervical cancer and high-grade lesions in Latin America and the Caribbean: systematic review and meta-analysis. PLoS One 2011; 6(10): e25493.
[http://dx.doi.org/10.1371/journal.pone.0025493] [PMID: 21991313]

[52] Smith JS, Lindsay L, Hoots B, *et al.* Human papillomavirus type distribution in invasive cervical cancer and high-grade cervical lesions: a meta-analysis update. Int J Cancer 2007; 121(3): 621-32.
[http://dx.doi.org/10.1002/ijc.22527] [PMID: 17405118]

[53] Kreimer AR, González P, Katki HA, *et al.* Efficacy of a bivalent HPV 16/18 vaccine against anal HPV 16/18 infection among young women: a nested analysis within the Costa Rica Vaccine Trial. Lancet Oncol 2011; 12(9): 862-70.
[http://dx.doi.org/10.1016/S1470-2045(11)70213-3] [PMID: 21865087]

[54] Herrero R, Quint W, Hildesheim A, *et al.* Reduced prevalence of oral human papillomavirus (HPV) 4 years after bivalent HPV vaccination in a randomized clinical trial in Costa Rica. PLoS One 2013; 8(7): e68329.
[http://dx.doi.org/10.1371/journal.pone.0068329] [PMID: 23873171]

[55] Giuliano AR, Palefsky JM, Goldstone S, *et al.* Efficacy of quadrivalent HPV vaccine against HPV Infection and disease in males. N Engl J Med 2011; 364(5): 401-11.
[http://dx.doi.org/10.1056/NEJMoa0909537] [PMID: 21288094]

[56] Miralles-Guri C, Bruni L, Cubilla AL, Castellsagué X, Bosch FX, de Sanjosé S. Human papillomavirus prevalence and type distribution in penile carcinoma. J Clin Pathol 2009; 62(10): 870-8.
[http://dx.doi.org/10.1136/jcp.2008.063149] [PMID: 19706632]

[57] Kreimer AR, Clifford GM, Boyle P, Franceschi S. Human papillomavirus types in head and neck squamous cell carcinomas worldwide: a systematic review. Cancer Epidemiol Biomarkers Prev 2005; 14(2): 467-75.
[http://dx.doi.org/10.1158/1055-9965.EPI-04-0551] [PMID: 15734974]

[58] Gonçalves AK, Cobucci RN, Rodrigues HM, de Melo AG, Giraldo PC. Safety, tolerability and side effects of human papillomavirus vaccines: a systematic quantitative review. Braz J Infect Dis 2014; 18(6): 651-9.
[http://dx.doi.org/10.1016/j.bjid.2014.02.005] [PMID: 24780368]

[59] Slade BA, Leidel L, Vellozzi C, *et al.* Postlicensure safety surveillance for quadrivalent human

papillomavirus recombinant vaccine. JAMA 2009; 302(7): 750-7. [http://dx.doi.org/10.1001/jama.2009.1201] [PMID: 19690307]

[60] Chao C, Klein NP, Velicer CM, *et al.* Surveillance of autoimmune conditions following routine use of quadrivalent human papillomavirus vaccine. J Intern Med 2012; 271(2): 193-203. [http://dx.doi.org/10.1111/j.1365-2796.2011.02467.x] [PMID: 21973261]

[61] Arnheim-Dahlström L, Pasternak B, Svanström H, Sparén P, Hviid A. Autoimmune, neurological, and venous thromboembolic adverse events after immunisation of adolescent girls with quadrivalent human papillomavirus vaccine in Denmark and Sweden: cohort study. BMJ 2013; 347: f5906. [http://dx.doi.org/10.1136/bmj.f5906] [PMID: 24108159]

CHAPTER 14

Therapeutic HPV Vaccines: Immunogenicity, Efficacy and Safety

Azam Bolhassani*

Department of Hepatitis and AIDS, Pasteur Institute of Iran, Tehran, Iran

Abstract: Up to now, a large number of HPV therapeutic vaccines have been developed targeting E6 and E7 oncoproteins including peptide/protein-based vaccines, live vector vaccines, cell-based vaccines and nucleic acid-based vaccines; each with advantages and disadvantages. These vaccines control HPV infection through cell-mediated immunity in preclinical and clinical trials, *e.g.*, adoptive T-cell therapy in patients with advanced cervical cancer and/or DNA-based vaccine in HPV-16 or HPV-18 positive CIN clinical trials. In this chapter, the potential use of therapeutic vaccines as safe and effective pharmacological tools in cervical diseases will be explained, focusing on vaccines that have been tested in clinical trials.

Keywords: HPV, Immunogenicity, Safety , Therapeutic vaccine.

INTRODUCTION

Immune mechanisms for protection against infection and for recovery from infection are not certainly similar; the first is the result of antibody production by HPV viral like particles (VLPs) and the latter is the result of cell-mediated immunity and the activation of cytotoxic effector cells induced by early proteins [1]. Systemic immunization with L1 VLPs generates antibody concentrations higher than in a natural infection, possibly because of high antigen concentration and delivery route that allows access to lymph nodes and spleen. The animal studies showed that anti-L2 antibodies are cross-neutralizing, but simple protein vaccines such as L2 are poorly immunogenic compared to the L1 VLPs. Strategies such as concatenating multiple L2 proteins increase immunogenicity and show cross-protection against HPVs 16, 18, 45 and 58 pseudovirions. In a natural infection, antibodies against L1 appear for 6-8 months following infection in about 50-70% of infected individuals. Other viral proteins such as E1, E2 and E6 do not elicit antibody responses. The IgM response occurs first and decays.

* **Corresponding author Azam Bolhassani:** Department of Hepatitis and AIDS, Pasteur Institute of Iran, Tehran, Iran; Tel: 66953311-20; E-mails: A_bolhasani@pasteur.ac.ir, azam.bolhassani@yahoo.com

The IgG1 response appears later and is more persistent [1]. High levels of IgA, IgG3 and IgG4 are detected, but IgG1 responses predominate. Two licensed vaccines (Cervarix and Gardasil) showed sero-conversion in virtually 100% of vaccines. Antibody titers in blood reach peaks 2-3 log higher than in natural infections, decline to levels several-fold lower than peak and then remain stable for years. Antibodies in the cervix are detectable at lower concentrations and vary with the menstrual cycle. Partial cross-protection against HPV31, HPV33 and HPV45 has been described, but although cross-neutralizing antibody concentrations are the same for both vaccines, data for the two vaccines regarding cross-protection vary [1]. The regression of HPV-established lesion is often associated with cellular immune responses against E6 and E7 oncoproteins. Currently, it is estimated that 32-43% of CIN2/3 lesions undergo spontaneous regression. The experimental data indicated that tissue-specific immune parameters may be highly informative as a therapeutic target in high-grade precancers of the cervix, anus and vagina. Two recent clinical trials testing HPV therapeutic vaccines in patients with vulvar epithelial hyperplasia showed complete responses in ~ 50% of subjects during 52 weeks of follow-up, against the expected 5% in unvaccinated individuals in the same period, despite modest systemic T cell responses [1]. Several immunotherapeutic strategies have been used in preclinical and clinical trials for cancer treatment with some promising results. Recently, to diminish the immunosuppressive effects of cancer microenvironment, the synergic combination of HPV therapeutic vaccines with radiotherapy, chemotherapy, immunomodulators or immune checkpoint inhibitors have been suggested in cervical cancer patients [2].

Therapeutic Vaccines

Generally, it is clear that T cells can recognize viral oncogene antigens in patients exposed to HPV infection, but their specific role in control of infection has not been proved. There are several preclinical and clinical studies (phases I and II) on peptides or proteins-, DNA plasmids- and different viral vectors-based vaccines [3, 4].

Peptides/Recombinant Proteins-based Vaccines

Therapeutic vaccination has been limited by inadequate antigen-specific immune responses. At present, the design of therapeutic vaccines to control the growth of HPV-induced tumors has focused on the use of E6 and E7 proteins or peptides as vaccine antigens [5]. Administered peptides and proteins derived from HPV antigens are taken up by DCs, processed and presented *via* MHC II and/or I to the $CD4^+/CD8^+$ T cells [6]. It is critical to predict immunodominant peptides of viral antigens associated with particular HLA allelic products which are recognized by human T cells. A recent study indicated that vaccination with longer peptides (22-35mer) harboring DC activating agents significantly generated both CD4 and CD8-specific T cell responses against HPV oncogenes compared to vaccination with minimal CTL epitopes [7, 8]. On the other hand, due to the poor immunogenicity of peptide vaccines, adjuvants were applied including chemokines, cytokines and Toll-like receptor ligands [9 - 15]. Several peptide vaccines have developed into clinical trials. For instance, administration of HPV16 E6 and E7 long peptides along with the adjuvant Montanide ISA-51 induced E6/E7-specific $CD4^+$ and $CD8^+$ immune responses in a phase I clinical trial of cervical cancer patients [16, 17]. The future of peptide-based vaccines relies on enhancement of their immunogenicity and identification of effective epitopes to prevent degradation and prolong antigen presentation. An E7 lipopeptide vaccine for special targeting DCs could significantly enhance the E7-specific $CD8^+$ activity in TC-1 tumor-bearing mice as compared to E7 peptide alone [18].

Recombinant proteins have the advantage over peptide approaches in delivery of all potential epitopes to the antigen processing cells of the immune system [19 - 21]. Due to their exogenous nature, protein-based vaccines are presented *via* MHC class II pathway generating an antibody response, thus it is required to create a bias for the MHC I presentation pathway producing a T-cell response. One of the most important strategies for inducing effective T cell responses is the use of adjuvants such as liposome-polycationic-DNA carrier particles and the saponin-based ISCOMATRIX [22 - 34]. In addition, generation of fusion proteins to target the antigen to DCs (*e.g.,* HPV16 E7 linked to adenylyl cyclase of *Bordetella pertussis*, the translocation domain of *Pseudomonas aeruginosa* exotoxin A, and heat shock proteins) can increase MHC I presentation and thus $CD8^+$ responses [22 - 34]. A protein-based vaccine that has progressed to clinical trials is TA-CIN containing a fusion protein composed of HPV16 L2, E6, and E7 that elicits both antibody and T cell-mediated responses [30, 34]. A study showed that vaccinated mice with the recombinant HPV16E7 linked to the N-terminal of glycoprotein 96 (rE7-NT-gp96), a member of heat shock protein 90 (HSP90) family, induced Th1 immunity and delayed the tumor occurrence and growth as compared to E7 protein, alone [35]. On the other hand, E7 co-delivered by Hp91 peptide derived from high mobility group box 1 (HMGB1) protein stimulated a strong Th1 cellular immune response and complete protection (100% survival) as compared to E7 co-injected with NT-gp96 protein (50-75% survival) after mice challenge with TC-1 tumor cell line [36]. Generally, Hp91 peptide and the full length of HMGB1 gene could be an effective adjuvant for improvement of therapeutic HPV protein- and DNA-based vaccines, respectively [37]. On the other hand, various vaccine delivery systems such as different routes of immunization and physical/chemical delivery methods have been used in cancer therapy to induce immunity against tumor-associated antigens (TAA) [38]. Recently, protein transduction domains (PTDs) or cell penetrating peptides (CPPs) as a linear or cyclic form have been shown to promote the delivery of therapeutic proteins or peptides into live cells. The successful delivery of proteins mainly depends on their physicochemical properties [39]. Up to now, several small protein transduction domains from viral proteins including Tat or VP22 could be fused to other peptides or proteins to entry them in various cell types at a dose-dependent approach. A major disadvantage of these PTD-fusion proteins is primary uptake into endosomal vesicles leading to inefficient release of the fusion proteins into the cytosol. Recently, non-covalent complex between proteins and CPPs has attracted a special interest to overcome some delivery limitations (*e.g.*, toxicity) [39]. Our group showed that the complexes of a short amphipathic peptide carrier, Pep-1 with the full-length HPV16 E7 protein (E7/Pep-1) form the stable nanoparticles (120-250 nm) through non-covalent binding and elicit high Th1 cellular immune response at a ratio of 1:20 in a murine tumor model. Therefore, Pep-1 CPP can be considered as a promising carrier for development of HPV protein vaccines [40].

Plasmid DNA-based Vaccines

The Naked plasmid DNA encoding an antigen is safe, stable, and capable of sustaining antigen expression in cells longer than RNA or protein vaccines [41, 42]. An important limitation of DNA vaccines is their low immunogenicity due to the lack of spread from transfected cells into surrounding cells *in vivo*. Different strategies have been developed to enhance DNA vaccine potency such as: (a) increasing the number of DCs expressing antigen; (b) enhancing antigen processing and presentation in DCs; and (c) improving the interaction between DCs and T cells [43, 44]. In strategy (a), the mode of plasmid DNA delivery to areas rich in DCs (*i.e.*, the Langerhans cells of the skin) is critical to make progress in DNA vaccination. For example, intradermal administration of DNA *via* gene gun [45, 46], the combination of intramuscular injection with electroporation (*e.g.*, VGX-3100, a DNA vaccine targeting HPV16 and HPV18 E6 and E7 in patients with CIN II/III) [47, 48], laser and microencapsulation of DNA [49, 50] are important approaches for increasing the number of DCs expressing antigen. Moreover, since DNA vaccines are unable to spread between cells, the use of delivery systems covalently or non-covalently allows the distribution of antigen in cells transfected with DNA. For example, the linkage of DNA encoding HPV16 E7 to herpes simplex virus 1 (HSV-1) VP22 [51], the complex formation between a peptide-polymer hybrid (PEI600-Tat conjugate) and HPV16 E7 DNA at a ratio of 10:50 (w/w) [52] and the use of MPG cell penetrating peptide condensing HPV16 E7 DNA into stable nanoparticles (180-210 nm) at an N/P ratio of 10:1 [53, 54] led to induce strong Th1 and CTL immune responses and protective effects against tumor growth in C57BL/6 mice. Other strategies to enhance DNA-encoded antigen uptake by DCs include linkage of HPV antigen to molecules which bind to scavenger receptors on the DC surface such as FMS-like tyrosine kinase 3 ligands and heat shock proteins [55, 56]. In addition, antigen expression can be increased through codon optimization of HPV DNAs and/or the use of demethylation agents (*e.g.,* 5-aza-2'-deoxycytidine) [57 - 61].

In strategy (b), HPV E7 DNA can be linked with molecules that localize antigen to the endoplasmic reticulum (ER) or that facilitate proteasome degradation to enhance MHC class I processing and cross-priming such as heat shock proteins (Hsp70, CRT, Gp96) and γ-tubulin inducing potent $CD8^+$ T cell immune responses. Moreover, the linkage of β2-microglobulin and MHCI heavy chain genes to HPV16 E6 epitope in DNA vaccine led to increase antigen processing and presentation, and induce E6-specific $CD8^+$ T cell immune responses and protection against TC-1 tumor cells in mice model [62 - 71]. On the other hand, DNA vaccine encoding E7 antigen linked to the sorting signal peptide of lysosomal-associated membrane protein 1 has been shown to generate E7-specific $CD4^+$ and $CD8^+$ cells and antitumor effects in vaccinated mice. Recent advances indicated that both MHC I and II expression are regulated by CIITA, and thus injection of CIITA DNA with CRT/E6 DNA leads to enhance E6-specific $CD8^+$ T cell immune responses in vaccinated mice [72 - 74]. In addition, a HPV E6/E7 DNA therapeutic vaccine (GX-188) was designed to facilitate the processing and presentation of HPV E6/E7 antigens by DCs through the co-expression of Fms-like tyrosine kinase-3 ligand (Flt3L). Vaccination with GX-188 by electroporation (GX-188E) significantly induced antigen-specific Th1 and CD8 T-cell immune responses in patients with CIN3 leading to complete regression of high-grade cervical lesions [75, 76].

On the other hand, the strategies to enhance DC and T cell interaction (strategy c) may rely on prolonging DC survival, increasing expression of cytokines and blocking DC inactivation. Prevention of the apoptosis of DCs can be achieved through the use of anti-apoptotic proteins or inhibition of proapoptotic proteins. For example, the use of siRNA targeting Bak and Bax proapoptotic proteins along with the E7 DNA vaccine improved DC resistance to apoptosis and enhanced anti-tumor effects in mice. Furthermore, a recent study showed that DNA vaccine encoding growth factor linked to E7 can prolong survival of DCs generating potent E7-specific antitumor responses without any oncogenic risk [77 - 79]. Preventing activated T-cell apoptosis is another way to increase $CD8^+$ responses. For instance, the use of DNA encoding small hairpin RNA to block Fas ligand co-administered with E7 DNA led to generate significant E7-specific $CD8^+$ responses and antitumor effects in vaccinated mice [80]. Also, further release of stimulatory cytokines from DCs improves DC and T cell interaction. For example, the combination of HPVE7 DNA vaccines with DNA encoding IL-2 and IL-12 as adjuvants caused tumor regression in mice through inducing E7-specific $CD8^+$ responses [81 - 84].

Several DNA vaccines have been evaluated in clinical trials such as a microencapsulated DNA vaccine encoding several HLA-A2-restricted HPV16 E7 epitopes (ZYC-101) in patients with CIN II/III [81 - 84], DNA vaccine encoding HPV16 and HPV18 E6 and E7-derived epitopes (ZYC-101a) in patients with CIN II/III lesions, DNA vaccine encoding HPV16 E7 linked to *M. tuberculosis* Hsp70 in women with CIN II/III [85, 86]. Our group showed that co-delivery of plasmids harboring HPV16 E7 and glycoprotein 96 (Gp96) as an adjuvant induces Th1 immune response compared to E7 DNA alone [68, 87]. In this line, other study demonstrated that the injection of plasmid DNA encoding HPV16 E7 linked to the C-terminal fragment of Gp96 (E7-CT-gp96) by electroporation significantly induces E7-specific IFN-γ immune responses as well as the best protective effects in vaccinated mice [88].

Naked RNA Replicon Vaccines

Naked RNA replicon vaccines derived from alphaviruses provide a novel approach for HPV vaccination. Self-replication of the RNA replicon allows a prolonged level of antigen expression enhancing immunogenicity significantly more than a DNA vaccine. However, RNA is less stable than DNA, thus attempts to overcome this problem led to use more stable "suicidal DNA" which is translated into RNA replicons within the transfected cell. These transfected cells undergo apoptosis leading to poor immunogenicity in DCs directly transfected with RNA replicons, a disadvantage associated with DNA vaccines. Apoptosis can be delayed by suicidal DNA encoding the E7 antigen linked to anti-apoptotic proteins (*e.g.,* Bcl-xL) inducing E7-specific $CD8^+$ T cell immune responses higher than E7 alone, due to prolonged survival of DCs. Another strategy is the development of the flavivirus Kunjin (KUN) vector to deliver replicons. For instance, DNA-launched KUN replicons encoding HPV16 E7 could generate E7-specific T cell responses and protect mice against E7-expressing tumor. Despite the relative success of RNA replicon-based vaccines in preclinical models, there is no progression to clinical trials [2, 89 - 96].

Live Vector-based Vaccines

Live vector-based vaccines cover both bacterial and viral vectors which are highly immunogenic as they replicate within host cells and facilitate spread of antigen. Vector-based vaccines can deliver the E6 and E7 antigens to DCs stimulating antigen presentation through MHC class I to $CD8^+$ cytotoxic T cells, and *via*

MHC class II to CD4+ helper T cells. However, a potential safety risk in immunocompromised individuals, limitation of repeated immunizations, and the pre-existing immunity to the vector are major disadvantages of the live vectors [6]. However, there is an urgent need for development of novel safe live vectors (*e.g.*, nonpathogenic parasites including *Leishmania tarentolae*, *Toxoplasma gondii* and *Trypanosoma cruzi*) that are capable of enhancing antigen presentation and eliciting potent immune responses [97]. Our group developed a novel live vaccine using the recombinant *Leishmania tarentolae* (*L.tar*) expressing E7-GFP fusion protein for mice protection against HPV-associated tumors [98]. Another study showed that subcutaneous administration of mice with the recombinant *L.tar* expressing E7 linked to the C-terminal of gp96 (*L.tar*-E7-CT-gp96) led to enhance the levels of IFN-γ and IgG2a as well as significant protective effects compared to group vaccinated with *L.tar*-E7 [99].

Bacterial Vectors

Attenuated bacteria can deliver genes or proteins of interest, such as E6 and E7, to antigen presenting cells (APCs). Different bacterial vectors have been used in HPV therapeutic vaccines including *Listeria* monocytogenes (Lm) [100, 101], *Lactobacillus* lactis [102, 103] and *Lactobacillus plantarum* [104]. *Listeria* is a promising vector due to its ability to infect monocytes and macrophages and secrete listeriolysin O (LLO) inducing $CD4^+$ and $CD8^+$ immune responses [105]. Three clinical trials were performed using a *Listeria*-based vaccine encoding HPV16 E7 (Lovaxin C), a *Listeria*-based vaccine expressing the fusion of lysteriolysin O with E7, and a safe live-attenuated *Listeria* vaccine secreting HPV16 E7 antigen fused to a fragment of listeriolysin O (Lm-LLO-E7: ADXS11-001) in women with advanced cervical cancer [106 - 108].

Viral Vector Vaccines

The levels of highly effective infection and expression of encoded antigen make viral vectors as a possible option in therapeutic HPV vaccines. Viruses that were used in HPV vaccine design include *adenovirus*, *adeno-associated virus*, *vaccinia virus*, and *alphaviruses* [6]. For example, a live recombinant *vaccinia virus* encoding HPV-16 and -18 E6 and E7 (TA-HPV) indicated the safety and immunogenicity in patients with advanced cervical carcinoma or vulval intraepithelial neoplasia. Moreover, *vaccinia* encoding fusion of E7 and calreticulin (CRT) could increase MHCI processing in DCs, and *vaccinia* encoding E7 and listeriolysin O could facilitate MHC I and II presentation [109 - 113]. On the other hand, vaccination with replication-deficient *adenoviruses* encoding CRT/E7 and/or hepatitis B surface antigen/E7 fusion proteins stimulated E7-specific antibody and $CD8^+$ T cell immune responses, and eradicated E7-

expressing tumors in mice model [114 - 116]. The *adeno-associated viruses* were also engineered to express E7 linked to *Mycobacterium tuberculosis* Hsp70 inducing CD8$^+$ T cell immune responses [117, 118]. Moreover, RNA viruses such as the *Semliki Forest virus* (SFV) expressing HPV16 E7 could be used as live vectors eliciting E7-specific CTL cells in HPV-transgenic mice [119]. This response could be further enhanced through the co-injection of IL-12 cytokine inhibiting tumor angiogenesis [120, 121]. A major problem is the generation of neutralizing antibodies upon first exposure to these vaccines. For instance, COX-2 inhibitors including Celecoxib can prevent the generation of neutralizing antibodies to *vaccinia* allowing repeated administration without losing infectivity [122].

Whole Cell-based Vaccines

These vaccines are divided into three strategies including dendritic cell-based vaccines, tumor-cell-based vaccines, and adoptive T-cell therapy (ACT) as mentioned in below sections.

Dendritic Cell-based Vaccines

Dendritic cells (DCs) have strong ability to control T-cell responses as ideal candidates for immunotherapy strategies. They can be divided into DCs pulsed with peptides/proteins, or transduced with DNA or viral vectors encoding target antigen. For example, a DC vaccine pulsed with the recombinant HPV16/18 E7 antigens and IL-2 could induce strong immunological responses but no clinical effect in patients with advanced cervical cancer. Also, several preclinical studies were performed with DC vaccines transduced by adenoviral vector carrying a mutated E7 protein with promising results [2].

Tumor Cell-based Vaccines

Delivery of whole tumor cells genetically modified with genes encoding cytokines (*e.g.,* IL-2, IL-12, and GM-CSF) could stimulate immune system to recognize tumor-associated antigens (TAA). However, the use of tumor cells harvested from patients is not considered in early stages of CIN due to safety concerns [2].

Adoptive T-Cell Therapy (ACT)

The ACT approach was used in chemotherapy-refractory metastatic cervical cancer. Tumor-infiltrating T-cells were collected from patients, expanded, and selected for HPV reactivity (HPVTILs). Single infusion of these TILs induced effective clinical response in patients with advanced cervical cancer [2].

Combinational Approaches

Combinational approaches use HPV therapeutic vaccines as well as other therapeutic modalities such as chemotherapy, radiotherapy or biotherapeutic agents. For example, apigenin, a chemotherapeutic agent inducing apoptotic death in tumor cells was tested in combination with HPV E7 DNA vaccine in mice bearing E7-expressing tumors. This regimen could enhance E7-specific $CD8^+$ responses and potent anti-tumor effects [2]. On the other hand, saffron and its components have been suggested as promising candidates for cancer prevention. Carotenoids (*e.g.*, crocin) and monoterpene aldehydes (*e.g.*, picrocrocin) are two potent ingredients of saffron. The anti-tumor effects of chemo-immunotherapy using saffron and its ingredients along with E7 DNA fused to the N-terminal fragment of Gp96 (E7-NT-gp96 DNA vaccine) indicated that 100% of mice treated with crocin were tumor-free, in contrast to DNA vaccine alone (~66.7%) and DNA + crocin (~33.3%) indicating the high potency of crocin as a chemotherapeutic agent. Interestingly, the multimodality treatment using DNA vaccine along with picrocrocin augmented the anti-tumor effects of picrocrocin [123]. In other study, three strategies including linkage to immunostimulatory molecules (NT-gp96), co-administration of chemokines (IP-10 or RANTES) and PEI600-Tat as non-viral gene delivery system were applied to enhance the efficiency of HPV16 E7 DNA vaccine. The data showed that co-administration of IP-10 with E7-NT-gp96 delivered by PEI600-Tat significantly elevated the levels of IFN-γ and IL-2 in the lymph nodes and suppressed TC-1 tumor growth in contrast to increased tumor growth by RANTES co-delivery. This approach suggests a combinational therapeutic strategy against HPV-related tumors [124].

Prime-Boost Vaccination Strategies

Prime-boost strategies are designed as a priming immunization (*e.g.*, DNA plasmid, viral vector or protein) followed by a heterologous boost with a different vector encoding the immunogen [125]. For example, the heterologous prime-boost immunization strategy of TA-CIN (HPV16 L2/E6/E7 fusion protein vaccine as a prime) with TA-HPV (recombinant *vaccinia virus* encoding HPV16/18 E6/E7 fusion protein as a booster) could enhance immunogenicity and induce antigen-specific T-cell immune responses in mice and also in patients with anogenital intraepithelial neoplasia [126 - 128]. Another example is a clinical trial using a DNA vaccine encoding a signaling peptide (Sig), the mutated E7 antigen [E7 (detox)], and Hsp70 [*i.e.*, pNGVL4a/Sig/E7 (detox)/Hsp70], boosted with TA-HPV in women with CIN II/III lesions as an effective strategy against viral infections [2].

CONCLUDING REMARKS

The effective vaccination against HPV infections provides an opportunity to treat and control HPV-associated cancers including cervical, vulvar, vaginal, anal, head and neck cancers. The FDA has approved two HPV prophylactic vaccines, but they do not exert therapeutic effects on pre-existing HPV-associated lesions. Thus, therapeutic vaccines are being developed to induce cell-mediated immune responses against the infected cells. Recently, several preclinical and clinical trials are underway to determine the best therapeutic regimens, *e.g.,* combinational approaches.

CONFLICT OF INTEREST

The author (editor) declares no conflict of interest, financial or otherwise.

ACKNOWLEDGEMENT

Declare none.

REFERENCES

[1] Bosch FX, Broker TR, Forman D, *et al.* Comprehensive control of human papillomavirus infections and related diseases. Vaccine 2013; 31 (Suppl. 5): F1-F31.
[http://dx.doi.org/10.1016/j.vaccine.2013.10.001] [PMID: 24331745]

[2] Vici P, Pizzuti L, Mariani L, *et al.* Targeting immune response with therapeutic vaccines in premalignant lesions and cervical cancer: hope or reality from clinical studies. Expert Rev Vaccines 2016; 15(10): 1327-36.
[http://dx.doi.org/10.1080/14760584.2016.1176533] [PMID: 27063030]

[3] Frazer IH. Prevention of cervical cancer through papillomavirus vaccination. Nat Rev Immunol 2004; 4(1): 46-54.
[http://dx.doi.org/10.1038/nri1260] [PMID: 14704767]

[4] Khallouf H, Grabowska AK, Riemer AB. Therapeutic vaccine strategies against human papillomavirus. Vaccines (Basel) 2014; 2(2): 422-62.
[http://dx.doi.org/10.3390/vaccines2020422] [PMID: 26344626]

[5] Bolhassani A, Mohit E, Rafati S. Different spectra of therapeutic vaccine development against HPV infections. Hum Vaccin 2009; 5(10): 671-89.
[http://dx.doi.org/10.4161/hv.5.10.9370] [PMID: 19684468]

[6] Lin K, Doolan K, Hung CF, Wu TC. Perspectives for preventive and therapeutic HPV vaccines. J Formos Med Assoc 2010; 109(1): 4-24.
[http://dx.doi.org/10.1016/S0929-6646(10)60017-4] [PMID: 20123582]

[7] Muderspach L, Wilczynski S, Roman L, *et al.* A phase I trial of a human papillomavirus (HPV) peptide vaccine for women with high-grade cervical and vulvar intraepithelial neoplasia who are HPV 16 positive. Clin Cancer Res 2000; 6(9): 3406-16.
[PMID: 10999722]

[8] Zwaveling S, Ferreira Mota SC, Nouta J, *et al.* Established human papillomavirus type 16-expressing tumors are effectively eradicated following vaccination with long peptides. J Immunol 2002; 169(1): 350-8.
[http://dx.doi.org/10.4049/jimmunol.169.1.350] [PMID: 12077264]

[9] Chang CL, Ma B, Pang X, Wu TC, Hung CF. Treatment with cyclooxygenase-2 inhibitors enables repeated administration of vaccinia virus for control of ovarian cancer. Mol Ther 2009; 17(8): 1365-72.
[http://dx.doi.org/10.1038/mt.2009.118] [PMID: 19471247]

[10] Vambutas A, DeVoti J, Nouri M, *et al.* Therapeutic vaccination with papillomavirus E6 and E7 long peptides results in the control of both established virus-induced lesions and latently infected sites in a pre-clinical cottontail rabbit papillomavirus model. Vaccine 2005; 23(45): 5271-80.
[http://dx.doi.org/10.1016/j.vaccine.2005.04.049] [PMID: 16054734]

[11] Zwaveling S, Ferreira Mota SC, Nouta J, *et al.* Established human papillomavirus type 16-expressing tumors are effectively eradicated following vaccination with long peptides. J Immunol 2002; 169(1): 350-8.
[http://dx.doi.org/10.4049/jimmunol.169.1.350] [PMID: 12077264]

[12] Sharma RK, Elpek KG, Yolcu ES, *et al.* Costimulation as a platform for the development of vaccines: a peptide-based vaccine containing a novel form of 4-1BB ligand eradicates established tumors. Cancer Res 2009; 69(10): 4319-26.
[http://dx.doi.org/10.1158/0008-5472.CAN-08-3141] [PMID: 19435920]

[13] Manuri PR, Nehete B, Nehete PN, *et al.* Intranasal immunization with synthetic peptides corresponding to the E6 and E7 oncoproteins of human papillomavirus type 16 induces systemic and mucosal cellular immune responses and tumor protection. Vaccine 2007; 25(17): 3302-10.
[http://dx.doi.org/10.1016/j.vaccine.2007.01.010] [PMID: 17291642]

[14] Chen YF, Lin CW, Tsao YP, Chen SL. Cytotoxic-T-lymphocyte human papillomavirus type 16 E5 peptide with CpG-oligodeoxynucleotide can eliminate tumor growth in C57BL/6 mice. J Virol 2004; 78(3): 1333-43.
[http://dx.doi.org/10.1128/JVI.78.3.1333-1343.2004] [PMID: 14722288]

[15] Daftarian P, Mansour M, Benoit AC, *et al.* Eradication of established HPV 16-expressing tumors by a single administration of a vaccine composed of a liposome-encapsulated CTL-T helper fusion peptide in a water-in-oil emulsion. Vaccine 2006; 24(24): 5235-44.
[http://dx.doi.org/10.1016/j.vaccine.2006.03.079] [PMID: 16675074]

[16] Kenter GG, Welters MJ, Valentijn AR, *et al.* Phase I immunotherapeutic trial with long peptides spanning the E6 and E7 sequences of high-risk human papillomavirus 16 in end-stage cervical cancer patients shows low toxicity and robust immunogenicity. Clin Cancer Res 2008; 14(1): 169-77.
[http://dx.doi.org/10.1158/1078-0432.CCR-07-1881] [PMID: 18172268]

[17] Welters MJ, Kenter GG, Piersma SJ, *et al.* Induction of tumor-specific CD4+ and CD8+ T-cell immunity in cervical cancer patients by a human papillomavirus type 16 E6 and E7 long peptides vaccine. Clin Cancer Res 2008; 14(1): 178-87.
[http://dx.doi.org/10.1158/1078-0432.CCR-07-1880] [PMID: 18172269]

[18] Chen W, Huang L. Induction of cytotoxic T-lymphocytes and antitumor activity by a liposomal lipopeptide vaccine. Mol Pharm 2008; 5(3): 464-71.
[http://dx.doi.org/10.1021/mp700126c] [PMID: 18266319]

[19] Goldstone SE, Palefsky JM, Winnett MT, Neefe JR. Activity of HspE7, a novel immunotherapy, in patients with anogenital warts. Dis Colon Rectum 2002; 45(4): 502-7.
[http://dx.doi.org/10.1007/s10350-004-6229-6] [PMID: 12006932]

[20] Santin AD, Bellone S, Gokden M, Cannon MJ, Parham GP. Vaccination with HPV-18 E7-pulsed dendritic cells in a patient with metastatic cervical cancer. N Engl J Med 2002; 346(22): 1752-3.
[http://dx.doi.org/10.1056/NEJM200205303462219] [PMID: 12037163]

[21] Stern PL. Immune control of human papillomavirus (HPV) associated anogenital disease and potential for vaccination. J Clin Virol 2005; 32 (Suppl. 1): S72-81.
[http://dx.doi.org/10.1016/j.jcv.2004.12.005] [PMID: 15753015]

[22] Cui Z, Huang L. Liposome-polycation-DNA (LPD) particle as a carrier and adjuvant for protein-based vaccines: therapeutic effect against cervical cancer. Cancer Immunol Immunother 2005; 54(12): 1180-90.
[http://dx.doi.org/10.1007/s00262-005-0685-2] [PMID: 15846491]

[23] Stewart TJ, Drane D, Malliaros J, *et al.* ISCOMATRIX adjuvant: an adjuvant suitable for use in anticancer vaccines. Vaccine 2004; 22(27-28): 3738-43.
[http://dx.doi.org/10.1016/j.vaccine.2004.03.026] [PMID: 15315854]

[24] Préville X, Ladant D, Timmerman B, Leclerc C. Eradication of established tumors by vaccination with recombinant *Bordetella pertussis* adenylate cyclase carrying the human papillomavirus 16 E7 oncoprotein. Cancer Res 2005; 65(2): 641-9.
[PMID: 15695409]

[25] Liao CW, Chen CA, Lee CN, *et al.* Fusion protein vaccine by domains of bacterial exotoxin linked with a tumor antigen generates potent immunologic responses and antitumor effects. Cancer Res 2005; 65(19): 9089-98.
[http://dx.doi.org/10.1158/0008-5472.CAN-05-0958] [PMID: 16204084]

[26] Walker KB, Keeble J, Colaco C. Mycobacterial heat shock proteins as vaccines - a model of facilitated antigen presentation. Curr Mol Med 2007; 7(4): 339-50.
[http://dx.doi.org/10.2174/156652407780831575] [PMID: 17584074]

[27] Chu NR, Wu HB, Wu T, Boux LJ, Siegel MI, Mizzen LA. Immunotherapy of a human papillomavirus (HPV) type 16 E7-expressing tumour by administration of fusion protein comprising Mycobacterium bovis bacille Calmette-Guérin (BCG) hsp65 and HPV16 E7. Clin Exp Immunol 2000; 121(2): 216-25.
[http://dx.doi.org/10.1046/j.1365-2249.2000.01293.x] [PMID: 10931134]

[28] Liu B, Ye D, Song X, *et al.* A novel therapeutic fusion protein vaccine by two different families of heat shock proteins linked with HPV16 E7 generates potent antitumor immunity and antiangiogenesis. Vaccine 2008; 26(10): 1387-96.
[http://dx.doi.org/10.1016/j.vaccine.2007.12.034] [PMID: 18272260]

[29] Einstein MH, Kadish AS, Burk RD, *et al.* Heat shock fusion protein-based immunotherapy for treatment of cervical intraepithelial neoplasia III. Gynecol Oncol 2007; 106(3): 453-60.
[http://dx.doi.org/10.1016/j.ygyno.2007.04.038] [PMID: 17586030]

[30] de Jong A, O'Neill T, Khan AY, *et al.* Enhancement of human papillomavirus (HPV) type 16 E6 and E7-specific T-cell immunity in healthy volunteers through vaccination with TA-CIN, an HPV16 L2E7E6 fusion protein vaccine. Vaccine 2002; 20(29-30): 3456-64.
[http://dx.doi.org/10.1016/S0264-410X(02)00350-X] [PMID: 12297390]

[31] Santin AD, Bellone S, Roman JJ, Burnett A, Cannon MJ, Pecorelli S. Therapeutic vaccines for cervical cancer: dendritic cell-based immunotherapy. Curr Pharm Des 2005; 11(27): 3485-500.
[http://dx.doi.org/10.2174/138161205774414565] [PMID: 16248803]

[32] Tillman BW, Hayes TL, DeGruijl TD, Douglas JT, Curiel DT. Adenoviral vectors targeted to CD40 enhance the efficacy of dendritic cell-based vaccination against human papillomavirus 16-induced tumor cells in a murine model. Cancer Res 2000; 60(19): 5456-63.
[PMID: 11034088]

[33] Mackova J, Kutinova L, Hainz P, *et al.* Adjuvant effect of dendritic cells transduced with recombinant vaccinia virus expressing HPV16-E7 is inhibited by co-expression of IL12. Int J Oncol 2004; 24(6): 1581-8.
[PMID: 15138603]

[34] Killock D. Therapeutic HPV vaccine holds promise. Nat Rev Clin Oncol 2015; 12(12): 686.
[http://dx.doi.org/10.1038/nrclinonc.2015.180] [PMID: 26462124]

[35] Mohit E, Bolhassani A, Zahedifard F, Taslimi Y, Rafati S. The contribution of NT-gp96 as an adjuvant for increasing HPV16 E7-specific immunity in C57BL/6 mouse model. Scand J Immunol

2012; 75(1): 27-37.
[http://dx.doi.org/10.1111/j.1365-3083.2011.02620.x] [PMID: 21916914]

[36] Talebi S, Bolhassani A, Azad TM, Arashkia A, Modaresi MH. Immuno-stimulating peptide derived from HMGB1 is more effective than the N-terminal domain of Gp96 as an endogenous adjuvant for improvement of protein vaccines. Protein Pept Lett 2017; 24(3): 190-6.
[http://dx.doi.org/10.2174/0929866523666161220111833] [PMID: 28000571]

[37] Talebi S, Bolhassani A, Sadat SM, Vahabpour R, Agi E, Shahbazi S. Hp91 immunoadjuvant: An HMGB1-derived peptide for development of therapeutic HPV vaccines. Biomed Pharmacother 2017; 85: 148-54.
[http://dx.doi.org/10.1016/j.biopha.2016.11.115] [PMID: 27930979]

[38] Bolhassani A, Safaiyan S, Rafati S. Improvement of different vaccine delivery systems for cancer therapy. Mol Cancer 2011; 10: 3.
[http://dx.doi.org/10.1186/1476-4598-10-3] [PMID: 21211062]

[39] Bolhassani A, Jafarzade BS, Mardani G. *In vitro* and *in vivo* delivery of therapeutic proteins using cell penetrating peptides. Peptides 2017; 87: 50-63.
[http://dx.doi.org/10.1016/j.peptides.2016.11.011] [PMID: 27887988]

[40] Mardani G, Bolhassani A, Agi E, Shahbazi S, Mehdi Sadat S. Protein vaccination with HPV16 E7/Pep-1 nanoparticles elicits a protective T-helper cell-mediated immune response. IUBMB Life 2016; 68(6): 459-67.
[http://dx.doi.org/10.1002/iub.1503] [PMID: 27094221]

[41] Garcia F, Petry KU, Muderspach L, *et al.* ZYC101a for treatment of high-grade cervical intraepithelial neoplasia: a randomized controlled trial. Obstet Gynecol 2004; 103(2): 317-26.
[http://dx.doi.org/10.1097/01.AOG.0000110246.93627.17] [PMID: 14754702]

[42] Kaisho T, Akira S. Regulation of dendritic cell function through toll-like receptors. Curr Mol Med 2003; 3(8): 759-71.
[http://dx.doi.org/10.2174/1566524033479366] [PMID: 14682496]

[43] Hung CF, Wu TC. Improving DNA vaccine potency *via* modification of professional antigen presenting cells. Curr Opin Mol Ther 2003; 5(1): 20-4.
[PMID: 12669466]

[44] Tsen SW, Paik AH, Hung CF, Wu TC. Enhancing DNA vaccine potency by modifying the properties of antigen-presenting cells. Expert Rev Vaccines 2007; 6(2): 227-39.
[http://dx.doi.org/10.1586/14760584.6.2.227] [PMID: 17408372]

[45] Trimble C, Lin CT, Hung CF, *et al.* Comparison of the CD8+ T cell responses and antitumor effects generated by DNA vaccine administered through gene gun, biojector, and syringe. Vaccine 2003; 21(25-26): 4036-42.
[http://dx.doi.org/10.1016/S0264-410X(03)00275-5] [PMID: 12922140]

[46] http://clinicaltrials.gov/ct2/show/NCT00685412?term2009.

[47] Babiuk LA, Babiuk SL. Immunization of animals: from DNA to the dinner plate. Vet Immunol Immunopathol 1999; 72(1-2): 189-202.
[http://dx.doi.org/10.1016/S0165-2427(99)00132-4] [PMID: 10614509]

[48] Best SR, Peng S, Juang CM, *et al.* Administration of HPV DNA vaccine *via* electroporation elicits the strongest CD8+ T cell immune responses compared to intramuscular injection and intradermal gene gun delivery. Vaccine 2009; 27(40): 5450-9.
[http://dx.doi.org/10.1016/j.vaccine.2009.07.005] [PMID: 19622402]

[49] Tsen SW, Wu CY, Meneshian A, Pai SI, Hung CF, Wu TC. Femtosecond laser treatment enhances DNA transfection efficiency *in vivo.* J Biomed Sci 2009; 16: 36.
[http://dx.doi.org/10.1186/1423-0127-16-36] [PMID: 19338665]

[50] Klencke B, Matijevic M, Urban RG, *et al.* Encapsulated plasmid DNA treatment for human

papillomavirus 16-associated anal dysplasia: a Phase I study of ZYC101. Clin Cancer Res 2002; 8(5): 1028-37.
[PMID: 12006515]

[51] Hung CF, Cheng WF, Chai CY, *et al.* Improving vaccine potency through intercellular spreading and enhanced MHC class I presentation of antigen. J Immunol 2001; 166(9): 5733-40.
[http://dx.doi.org/10.4049/jimmunol.166.9.5733] [PMID: 11313416]

[52] Bolhassani A, Ghasemi N, Servis C, Taghikhani M, Rafati S. The efficiency of a novel delivery system (PEI600-Tat) in development of potent DNA vaccine using HPV16 E7 as a model antigen. Drug Deliv 2009; 16(4): 196-204.
[http://dx.doi.org/10.1080/10717540902757721] [PMID: 19514980]

[53] Bolhassani A. Potential efficacy of cell-penetrating peptides for nucleic acid and drug delivery in cancer. Biochim Biophys Acta 2011; 1816(2): 232-46.
[PMID: 21840374]

[54] Saleh T, Bolhassani A, Shojaosadati SA, Aghasadeghi MR. MPG-based nanoparticle: An efficient delivery system for enhancing the potency of DNA vaccine expressing HPV16E7. Vaccine 2015; 33(28): 3164-70.
[http://dx.doi.org/10.1016/j.vaccine.2015.05.015] [PMID: 26001433]

[55] Hung CF, Hsu KF, Cheng WF, *et al.* Enhancement of DNA vaccine potency by linkage of antigen gene to a gene encoding the extracellular domain of Fms-like tyrosine kinase 3-ligand. Cancer Res 2001; 61(3): 1080-8.
[PMID: 11221836]

[56] Hauser H, Chen SY. Augmentation of DNA vaccine potency through secretory heat shock protein-mediated antigen targeting. Methods 2003; 31(3): 225-31.
[http://dx.doi.org/10.1016/S1046-2023(03)00136-1] [PMID: 14511955]

[57] Cheung YK, Cheng SC, Sin FW, Xie Y. Plasmid encoding papillomavirus Type 16 (HPV16) DNA constructed with codon optimization improved the immunogenicity against HPV infection. Vaccine 2004; 23(5): 629-38.
[http://dx.doi.org/10.1016/j.vaccine.2004.07.010] [PMID: 15542183]

[58] Liu W, Gao F, Zhao KN, *et al.* Codon modified human papillomavirus type 16 E7 DNA vaccine enhances cytotoxic T-lymphocyte induction and anti-tumour activity. Virology 2002; 301(1): 43-52.
[http://dx.doi.org/10.1006/viro.2002.1584] [PMID: 12359445]

[59] Lin CT, Tsai YC, He L, *et al.* A DNA vaccine encoding a codon-optimized human papillomavirus type 16 E6 gene enhances CTL response and anti-tumor activity. J Biomed Sci 2006; 13(4): 481-8.
[http://dx.doi.org/10.1007/s11373-006-9086-6] [PMID: 16649071]

[60] Ohlschläger P, Quetting M, Alvarez G, Dürst M, Gissmann L, Kaufmann AM. Enhancement of immunogenicity of a therapeutic cervical cancer DNA-based vaccine by co-application of sequence-optimized genetic adjuvants. Int J Cancer 2009; 125(1): 189-98.
[http://dx.doi.org/10.1002/ijc.24333] [PMID: 19358269]

[61] Lu D, Hoory T, Monie A, Wu A, Wang MC, Hung CF. Treatment with demethylating agent, 5-aza--'-deoxycytidine enhances therapeutic HPV DNA vaccine potency. Vaccine 2009; 27(32): 4363-9.
[http://dx.doi.org/10.1016/j.vaccine.2009.02.041] [PMID: 19481843]

[62] Smahel M, Poláková I, Pokorná D, Ludvíková V, Dusková M, Vlasák J. Enhancement of T cell-mediated and humoral immunity of β-glucuronidase-based DNA vaccines against HPV16 E7 oncoprotein. Int J Oncol 2008; 33(1): 93-101.
[PMID: 18575754]

[63] Massa S, Simeone P, Muller A, Benvenuto E, Venuti A, Franconi R. Antitumor activity of DNA vaccines based on the human papillomavirus-16 E7 protein genetically fused to a plant virus coat protein. Hum Gene Ther 2008; 19(4): 354-64.
[http://dx.doi.org/10.1089/hum.2007.122] [PMID: 18439124]

[64] Chen CH, Wang TL, Hung CF, *et al.* Enhancement of DNA vaccine potency by linkage of antigen gene to an HSP70 gene. Cancer Res 2000; 60(4): 1035-42. [PMID: 10706121]

[65] Cheng WF, Hung CF, Chai CY, *et al.* Tumor-specific immunity and antiangiogenesis generated by a DNA vaccine encoding calreticulin linked to a tumor antigen. J Clin Invest 2001; 108(5): 669-78. [http://dx.doi.org/10.1172/JCI200112346] [PMID: 11544272]

[66] Kim JW, Hung CF, Juang J, *et al.* Comparison of HPV DNA vaccines employing intracellular targeting strategies. Gene Ther 2004; 11(12): 1011-8. [http://dx.doi.org/10.1038/sj.gt.3302252] [PMID: 14985791]

[67] Peng S, Ji H, Trimble C, *et al.* Development of a DNA vaccine targeting human papillomavirus type 16 oncoprotein E6. J Virol 2004; 78(16): 8468-76. [http://dx.doi.org/10.1128/JVI.78.16.8468-8476.2004] [PMID: 15280455]

[68] Enhanced immunogenicity of HPV16E7 accompanied by Gp96 as an adjuvant in two vaccination strategies. Vaccine 2008; 26:3362–70.

[69] Hung CF, Cheng WF, Hsu KF, *et al.* Cancer immunotherapy using a DNA vaccine encoding the translocation domain of a bacterial toxin linked to a tumor antigen. Cancer Res 2001; 61(9): 3698-703. [PMID: 11325841]

[70] Hung CF, Cheng WF, He L, *et al.* Enhancing major histocompatibility complex class I antigen presentation by targeting antigen to centrosomes. Cancer Res 2003; 63(10): 2393-8. [PMID: 12750257]

[71] Huang CH, Peng S, He L, *et al.* Cancer immunotherapy using a DNA vaccine encoding a single-chain trimer of MHC class I linked to an HPV-16 E6 immunodominant CTL epitope. Gene Ther 2005; 12(15): 1180-6. [http://dx.doi.org/10.1038/sj.gt.3302519] [PMID: 15800656]

[72] Ji H, Wang TL, Chen CH, *et al.* Targeting human papillomavirus type 16 E7 to the endosomal/lysosomal compartment enhances the antitumor immunity of DNA vaccines against murine human papillomavirus type 16 E7-expressing tumors. Hum Gene Ther 1999; 10(17): 2727-40. [http://dx.doi.org/10.1089/10430349950016474] [PMID: 10584920]

[73] Hung CF, Tsai YC, He L, Wu TC. DNA vaccines encoding Ii-PADRE generates potent PADRE-specific CD4+ T-cell immune responses and enhances vaccine potency. Mol Ther 2007; 15(6): 1211-9. [http://dx.doi.org/10.1038/sj.mt.6300121] [PMID: 17356542]

[74] Kim D, Hoory T, Monie A, Ting JP, Hung CF, Wu TC. Enhancement of DNA vaccine potency through coadministration of CIITA DNA with DNA vaccines *via* gene gun. J Immunol 2008; 180(10): 7019-27. [http://dx.doi.org/10.4049/jimmunol.180.10.7019] [PMID: 18453624]

[75] Yang A, Farmer E, Wu TC, Hung CF. Perspectives for therapeutic HPV vaccine development. J Biomed Sci 2016; 23(1): 75. [http://dx.doi.org/10.1186/s12929-016-0293-9] [PMID: 27809842]

[76] Kim TJ, Jin HT, Hur SY, *et al.* Clearance of persistent HPV infection and cervical lesion by therapeutic DNA vaccine in CIN3 patients. Nat Commun 2014; 5: 5317. [http://dx.doi.org/10.1038/ncomms6317] [PMID: 25354725]

[77] Kim TW, Hung CF, Boyd D, *et al.* Enhancing DNA vaccine potency by combining a strategy to prolong dendritic cell life with intracellular targeting strategies. J Immunol 2003; 171(6): 2970-6. [http://dx.doi.org/10.4049/jimmunol.171.6.2970] [PMID: 12960321]

[78] Kim TW, Lee JH, He L, *et al.* Modification of professional antigen-presenting cells with small interfering RNA *in vivo* to enhance cancer vaccine potency. Cancer Res 2005; 65(1): 309-16. [PMID: 15665308]

[79] Cheng WF, Chang MC, Sun WZ, *et al.* Connective tissue growth factor linked to the E7 tumor antigen generates potent antitumor immune responses mediated by an antiapoptotic mechanism. Gene Ther 2008; 15(13): 1007-16.
[http://dx.doi.org/10.1038/gt.2008.25] [PMID: 18356819]

[80] Huang B, Mao CP, Peng S, Hung CF, Wu TC. RNA interference-mediated *in vivo* silencing of fas ligand as a strategy for the enhancement of DNA vaccine potency. Hum Gene Ther 2008; 19(8): 763-73.
[http://dx.doi.org/10.1089/hum.2007.059] [PMID: 18627219]

[81] Leachman SA, Tigelaar RE, Shlyankevich M, *et al.* Granulocyte-macrophage colony-stimulating factor priming plus papillomavirus E6 DNA vaccination: effects on papilloma formation and regression in the cottontail rabbit papillomavirus--rabbit model. J Virol 2000; 74(18): 8700-8.
[http://dx.doi.org/10.1128/JVI.74.18.8700-8708.2000] [PMID: 10954571]

[82] Chen CH, Wu TC. Experimental vaccine strategies for cancer immunotherapy. J Biomed Sci 1998; 5(4): 231-52.
[http://dx.doi.org/10.1007/BF02255855] [PMID: 9691216]

[83] Kim MS, Sin JI. Both antigen optimization and lysosomal targeting are required for enhanced anti-tumour protective immunity in a human papillomavirus E7-expressing animal tumour model. Immunology 2005; 116(2): 255-66.
[http://dx.doi.org/10.1111/j.1365-2567.2005.02219.x] [PMID: 16162274]

[84] Sheets EE, Urban RG, Crum CP, *et al.* Immunotherapy of human cervical high-grade cervical intraepithelial neoplasia with microparticle-delivered human papillomavirus 16 E7 plasmid DNA. Am J Obstet Gynecol 2003; 188(4): 916-26.
[http://dx.doi.org/10.1067/mob.2003.256] [PMID: 12712086]

[85] Garcia F, Petry KU, Muderspach L, *et al.* ZYC101a for treatment of high-grade cervical intraepithelial neoplasia: a randomized controlled trial. Obstet Gynecol 2004; 103(2): 317-26.
[http://dx.doi.org/10.1097/01.AOG.0000110246.93627.17] [PMID: 14754702]

[86] Trimble CL, Peng S, Kos F, *et al.* A phase I trial of a human papillomavirus DNA vaccine for HPV16+ cervical intraepithelial neoplasia 2/3. Clin Cancer Res 2009; 15(1): 361-7.
[http://dx.doi.org/10.1158/1078-0432.CCR-08-1725] [PMID: 19118066]

[87] Bolhassani A, Rafati S. Heat-shock proteins as powerful weapons in vaccine development. Expert Rev Vaccines 2008; 7(8): 1185-99.
[http://dx.doi.org/10.1586/14760584.7.8.1185] [PMID: 18844593]

[88] Daemi A, Bolhassani A, Rafati S, Zahedifard F, Hosseinzadeh S, Doustdari F. Different domains of glycoprotein 96 influence HPV16 E7 DNA vaccine potency *via* electroporation mediated delivery in tumor mice model. Immunol Lett 2012; 148(2): 117-25.
[http://dx.doi.org/10.1016/j.imlet.2012.10.003] [PMID: 23085605]

[89] Hariharan MJ, Driver DA, Townsend K, *et al.* DNA immunization against herpes simplex virus: enhanced efficacy using a Sindbis virus-based vector. J Virol 1998; 72(2): 950-8.
[PMID: 9444987]

[90] Cheng WF, Hung CF, Hsu KF, *et al.* Cancer immunotherapy using Sindbis virus replicon particles encoding a VP22-antigen fusion. Hum Gene Ther 2002; 13(4): 553-68.
[http://dx.doi.org/10.1089/10430340252809847] [PMID: 11874633]

[91] Berglund P, Quesada-Rolander M, Putkonen P, Biberfeld G, Thorstensson R, Liljeström P. Outcome of immunization of cynomolgus monkeys with recombinant Semliki Forest virus encoding human immunodeficiency virus type 1 envelope protein and challenge with a high dose of SHIV-4 virus. AIDS Res Hum Retroviruses 1997; 13(17): 1487-95.
[http://dx.doi.org/10.1089/aid.1997.13.1487] [PMID: 9390747]

[92] Pushko P, Parker M, Ludwig GV, Davis NL, Johnston RE, Smith JF. Replicon-helper systems from

attenuated Venezuelan equine encephalitis virus: expression of heterologous genes *in vitro* and immunization against heterologous pathogens *in vivo*. Virology 1997; 239(2): 389-401. [http://dx.doi.org/10.1006/viro.1997.8878] [PMID: 9434729]

[93] Kim TW, Hung CF, Juang J, He L, Hardwick JM, Wu TC. Enhancement of suicidal DNA vaccine potency by delaying suicidal DNA-induced cell death. Gene Ther 2004; 11(3): 336-42. [http://dx.doi.org/10.1038/sj.gt.3302164] [PMID: 14737094]

[94] Herd KA, Harvey T, Khromykh AA, Tindle RW. Recombinant Kunjin virus replicon vaccines induce protective T-cell immunity against human papillomavirus 16 E7-expressing tumour. Virology 2004; 319(2): 237-48. [http://dx.doi.org/10.1016/j.virol.2003.10.032] [PMID: 14980484]

[95] Cheng WF, Hung CH, Chai CY, *et al.* Enhancement of sindbis virus self-replicating RNA vaccine potency by linkage of herpes simplex virus type 1 VP22 protein to antigen. J Virol 2001; 75(5): 2368-76. [http://dx.doi.org/10.1128/JVI.75.5.2368-2376.2001] [PMID: 11160740]

[96] Cheng WF, Hung CF, Hsu KF, *et al.* Enhancement of sindbis virus self-replicating RNA vaccine potency by targeting antigen to endosomal/lysosomal compartments. Hum Gene Ther 2001; 12(3): 235-52. [http://dx.doi.org/10.1089/10430340150218387] [PMID: 11177561]

[97] Bolhassani A, Zahedifard F. Therapeutic live vaccines as a potential anticancer strategy. Int J Cancer 2012; 131(8): 1733-43. [http://dx.doi.org/10.1002/ijc.27640] [PMID: 22610886]

[98] Salehi M, Taheri T, Mohit E, *et al.* Recombinant *Leishmania tarentolae* encoding the HPV type 16 E7 gene in tumor mice model. Immunotherapy 2012; 4(11): 1107-20. [http://dx.doi.org/10.2217/imt.12.110] [PMID: 23194361]

[99] Hosseinzadeh S, Bolhassani A, Rafati S, *et al.* A non-pathogenic live vector as an efficient delivery system in vaccine design for the prevention of HPV16 E7-overexpressing cancers. Drug Deliv 2013; 20(3-4): 190-8. [http://dx.doi.org/10.3109/10717544.2013.801534] [PMID: 23745741]

[100] Sewell DA, Pan ZK, Paterson Y. Listeria-based HPV-16 E7 vaccines limit autochthonous tumor growth in a transgenic mouse model for HPV-16 transformed tumors. Vaccine 2008; 26(41): 5315-20. [http://dx.doi.org/10.1016/j.vaccine.2008.07.036] [PMID: 18680778]

[101] Souders NC, Sewell DA, Pan ZK, *et al.* Listeria-based vaccines can overcome tolerance by expanding low avidity CD8+ T cells capable of eradicating a solid tumor in a transgenic mouse model of cancer. Cancer Immun 2007; 7: 2. [PMID: 17279610]

[102] Bermúdez-Humarán LG, Langella P, Miyoshi A, *et al.* Production of human papillomavirus type 16 E7 protein in Lactococcus lactis. Appl Environ Microbiol 2002; 68(2): 917-22. [http://dx.doi.org/10.1128/AEM.68.2.917-922.2002] [PMID: 11823236]

[103] Bermúdez-Humarán LG, Cortes-Perez NG, Le Loir Y, *et al.* An inducible surface presentation system improves cellular immunity against human papillomavirus type 16 E7 antigen in mice after nasal administration with recombinant lactococci. J Med Microbiol 2004; 53(Pt 5): 427-33. [http://dx.doi.org/10.1099/jmm.0.05472-0] [PMID: 15096553]

[104] Cortes-Perez NG, Azevedo V, Alcocer-González JM, *et al.* Cell-surface display of E7 antigen from human papillomavirus type-16 in Lactococcus lactis and in Lactobacillus plantarum using a new cell-wall anchor from lactobacilli. J Drug Target 2005; 13(2): 89-98. [http://dx.doi.org/10.1080/10611860400024219] [PMID: 15823960]

[105] Peters C, Paterson Y. Enhancing the immunogenicity of bioengineered Listeria monocytogenes by passaging through live animal hosts. Vaccine 2003; 21(11-12): 1187-94. [http://dx.doi.org/10.1016/S0264-410X(02)00554-6] [PMID: 12559797]

[106] Lowry F. Live Listeria vaccine proves safe against endstage cervical cancer in human trial. Ob Gyn News 2008.

[107] Sewell DA, Shahabi V, Gunn GR III, Pan ZK, Dominiecki ME, Paterson Y. Recombinant Listeria vaccines containing PEST sequences are potent immune adjuvants for the tumor-associated antigen human papillomavirus-16 E7. Cancer Res 2004; 64(24): 8821-5.
[http://dx.doi.org/10.1158/0008-5472.CAN-04-1958] [PMID: 15604239]

[108] Maciag PC, Radulovic S, Rothman J. The first clinical use of a live-attenuated Listeria monocytogenes vaccine: a Phase I safety study of Lm-LLO-E7 in patients with advanced carcinoma of the cervix. Vaccine 2009; 27(30): 3975-83.
[http://dx.doi.org/10.1016/j.vaccine.2009.04.041] [PMID: 19389451]

[109] Kaufmann AM, Stern PL, Rankin EM, *et al.* Safety and immunogenicity of TA-HPV, a recombinant vaccinia virus expressing modified human papillomavirus (HPV)-16 and HPV-18 E6 and E7 genes, in women with progressive cervical cancer. Clin Cancer Res 2002; 8(12): 3676-85.
[PMID: 12473576]

[110] Davidson EJ, Boswell CM, Sehr P, *et al.* Immunological and clinical responses in women with vulval intraepithelial neoplasia with a vaccinia virus encoding HPV 16/18 oncoproteins. Cancer Res 2003; 63: 6032-41.
[PMID: 14522932]

[111] Hsieh CJ, Kim TW, Hung CF, *et al.* Enhancement of vaccinia vaccine potency by linkage of tumor antigen gene to gene encoding calreticulin. Vaccine 2004; 22(29-30): 3993-4001.
[http://dx.doi.org/10.1016/j.vaccine.2004.03.057] [PMID: 15364449]

[112] Lamikanra A, Pan ZK, Isaacs SN, Wu TC, Paterson Y. Regression of established human papillomavirus type 16 (HPV-16) immortalized tumors in vivo by vaccinia viruses expressing different forms of HPV-16 E7 correlates with enhanced CD8(+) T-cell responses that home to the tumor site. J Virol 2001; 75(20): 9654-64.
[http://dx.doi.org/10.1128/JVI.75.20.9654-9664.2001] [PMID: 11559797]

[113] Kaufmann AM, Stern PL, Rankin EM, *et al.* Safety and immunogenicity of TA-HPV, a recombinant vaccinia virus expressing modified human papillomavirus (HPV)-16 and HPV-18 E6 and E7 genes, in women with progressive cervical cancer. Clin Cancer Res 2002; 8(12): 3676-85.
[PMID: 12473576]

[114] Trimble CL, Frazer IH. Development of therapeutic HPV vaccines. Lancet Oncol 2009; 10(10): 975-80.
[http://dx.doi.org/10.1016/S1470-2045(09)70227-X] [PMID: 19796749]

[115] Gomez-Gutierrez JG, Elpek KG, Montes de Oca-Luna R, Shirwan H, Sam Zhou H, McMasters KM. Vaccination with an adenoviral vector expressing calreticulin-human papillomavirus 16 E7 fusion protein eradicates E7 expressing established tumors in mice. Cancer Immunol Immunother 2007; 56(7): 997-1007.
[http://dx.doi.org/10.1007/s00262-006-0247-2] [PMID: 17146630]

[116] Báez-Astúa A, Herráez-Hernández E, Garbi N, *et al.* Low-dose adenovirus vaccine encoding chimeric hepatitis B virus surface antigen-human papillomavirus type 16 E7 proteins induces enhanced E7-specific antibody and cytotoxic T-cell responses. J Virol 2005; 79(20): 12807-17.
[http://dx.doi.org/10.1128/JVI.79.20.12807-12817.2005] [PMID: 16188983]

[117] Brodsky JL. Post-translational protein translocation: not all hsc70s are created equal. Trends Biochem Sci 1996; 21(4): 122-6.
[http://dx.doi.org/10.1016/S0968-0004(96)80163-0] [PMID: 8701466]

[118] Cyr DM, Neupert W. Roles for hsp70 in protein translocation across membranes of organelles. In: Feige U RIM, Yahara I, and Polla BS, eds. Stress-inducible cellular responses. Switzerland: Birkhauser, 1996: 25-40.
[http://dx.doi.org/10.1007/978-3-0348-9088-5_3]

[119] Riezebos-Brilman A, Regts J, Freyschmidt EJ, Dontje B, Wilschut J, Daemen T. Induction of human papilloma virus E6/E7-specific cytotoxic T-lymphocyte activity in immune-tolerant, E6/E7-transgenic mice. Gene Ther 2005; 12(18): 1410-4.
[http://dx.doi.org/10.1038/sj.gt.3302536] [PMID: 15843807]

[120] Riezebos-Brilman A, Regts J, Chen M, Wilschut J, Daemen T. Augmentation of alphavirus vector-induced human papilloma virus-specific immune and anti-tumour responses by co-expression of interleukin-12. Vaccine 2009; 27(5): 701-7.
[http://dx.doi.org/10.1016/j.vaccine.2008.11.032] [PMID: 19041356]

[121] Voest EE, Kenyon BM, O'Reilly MS, Truitt G, D'Amato RJ, Folkman J. Inhibition of angiogenesis *in vivo* by interleukin 12. J Natl Cancer Inst 1995; 87(8): 581-6.
[http://dx.doi.org/10.1093/jnci/87.8.581] [PMID: 7538593]

[122] Chang CL, Ma B, Pang X, Wu TC, Hung CF. Treatment with cyclooxygenase-2 inhibitors enables repeated administration of vaccinia virus for control of ovarian cancer. Mol Ther 2009; 17(8): 1365-72.
[http://dx.doi.org/10.1038/mt.2009.118] [PMID: 19471247]

[123] Khavari A, Bolhassani A, Alizadeh F, *et al.* Chemo-immunotherapy using saffron and its ingredients followed by E7-NT (gp96) DNA vaccine generates different anti-tumor effects against tumors expressing the E7 protein of human papillomavirus. Arch Virol 2015; 160(2): 499-508.
[http://dx.doi.org/10.1007/s00705-014-2250-9] [PMID: 25395243]

[124] Mohit E, Bolhassani A, Zahedifard F, *et al.* Immunomodulatory effects of IP-10 chemokine along with PEI600-Tat delivery system in DNA vaccination against HPV infections. Mol Immunol 2013; 53(1-2): 149-60.
[http://dx.doi.org/10.1016/j.molimm.2012.07.011] [PMID: 22926003]

[125] Woodland DL. Jump-starting the immune system: prime-boosting comes of age. Trends Immunol 2004; 25(2): 98-104.
[http://dx.doi.org/10.1016/j.it.2003.11.009] [PMID: 15102369]

[126] van der Burg SH, Kwappenberg KM, O'Neill T, *et al.* Pre-clinical safety and efficacy of TA-CIN, a recombinant HPV16 L2E6E7 fusion protein vaccine, in homologous and heterologous prime-boost regimens. Vaccine 2001; 19(27): 3652-60. b
[http://dx.doi.org/10.1016/S0264-410X(01)00086-X] [PMID: 11395199]

[127] de Jong A, O'Neill T, Khan AY, *et al.* Enhancement of human papillomavirus (HPV) type 16 E6 and E7-specific T-cell immunity in healthy volunteers through vaccination with TA-CIN, an HPV16 L2E7E6 fusion protein vaccine. Vaccine 2002; 20(29-30): 3456-64.
[http://dx.doi.org/10.1016/S0264-410X(02)00350-X] [PMID: 12297390]

[128] Smyth LJ, Van Poelgeest MI, Davidson EJ, *et al.* Immunological responses in women with HPV16 associated lower genital intraepitelial neoplasia (LGIN) following induced by heterologous prime-boost HPV16 oncogene vaccination. Clin Cancer Res 2004; 10: 2954-61.
[http://dx.doi.org/10.1158/1078-0432.CCR-03-0703] [PMID: 15131030]

CHAPTER 15

Preclinical and Clinical Experiments on HPV Vaccines

Azam Bolhassani* and **Afshin Khavari**

Department of Hepatitis and AIDS, Pasteur Institute of Iran, Tehran, Iran

Abstract: Persistent infection with human papillomavirus (HPV) is a key factor in the development of precancerous lesions and invasive cervical cancer. Prophylactic vaccines are an effective approach to reduce HPV-related disease burden. Regarding the studies, at least 110-120 countries have implemented Cervarix™ and Gardasil™ for induction of protective effects against HPV infections. On the other hand, several clinical trials are underway for therapeutic HPV vaccination. Special approaches is considered to increase the potency of therapeutic vaccines including the use of effective adjuvant, selection of strong immunogen and combination therapies to overcome tumor immune suppression. In this chapter, we will summarize main preventive and therapeutic HPV vaccines in preclinical and clinical trials.

Keywords: Clinical study, HPV infection, Preclinical study, Prophylactic vaccine, Therapeutic vaccine.

INTRODUCTION

Preclinical model systems to study multiple features of the papillomavirus life cycle have greatly helped our understanding of HPV biology, disease progression and treatments. However, these models are both species and tissue restricted. Thus, fundamental properties of HPV viral proteins can be assessed in specialized cell culture systems but host responses that involve innate immunity and host restriction factors require preclinical models. Fortunately, there are new animal models of papillomavirus infections that are available to the PV research community. Old models that continue to have value include canine, bovine and rabbit PV models and new rodent models are in place to better assess host-virus interactions [1]. The studies showed that beside prophylactic strategies, the use of therapeutic vaccine for HPV-associated cancers can be useful in treatment of premalignant lesions. It has been shown that chimeric VLPs harboring HPV16 E7

* **Corresponding author Azam Bolhassani:** Department of Hepatitis and AIDS, Pasteur Institute of Iran, Tehran, Iran; Tel: 66953311-20; E-mails: A_bolhasani@pasteur.ac.ir, azam.bolhassani@yahoo.com

can activate DCs and generate T-cell responses to E7 as well as neutralizing antibodies to viral capsids as an effective treatment against persistent HPV infection [2].

Preclinical and Clinical Trials of HPV Prophylactic Vaccines

Up to now, two distinct preventive vaccines have been approved by the FDA including Gardasil® (Merck &Co.,Whitehouse Station, NJUSA), a quadrivalent vaccine containing VLPs of types 6, 11, 16 and 18, and Cervarix® (GlaxoSmithKline Biologicals, Rixensart, Belgium), a bivalent vaccine containing VLPs of types 16 and 18 [3]. Both vaccines demonstrated high and similar protective effects against the vaccine-targeted types for a range of cervical disorders from persistent infection to CIN3, genital warts, vulvar/vaginal neoplasia and anal infections in women. These vaccines had no therapeutic effects against established infection or CIN. Moreover, both vaccines showed some degree of cross-protection for both HPV infection and lesions related to non-vaccine types. Cross-protection was restricted to HPV31 for Gardasil® and to HPVs 31, 33, 52, 45 and 51 for Cervarix®. On the other hand, both vaccines, given as three parenteral doses over a six-month period, exhibited excellent safety in the clinical trials, but had no effect on pre-existing infections [3, 4]. The greater cross-protection of the bivalent vaccine may be due to differences in the adjuvants and/or in the manufacturing process (*i.e.,* disassembly-reassembly steps) of the two vaccines. The bivalent vaccine (Cervarix) uses AS04 composed of monophosphoryl lipid A (a TLR4 agonist) and alum, while the quadrivalent vaccine (Gardasil) uses alum adjuvant. Moreover, the VLPs for Cervarix are produced in insect cells, while those for Gardasil are generated in yeast [5, 6]. Several second-generation prophylactic vaccines have been developed to resolve some of the limitations of Gardasil and Cervarix vaccines. Recently, a nonavalent vaccine containing L1 VLPs of types 6, 11, 16, 18, 31, 33, 45, 52, 58 is in the advanced stage of phase III efficacy trials. Other second- generation vaccines were based on L1-pentameric subunits, and the minor virion protein L2 with promising results in preclinical studies [7, 8]. The L2-based vaccines could produce broader cross-type protective immunity with lower cost as compared to L1 VLP immunization [9, 10]. Several studies have shown that the N-terminal region of L2 elicits neutralizing antibodies against different HPV types [11 - 13]. However, the immunogenicity of recombinant L2 protein is poor, thus, different formulations are necessary to increase its potency such as the multivalent display of an L2 epitope on the surface of a recombinant bacteriophage PP7 coat protein VLP [11, 14, 15], the generation of a concatenated multimeric L2 fusion protein containing N-terminal L2 peptides derived from 3 to 22 HPV types [11, 16, 17], and the use of a mixture of eight L2-PP7 VLPs displaying L2 sequence from various HPV types [11, 14]. Generally, high-titer neutralizing antibody responses have been induced by fusion VLPs compared to the particles expressing a single epitope [15].

In 2017, Yin *et al.* investigated the immunogenicity and dosage effect of a trivalent HPV 16/18/58 vaccine (3vHPV) produced in *Escherichia coli* (*E. coli*), with Gardasil quadrivalent vaccine (4vHPV, Merck & Co.) as a positive control in rhesus macaques. Strong immune responses against HPV16/18/58 were successfully induced in macaques receiving 3vHPV vaccine. Generally, HPV16/18-specific neutralizing antibody and total IgG antibody responses in rhesus macaques receiving 3vHPV were non-inferior to those observed in rhesus macaques receiving 4vHPV. Moreover, the durability of antibody responses specific to HPV 16/18 elicited by 3vHPV vaccines was non-inferior to that associated with Gardasil 4vHPV [18]. On the other hand, immunization of rabbits with short synthetic L2 peptides coupled to Keyhole Limpet Hemocyanin (KLH) protected them against experimental challenge with the cottontail rabbit papillomavirus (CRPV) and the rabbit oral PV (ROPV) at both mucosal and cutaneous sites [19]. Campo's laboratory showed protection of cattle from BPV4 challenge after vaccination with three immunodominant L2 peptides comprising residues 101-120, 131-151 and 151-170 in alum [20]. Also, Kawana *et al.* found that intranasal vaccination of BALB/c mice with HPV16 L2 108-120 could induce IgG and IgA antibodies, and neutralize HPV16 and several other HPV genotypes [21]. On the other hand, the studies showed that the L2 residues 17-36 could protect naive mice from cutaneous challenge with HPV16 pseudovirions as a promising candidate for a preventive vaccine [22]. Alphs *et al.* produced a synthetic vaccine candidate containing the target epitope (HPV16 L2 17-36) along with the TLR2 ligand Pam2Cys (P2C) and a free T helper epitope (P25) in a simple branched structure as an effective strategy compared to poorly immunogenic self-epitope vaccine [23 - 26]. Other study also showed that immunization with L2 residues 11-200 could protect cattle and rabbits against viral challenge at mucosal or cutaneous sites [27 - 30]. The researchers examined concatenated fusion proteins containing several homologous L2 peptides (residues 11-200, 11-88, 17-36) derived from different HPV genotypes (HPV-1, -5, -6, -16 and -18) for generation of a broadly protective HPV vaccine. The data indicated that the L2 residues 11-88 generated higher neutralizing antibody titers than other constructs [31]. In addition, immunization with the L2 residues 11-200 formulated in alum + immuno-stimulatory sequence (ISS) 1018 was more effective than the L2 residues 11-200, alone suggesting the use of a potent adjuvant to maintain long-term protection after vaccination with multi-type L2 regimen [31 - 35]. Regarding the high immunogenicity of L1 VLPs [36, 37], several groups have replaced the surface loops comprising the L1 immunodominant neutralizing epitopes with L2 epitopes (*i.e.,* HPV16 L2 65-81 and 108-120). These chimeras were immunogenic and generated low, but measurable, L2-specific neutralizing antibody titers in mice [38, 39]. In this line, Palmer *et al.* utilized the recombinant tobacco mosaic virus to display the L2 94-122 epitope of ROPV and CRPV by insertion between residues 155 and 156, of the U1 coat protein. Vaccination with these constructs in RIBI adjuvant (a stable oil-in-water emulsion) could protect rabbits against experimental CRPV challenge [40, 41]. Up to now, several chimeric VLPs were generated by inserting L2 epitopes within the DE loop and/or C-terminal region of L1. The chimeric L1/L2 VLP containing HPV18 L1 with insertions of HPV33 L2 (residues 17-36; L1 DE loop) and HPV58 L2 (residues 56-75; L1 C-terminus) could stimulate stable immune responses and protect animals against different HPVs (*i.e.,* HPV-6, -11, -16, -31, -35, -39, -45, -58, -59 pseudovirions) in both mouse and rabbit challenge models [42].

Preclinical and Clinical Therapeutic Vaccines

As known, HPV E6 and E7 oncoproteins are promising targets for therapeutic vaccines, *e.g.*, naked DNA- and protein-based HPV vaccines, against HPV-related tumor models. The studies demonstrated that the heterologous DNA prime/ protein boost vaccination is well tolerated by mice and can significantly induce antigen-specific $CD8^+$ T cell responses [43]. In addition, a therapeutic HPV vaccine composed of the recombinant HPV-16 and HPV-18 E7 proteins fused to catalytically inactive *Bordetella pertussis* CyaA (GTL001) could prevent high-grade lesions in HPV-infected women. The data showed that the group receiving GTL001+imiquimod increased antigen-specific T-cell responses and decreased HPV16/18 viral load [44]. Induction of cellular immunity is important to design therapeutic vaccines. This immunity is regulated by both activation signals (co-stimulatory molecules) and inhibition signals (immune checkpoints). Indeed, immune suppressive milieu is observed inside tumor microenvironment [45, 46]. Thus, inhibition of immune checkpoint is suggested as one potential method to enhance anti-tumor immunity. Among a variety of immune checkpoint, cytotoxic T lymphocyte-associated antigen 4 (CTLA-4) and programmed death receptor (PD-1) were known as powerful immune suppressors. In HPV-associated head and neck cancer, a higher percentage of PD-1 expressing $CD8^+$ T cell was observed in tumor tissue than in the peripheral blood suggesting that $CD8^+$ T cells begin to express PD-1 receptor after entering tumor environment. Human antibodies against CTLA-4 (Ipilimumab, NCT01711515) and PD-1 (Nivolumab, NCT02257528) were approved by FDA in 2011 and 2014, respectively [45, 46]. Several clinical trials were designed to incorporate these therapeutic agents into therapeutic regimens against HPV-related cancers. For instance, a phase I trial of Ipilimumab and a phase II trial of Nivolumab are currently underway in patients with advanced cervical cancer. Other molecules inhibiting immune functions in the tumor microenvironment include regulatory T cell, indoleamine 2, 3-dioxygenase, arginase, nitric oxide synthase, IL-4, IL-10 and TGF-β. Thus, the ability to overcome this immune suppression may further enhance the potency of immunotherapy against HPV-associated cancers [47]. There are many different preclinical trials for therapeutic vaccines. Some of them have been achieved to clinical trials at different phases such as NCT02128126, NCT02481414, NCT02065973, NCT01653249, NCT00676949, NCT00054041, NCT02529930, NCT00788164, NCT00988559, NCT02172911, NCT02411019, NCT01266460 and NCT01022346 [46 - 49]. Tables **1** and **2** indicate the recent and ongoing clinical trials for therapeutic vaccines.

Table 1. The recent therapeutic HPV vaccines in clinical trials [48, 49].

Vaccine	Antigen(s)	Construct	Organization	Trial design	Outcome	Side effects
Bacterial Vector Based						
Lm-LLo-E7 (ADXS11-001; ADXS-HPV)	HPV-16 E7	prfA-defective Listeria monocytogenes strain transformed with plasmid encoding HPV-16 E7 antigen fused to a f ragment of nonhemolytic listeriolysin O (LLO)	Advaxis, Inc.	Phase I in patients with metastatic, refractory or recurrent, advanced squamous cell carcinoma of the cervix (15 patients)	Increase in E7-specific T cells detected in PBMCs of three patients. Reduction in tumor size observed in 4 patients.	Pyrexia, vomiting, chills, headache, anemia, nausea, tachycardia, muscle and skeletal pain.
GLBL101c	HPV16-E7	Recombinant *Lactobacillus casei* expressing modified version of HPV16-E7	GENOLAC BL Corp	Phase I/IIa in HPV16+ CIN3 patients (17 patients)	Significant increase in E7-CMI in cervical vaginal tract. 9 patients experienced disease regression to CIN2, and 5 further regressed to LSIL	No major side effects observed.
Viral Vector Based						
TA-HPV	HPV-16/18 E6/E7	Recombinant Vaccinia virus	European Organization for Research and Treatment of Cancer (EORTC)	Phase I/II in patients with advanced stage of cervical cancer (8 patients)	Vaccination induced HPV-specific cytotoxic T lymphocyte immune response in 28 % of participants (3 out of 8). 2 patients showed tumor free condition at 15 and 21 months after vaccination.	Single dose generated mild and tolerable toxicity
				Phase I in patients with clinical International Federation of Gynecology and Obstetrics (FIGO) stage Ib or IIa cervical cancer who will undergo radical hysterectomy (29 patients)	After a single vaccination HPV-specific CTLs were found in 4 patients. 8 patients (28 %) developed HPV-specific serological responses.	Mild to moderate local toxicity
				Phase II in patients ages 42–54 with high-grade HPV-positive vulval or vaginal intraepithelial neoplasia of up to 15 years duration (12 patients)	5 of 12 (42 %) patients showed at least 50 % reduction in total lesion diameter over 24 weeks with 1 patient showing complete regression of lesion. Overall, 83 % of women showed some average decrease in lesion size of 40 %. All patients showed an increased IgG titer and T-cell response to the vaccinia virus.	A local reaction at the site of vaccination between day 7–10 was common and 2 patients had temporarily limited arm movement.
TG4001	HPV-16 E6/E7	Recombinant modified vaccinia Ankara-expressing HPV-16 E6, E7, and IL-2	Transgene/roche	Phase I in HPV16+ CIN2/3 patients (21 patients)	Ten of 21 (48 %) showed disease regression, HPV DNA clearance in eight patients and mRNA clearance in seven patients	Inflammation, pruritus, edema, lymphadenopathy, fever, headache, asthenia, bone pain, vaginal discharge
MVA E2	HPV-16 E2	Recombinant Modified Vaccinia Ankara encoding E2 from BPV	Instituto Mexicano del Seguro Social	Phase III in patients with HPV-induced AGIN (1176	90 % lesion clearance in female treated patient and 100 % lesion clearance in male	Headache, flu-like symptom, fever,

(Table 1) contd.....

				female patients and 180 male patients)	treated patients. Antibody and T cell responses observed in all tested patients.	chills, abdominal pain, joint pain.
Peptide/Protein Based						
HPV16-SLP	HPV-16 E6/E7	Combination of nine HPV-16 E6 and four HPV-16 E7 synthetic peptides with incomplete Freund's adjuvant	ISA Pharmaceuticals	Phase II in patients with HPV16+ VIN3 (20 patients)	15 patients had objective clinical response at 12 months. 9 complete responses and 6 partial response. 85 % with circulating HPV-16 specific T cells. 83 % had CMI against HPV-16.	Local swelling, redness, increased skin temperature, pain at vaccination site, fever, flu like symptoms, chills, and tiredness.
				Phase II study in patients with HPV16+ HSIL (9 patients)	All vaccinated patients showed strong HPV-specific T cell response after vaccination. Change in patterns of immune infiltrate.	Itching, redness, swelling, and pain at injection site, headache, diarrhea, fatigue/dizziness, nausea, chills, myalgia, rash, fever, urticarial, edema.
				Phase II in patients HPV16+ advanced or recurrent gynecological carcinoma (20 patients)	9 patients with HPV-16 specific immune response. Duration of survival correlates with magnitude of T cell response.	Injection site reaction, fever, chills, fatigue, nausea, flue-like symptom
				Phase II in patients with low-grade abnormalities of the cervix (50 patients)	97 % of vaccinated patients generated HPV 16-specific CMI	Flu-like symptom, injection site reaction.
				Observational study in patients with advanced, recurrent, or metastatic cervical cancer scheduled to receive standard Carboplatin/Paclitaxel chemotherapy (18 patients).	11 of 12 vaccinated patients induced proliferative T cell responses	Chemotherapy related anemia, thrombocytopenia, leucopenia, neutropenia, and alopecia. Cancer related shortness of breath, pulmonary embolism, abdominal pain, gastroenteritis, erysipelas, hydronephrosis
GL-0810	HPV-16 antigen	HPV-16 immunomodulatory peptide with adjuvant Montanide and GM-CSF	Gliknik Inc.	Phase I in patients with recurrent/metastatic squamous cell carcinoma of the head and neck (5 patients)	80 % of patients who received four vaccinated developed T cell and antibody response. Progression free and overall survival is 8- to 196 days respectively	Erythema, itching, and pain at injection site
Pepcan + Candin	HPV-16 E6	HPV16 E6 peptides combined with Candida skin testing reagent candin.	University of Arkansas	Phase I study in patients with biopsy-confirmed HSIL (31 patients)	45 % patients experienced histological disease regression.	Mild to moderate injection site reaction.
GTL001 (ProCervix)	HPV-16 and HPV-18	Recombinant HPV16 and HPV18 E7 proteins fused to catalytically inactive	Genticel	Phase I trial in patients positive for HPV-16 or HPV-18 infection but with	Patients in cohort 4 ($n = 9$) who received 600ug GTL001 powder + imiquimod	Injection site reactions including pain, swelling, induration, tenderness, and itching

(Table 1) contd.....

		Bordetella pertussis CyaA expressed in *E. coli*		normal cytology (47 patients)	experienced the highest HPV16/18 clearance rate.	
TA-CIN	HPV-16 E6/E7/L2	HPV16 E6E7L2 fusion protein	Xenova Research Limited	Phase I in healthy patients (40 subjects)	TA-CIN specific IgG in 24 of 32 vaccinated patients. 25 of 32 vaccinated patients generated CMI.	Injection site reaction, tenderness. Headache and fatigue
				Phase II with VIN2/3 patients (19 patients)	63 % lesion response 1 year after vaccination. Significant increase. Significant CMI observed in lesion responders.	Local reaction associated with imiquimod.
TA-CIN + TA-HPV	HPV-16/18 E6/E7/L2	HPV16 E6E7L2 fusion protein and vaccinia virus with HPV16/18 E6/E7	Celtic Pharma	Phase I with HPV16+ VIN patient (10 patients)	Partial or complete clinical response in 2 patients. All but 1 patient showed HPV-16 specific IgG and/or T cell responses.	Pain at injection site.
				Phase II with HPV16+ high-grade AGIN Patients (29 patients)	17 patients showed TA-CIN induced T cell responses. 11 generated HPV-16/18 E6 and/or E7 specific T cells. 14 with IgG response to HPV-16 E7.	N/A
Nucleotide Based						
pNGVL4a-sig/E7(detox)/HSP70+ TA-HPV	HPV-16/18 E6/E7	Plasmid encoding mutated form of HPV16-E7 linked to sig and HSP70 and vaccinia virus with HPV16/18 E6/E7	Sidney Kimmel Comprehensive Cancer Center	Phase I with HPV16+ CIN3 Patients (12 patients)	58 % vaccinated patients have generated HPV-16 E7-specific CMI. Increase CD8+ T cell infiltration to lesions.	Tenderness, local site reaction, blister, erythema, pruritus
pNGVL4a-CRT/E7(detox)	HPV-16 E7	Plasmid encoding mutated form of HPV16-E7 linked to CRT	Sidney Kimmel Comprehensive Cancer Center	Phase I with HPV16+ CIN2/3 Patients (32 patients)	30 % vaccinated patients experienced histological regression to CIN1 or less. Increase in intraepithelial C8+ T cells infiltrate after vaccination.	Injection site reaction.
GX-188E	HPV-16/18 E6/E7	Plasmid encoding fusion protein of HPV 16/18 E6/E7 linked to Flt3L and tpa	Genexine, Inc	Phase I in patients with HPV 16/18+ CIN3 (9 patients)	All patients displayed enhanced HPV-specific CMI. 7 patients demonstrated complete lesion regression by the end of the trial.	Chills, injection site pain, swelling, hypoesthesia, headache, fatigue, rhinitis
VGX-3100	HPV-16/18 E6/E7	Mixture of two plasmids encoding optimized consensus of E6 and E7 antigen of HPV 16 and 18	Inovio Pharmaceuticals	Phase I with HPV16/18+CIN2/3 Patients (18 patients)	HPV-specific CMI observed in 78 % patients and HPV-specific humoral response observed in all patients.	Injection site reaction, pain, fever, tenderness.
				Phase IIb with HPV16/18+CIN2/3 Patients (167 patients)	49.5 % vaccinated patient demonstrated regression compared to 30.6 % in placebo group. Vaccinations	Injection site reaction, fatigues, headache, lyalgia, nausea, arthralgia, erythema

Abbreviations: CIN, Cervical intraepithelial neoplasia; AGIN, Anogenital intraepithelial neoplasia; HSIL: High-grade squamous intraepithelial lesion; VIN, vulvar intraepithelial neoplasia.

Combined Prophylactic/Therapeutic Vaccines

A preventive and therapeutic vaccine can be highly effective to protect women against cervical cancer for the future. The most advanced candidates for this type of vaccine are chimeric VLPs which incorporate peptides of early proteins (*i.e.*, E6 or E7) as fusions of L1 or L2 [50, 51]. Chimeric VLPs induced both neutralizing antibodies to L1 and T-cell responses to the peptides of early protein in mouse model. For example, a combined vaccine tested in clinical trials was

TA-CIN containing an HPV16 L2-E6-E7 fusion protein. The safety and T-cell responses to this vaccine were established in a phase-I clinical trial. The therapeutic efficiency of this vaccine has been further enhanced as part of a heterologous prime/boost strategy with a recombinant *vaccinia virus* that expresses E6 and E7 from HPV-16 and -18. In addition, it is possible to combine an effective therapeutic vaccine with the VLPs. VLPs can provide a potent adjuvant effect in that they activate professional APCs and induce a potent T-helper response in humans [51].

Table 2. Ongoing therapeutic HPV vaccines in clinical trials.

Vaccine	Antigen(s)	Construct	Organization	Trial Design	Estimated Date of Trial Completion	Clinical Trials.gov Identifier
Persistent HPV Infection and Low-Grade Squamous Intraepithelial Lesion						
PDS0101	HPV-16 E6/E7	R-enantiomer of 1,2-dioleoyl-3-trimethylammonium-propane chloride + Peptides HPV-16 E6 and E7	PDS Biotechnology Corp.	Phase I in female patients with high risk HPV infection or CIN1 (18 estimated patients)	Information not provided	NCT02065973
ProCervix	HPV-16/18 E7	2 recombinant adenylate cyclase (CyaA) proteins. CyaA-HPV 16E7 & CyaA-HPV 18E7	Genticel	Phase II in female patients with HPV16/18+ infection or ASCUS/LSIL (220 estimated patients)	December 2016	NCT01957878
Cervical Intraepithelial Neoplasia (CIN)/High-Grade Squamous Intraepithelial Lesion						
GX-188E	HPV-16/18 E6/E7	Plasmid encoding fusion protein of HPV 16/18 E6/E7 linked to Flt3L and tpa	Genexine, Inc	Phase II in HPV 16/18+ CIN2, CIN2/3, and CIN3 patients in Eastern Europe (120 estimated patients)	December 2017	NCT02596243
				Phase II in HPV 16/18+ CIN3 patients in South Korea (72 estimated patients)	October 2016	NCT02139267
pNGVL4a-CRT/E7(detox)	HPV-16 E7	Plasmid encoding mutated form of HPV16-E7 linked to calreticulin	Sidney Kimmel Comprehensive Cancer Center	Phase I in patients with HPV16+ CIN2/3 (39 estimated patients)	March 2017	NCT00988559
pNGVL4a-sig/E7(detox)/ HSP70 + TA-HPV	HPV-16/18 E6/E7	Plasmid encoding mutated form of HPV16-E7 linked to sig and HSP70 and vaccinia virus with HPV16/18 E6/E7		Phase I in patients with HPV16+ CIN3 in combination with topical imiquimod (48 estimated patients)	December 2016	NCT00788164
TVGV-1 + GPI-0100	HPV-16 E7	Fusion protein of HPV-16 E7 and ER targeting sequence	THEVAX Genetics Vaccine Co.	Phase IIa in patients with HPV induced cervical HSIL (51 estimated patients)	June 2017	NCT02576561
Pepcan + Candin	HPV-16 E6	HPV16 E6 peptides combined with Candida skin testing reagent candin.	University of Arkansas	Phase II in patients with cervical HSIL (125 estimated patients)	August 2020	NCT02481414
Anal Intraepithelial Neoplasia (AIN)						
ISA101 (SLP-HPV-01, HPV16-SLP)	HPV-16 E6/E7	Combination of nine HPV-16 E6 and four HPV-16 E7 synthetic peptides with incomplete Freund's adjuvant	ISA Pharmaceuticals	Phase I/II in HIV+ male patients with HPV-16+ AIN2/3 (45 estimated patients)	February 2018	NCT01923116
ADXS11-001 (Lm-LLo-E7)	HPV-16-E7		Advaxis, Inc.		March 2017	NCT02399813

(Table 2) contd.....

		prfA-defective Listeria monocytogenes strain transformed with plasmid encoding HPV-16 E7 antigen fused to a fragment of nonhemolytic listeriolysin O (LLO)		Phase II trial in patients with persistent, recurrent, loco-regional, or metastatic anal cancer or HPV+ squamous cell carcinoma of the rectum that are either treatment naïve in the metastatic setting or have progressed or become intolerant to platinum based therapy (55 estimated patients)		
HPV-Associated Incurable Solid Tumors						
ISA101 (SLP-HPV-01; HPV16-SLP)	HPV-16 E6/E7	Combination of nine HPV-16 E6 and four HPV-16 E7 synthetic peptides with incomplete Freund's adjuvant	ISA Pharmaceuticals	Phase II in patients with HPV-16+ Incurable solid tumors (oropharyngeal squamous cell carcinoma, cervical, vulvar, vaginal, anal, and penile cancer) as combination therapy with Nivolumab (28 estimated patients)	December 2018	NCT02426892
DPX-E7	HPV-16 E7	HPV16-E711-19 nanomer	Dana-Farber Cancer Institute	Phase Ib/II trial in HLA-A*02 positive patients with incurable HPV 16-related oropharyngeal, cervical and anal cancer (44 estimated patients)	May 2023	NCT02865135
Head and Neck Cancer						
ADXS11-001 (Lm-LLo-E7)	HPV-16-E7	prfA-defective Listeria monocytogenes strain transformed with plasmid encoding HPV-16 E7 antigen fused to a fragment of nonhemolytic listeriolysin O (LLO)	Advaxis, Inc.	Phase II in patients with HPV+ Oropharyngeal Squamous Cell Carcinoma before robot-assisted resection (30 estimated patients)	March 2017	NCT02002182
				Phase I/II in patients with locally advanced or metastatic cervical or HPV+ Head and nack cancer with or without MED14736 chemoblie (66 estimated patients)	December 2019	NCT02291055
INO-3112 (VGX-3100 + INO-9012)	HPV-16/18 E6/E7	Mixture of three plasmids encoding optimized consensus of E6 and E7 antigen of HPV 16 and 18 and proprietary immune activator expressing IL-12	Inovio Pharmaceuticals	Phase I/IIA in patients with HPV associated head and neck squamous cell carcinoma (25 estimated patients)	December 2017	NCT02163057
Cervical Cancer						
ADXS11-001 (Lm-LLo-E7)	HPV-16-E7	prfA-defective Listeria monocytogenes strain transformed with plasmid encoding HPV-16 E7 antigen fused to a fragment of nonhemolytic listeriolysin O (LLO)	Advaxis, Inc.	Phase II in patients with persistent or recurrent squamous or non-squamous cell carcinoma of the cervix (67 estimated patients)	October 2018	NCT01266460
INO-3112 (VGX-3100 + INO-9012)	HPV-16/18 E6/E7	Mixture of three plasmids encoding optimized consensus of E6 and E7 antigen of HPV 16 and 18	Inovio Pharmaceuticals	Phase I/IIA in female patients with new, recurrent, or persistent cervical cancer (30 estimated patients)	April 2019	NCT02172911
		and proprietary immune activator expressing IL-12		Phase II in patients with locally advanced cervical cancer as combination therapy with chemoradiation (126 estimated patients)	May 2021	NCT02501278
ISA101 (SLP-HPV-01; HPV16-SLP)	HPV-16 E6/E7	Combination of nine HPV-16 E6 and four HPV-16 E7 synthetic peptides with incomplete Freund's adjuvant	ISA Pharmaceuticals	Phase I/II in female patients with HPV-16+ advanced or recurrent cervical cancer (48 estimated patients)	December 2016	NCT02128126
TA-CIN + GPI-0100	HPV-16 E6/ E7/L2	HPV16 E6E7L2 fusion protein + GPI-0100 adjuvant	Sidney Kimmel Comprehensive Cancer Center	Phase I in patients with HPV16 associated cervical cancer (30 estimated patients)	May 2020	NCT02405221

Abbreviations: AGIN, Anogenital intraepithelial neoplasia; AIN, Anal intraepithelial neoplasia; ASCUC: Atypical squamous cells of undetermined significance; CIN, Cervical intraepithelial neoplasia; ER: Endoplasmic reticulum; HSIL: High-grade squamous intraepithelial lesion; LSIL: Low-grade squamous intraepithelial lesion; HPV: Human papillomavirus; HIV: Human immunodeficiency virus.

CONCLUDING REMARKS

Generally, two HPV vaccines (Cervarix and Gardasil) have been proven to be safe and effective in worldwide; but however, it is necessary to improve low-cost, effective and stable prophylactic vaccines that are able to stimulate broader protection against different HPV genotypes and also suitable for low-resource areas.

On the other hand, further studies should be performed to develop therapeutic vaccines in clinical trials. Recently, immune checkpoint inhibitors were incorporated into clinical trials to reduce disease burden associated with HPV infections and improve the living quality of the patients.

CONFLICT OF INTEREST

The author (editor) declares no conflict of interest, financial or otherwise.

ACKNOWLEDGEMENT

Declare none.

REFERENCES

[1] Christensen ND, Budgeon LR, Cladel NM, Hu J. Recent advances in preclinical model systems for papillomaviruses. Virus Res 2017; 231: 108-18. [http://dx.doi.org/10.1016/j.virusres.2016.12.004] [PMID: 27956145]

[2] Stern PL. Immune control of human papillomavirus (HPV) associated anogenital disease and potential for vaccination. J Clin Virol 2005; 32 (Suppl. 1): S72-81. [http://dx.doi.org/10.1016/j.jcv.2004.12.005] [PMID: 15753015]

[3] Bosch FX, Broker TR, Forman D, *et al.* Comprehensive control of human papillomavirus infections and related diseases. Vaccine 2013; 31 (Suppl. 5): F1-F31. [http://dx.doi.org/10.1016/j.vaccine.2013.10.001] [PMID: 24331745]

[4] Schiller JT, Castellsagué X, Garland SM. A review of clinical trials of human papillomavirus prophylactic vaccines. Vaccine 2012; 30(5) (Suppl. 5): F123-38. [http://dx.doi.org/10.1016/j.vaccine.2012.04.108] [PMID: 23199956]

[5] Einstein MH, Takacs P, Chatterjee A, *et al.* Comparison of long-term immunogenicity and safety of human papillomavirus (HPV)-16/18 AS04-adjuvanted vaccine and HPV-6/11/16/18 vaccine in healthy women aged 18-45 years: end-of-study analysis of a Phase III randomized trial. Hum Vaccin Immunother 2014; 10(12): 3435-45. [http://dx.doi.org/10.4161/hv.36121] [PMID: 25483701]

[6] Lowy DR. HPV vaccination to prevent cervical cancer and other HPV-associated disease: from basic science to effective interventions. J Clin Invest 2016; 126(1): 5-11. [http://dx.doi.org/10.1172/JCI85446] [PMID: 26727228]

[7] Brabin L, Kitchener HC, Stern PL. Implementation of prophylactic HPV vaccination: progress and future challenges. Expert Rev Obstet Gynecol 2010; 5: 591-603. [http://dx.doi.org/10.1586/eog.10.42]

[8] Poljak M. Prophylactic human papillomavirus vaccination and primary prevention of cervical cancer: issues and challenges. Clin Microbiol Infect 2012; 18(5) (Suppl. 5): 64-9. [http://dx.doi.org/10.1111/j.1469-0691.2012.03946.x] [PMID: 22862799]

[9] Wang JW, Roden RB. Virus-like particles for the prevention of human papillomavirus-associated malignancies. Expert Rev Vaccines 2013; 12(2): 129-41. [http://dx.doi.org/10.1586/erv.12.151] [PMID: 23414405]

[10] Karanam B, Jagu S, Huh WK, Roden RB. Developing vaccines against minor capsid antigen L2 to prevent papillomavirus infection. Immunol Cell Biol 2009; 87(4): 287-99. [http://dx.doi.org/10.1038/icb.2009.13] [PMID: 19421199]

[11] Tumban E, Peabody J, Tyler M, Peabody DS, Chackerian B. VLPs displaying a single L2 epitope induce broadly cross-neutralizing antibodies against human papillomavirus. PLoS One 2012; 7(11): e49751. [http://dx.doi.org/10.1371/journal.pone.0049751] [PMID: 23185426]

[12] Roden RB, Yutzy WH IV, Fallon R, Inglis S, Lowy DR, Schiller JT. Minor capsid protein of human genital papillomaviruses contains subdominant, cross-neutralizing epitopes. Virology 2000; 270(2): 254-7. [http://dx.doi.org/10.1006/viro.2000.0272] [PMID: 10792983]

[13] Christensen ND, Kreider JW, Kan NC, DiAngelo SL. The open reading frame L2 of cottontail rabbit papillomavirus contains antibody-inducing neutralizing epitopes. Virology 1991; 181(2): 572-9. [http://dx.doi.org/10.1016/0042-6822(91)90890-N] [PMID: 1707567]

[14] Tumban E, Peabody J, Peabody DS, Chackerian B. A pan-HPV vaccine based on bacteriophage PP7 VLPs displaying broadly cross-neutralizing epitopes from the HPV minor capsid protein, L2. PLoS One 2011; 6(8): e23310. [http://dx.doi.org/10.1371/journal.pone.0023310] [PMID: 21858066]

[15] Tyler M, Tumban E, Peabody DS, Chackerian B. The use of hybrid virus-like particles to enhance the immunogenicity of a broadly protective HPV vaccine. Biotechnol Bioeng 2014; 111(12): 2398-406. [http://dx.doi.org/10.1002/bit.25311] [PMID: 24917327]

[16] Jagu S, Karanam B, Gambhira R, *et al.* Concatenated multitype L2 fusion proteins as candidate prophylactic pan-human papillomavirus vaccines. J Natl Cancer Inst 2009; 101(11): 782-92. [http://dx.doi.org/10.1093/jnci/djp106] [PMID: 19470949]

[17] Tyler M, Tumban E, Dziduszko A, Ozbun MA, Peabody DS, Chackerian B. Immunization with a consensus epitope from human papillomavirus L2 induces antibodies that are broadly neutralizing. Vaccine 2014; 32(34): 4267-74. [http://dx.doi.org/10.1016/j.vaccine.2014.06.054] [PMID: 24962748]

[18] Yin F, Wang Y, Chen N, *et al.* A novel trivalent HPV 16/18/58 vaccine with anti-HPV 16 and 18 neutralizing antibody responses comparable to those induced by the Gardasil quadrivalent vaccine in rhesus macaque model. Papillomavirus Res 2017; 3: 85-90. [http://dx.doi.org/10.1016/j.pvr.2017.02.005] [PMID: 28720462]

[19] Embers ME, Budgeon LR, Pickel M, Christensen ND. Protective immunity to rabbit oral and cutaneous papillomaviruses by immunization with short peptides of L2, the minor capsid protein. J Virol 2002; 76(19): 9798-805. [http://dx.doi.org/10.1128/JVI.76.19.9798-9805.2002] [PMID: 12208958]

[20] Campo MS, O'Neil BW, Grindlay GJ, Curtis F, Knowles G, Chandrachud L. A peptide encoding a B-cell epitope from the N-terminus of the capsid protein L2 of bovine papillomavirus-4 prevents disease. Virology 1997; 234(2): 261-6. [http://dx.doi.org/10.1006/viro.1997.8649] [PMID: 9268157]

[21] Kawana K, Kawana Y, Yoshikawa H, Taketani Y, Yoshiike K, Kanda T. Nasal immunization of mice with peptide having a cross-neutralization epitope on minor capsid protein L2 of human papillomavirus type 16 elicit systemic and mucosal antibodies. Vaccine 2001; 19(11-12): 1496-502. [http://dx.doi.org/10.1016/S0264-410X(00)00367-4] [PMID: 11163673]

[22] Gambhira R, Karanam B, Jagu S, *et al.* A protective and broadly cross-neutralizing epitope of human papillomavirus L2. J Virol 2007; 81(24): 13927-31. [http://dx.doi.org/10.1128/JVI.00936-07] [PMID: 17928339]

[23] Alphs HH, Gambhira R, Karanam B, *et al.* Protection against heterologous human papillomavirus

challenge by a synthetic lipopeptide vaccine containing a broadly cross-neutralizing epitope of L2. Proc Natl Acad Sci USA 2008; 105(15): 5850-5.
[http://dx.doi.org/10.1073/pnas.0800868105] [PMID: 18413606]

[24] Jackson DC, Lau YF, Le T, *et al.* A totally synthetic vaccine of generic structure that targets Toll-like receptor 2 on dendritic cells and promotes antibody or cytotoxic T cell responses. Proc Natl Acad Sci USA 2004; 101(43): 15440-5.
[http://dx.doi.org/10.1073/pnas.0406740101] [PMID: 15489266]

[25] Jackson DC, Purcell AW, Fitzmaurice CJ, Zeng W, Hart DN. The central role played by peptides in the immune response and the design of peptide-based vaccines against infectious diseases and cancer. Curr Drug Targets 2002; 3(2): 175-96.
[http://dx.doi.org/10.2174/1389450024605436] [PMID: 11958299]

[26] Nardelli-Haefliger D, Lurati F, Wirthner D, *et al.* Immune responses induced by lower airway mucosal immunisation with a human papillomavirus type 16 virus-like particle vaccine. Vaccine 2005; 23(28): 3634-41.
[http://dx.doi.org/10.1016/j.vaccine.2005.02.019] [PMID: 15882523]

[27] Chandrachud LM, Grindlay GJ, McGarvie GM, *et al.* Vaccination of cattle with the N-terminus of L2 is necessary and sufficient for preventing infection by bovine papillomavirus-4. Virology 1995; 211(1): 204-8.
[http://dx.doi.org/10.1006/viro.1995.1392] [PMID: 7544045]

[28] Gaukroger JM, Chandrachud LM, O'Neil BW, Grindlay GJ, Knowles G, Campo MS. Vaccination of cattle with bovine papillomavirus type 4 L2 elicits the production of virus-neutralizing antibodies. J Gen Virol 1996; 77(Pt 7): 1577-83.
[http://dx.doi.org/10.1099/0022-1317-77-7-1577] [PMID: 8758002]

[29] Gambhira R, Jagu S, Karanam B, *et al.* Protection of rabbits against challenge with rabbit papillomaviruses by immunization with the N-terminus of HPV16 minor capsid antigen L2. J Virol 2007; 81: 13927-31.
[http://dx.doi.org/10.1128/JVI.00936-07] [PMID: 17928339]

[30] Pastrana DV, Gambhira R, Buck CB, *et al.* Cross-neutralization of cutaneous and mucosal Papillomavirus types with anti-sera to the amino terminus of L2. Virology 2005; 337(2): 365-72.
[http://dx.doi.org/10.1016/j.virol.2005.04.011] [PMID: 15885736]

[31] Jagu S, Karanam B, Gambhira R, *et al.* Concatenated multitype L2 fusion proteins as candidate prophylactic pan-human papillomavirus vaccines. J Natl Cancer Inst 2009; 101(11): 782-92.
[http://dx.doi.org/10.1093/jnci/djp106] [PMID: 19470949]

[32] de Villiers EM, Fauquet C, Broker TR, Bernard HU, zur Hausen H. Classification of papillomaviruses. Virology 2004; 324(1): 17-27.
[http://dx.doi.org/10.1016/j.virol.2004.03.033] [PMID: 15183049]

[33] Hangartner L, Zinkernagel RM, Hengartner H. Antiviral antibody responses: the two extremes of a wide spectrum. Nat Rev Immunol 2006; 6(3): 231-43.
[http://dx.doi.org/10.1038/nri1783] [PMID: 16498452]

[34] Bachmann MF, Kalinke U, Althage A, *et al.* The role of antibody concentration and avidity in antiviral protection. Science 1997; 276(5321): 2024-7.
[http://dx.doi.org/10.1126/science.276.5321.2024] [PMID: 9197261]

[35] Chackerian B, Lenz P, Lowy DR, Schiller JT. Determinants of autoantibody induction by conjugated papillomavirus virus-like particles. J Immunol 2002; 169(11): 6120-6.
[http://dx.doi.org/10.4049/jimmunol.169.11.6120] [PMID: 12444114]

[36] Lenz P, Day PM, Pang YY, *et al.* Papillomavirus-like particles induce acute activation of dendritic cells. J Immunol 2001; 166(9): 5346-55.
[http://dx.doi.org/10.4049/jimmunol.166.9.5346] [PMID: 11313370]

[37] Lenz P, Thompson CD, Day PM, Bacot SM, Lowy DR, Schiller JT. Interaction of papillomavirus virus-like particles with human myeloid antigen-presenting cells. Clin Immunol 2003; 106(3): 231-7. [http://dx.doi.org/10.1016/S1521-6616(02)00039-6] [PMID: 12706410]

[38] Varsani A, Williamson AL, de Villiers D, Becker I, Christensen ND, Rybicki EP. Chimeric human papillomavirus type 16 (HPV-16) L1 particles presenting the common neutralizing epitope for the L2 minor capsid protein of HPV-6 and HPV-16. J Virol 2003; 77(15): 8386-93. [http://dx.doi.org/10.1128/JVI.77.15.8386-8393.2003] [PMID: 12857908]

[39] Slupetzky K, Gambhira R, Culp TD, *et al.* A papillomavirus-like particle (VLP) vaccine displaying HPV16 L2 epitopes induces cross-neutralizing antibodies to HPV11. Vaccine 2007; 25(11): 2001-10. [http://dx.doi.org/10.1016/j.vaccine.2006.11.049] [PMID: 17239496]

[40] Palmer KE, Benko A, Doucette SA, *et al.* Protection of rabbits against cutaneous papillomavirus infection using recombinant tobacco mosaic virus containing L2 capsid epitopes. Vaccine 2006; 24(26): 5516-25. [http://dx.doi.org/10.1016/j.vaccine.2006.04.058] [PMID: 16725236]

[41] Karanam B, Jagu S, Huh WK, Roden RB. Developing vaccines against minor capsid antigen L2 to prevent papillomavirus infection. Immunol Cell Biol 2009; 87(4): 287-99. [http://dx.doi.org/10.1038/icb.2009.13] [PMID: 19421199]

[42] Boxus M, Fochesato M, Miseur A, *et al.* Broad cross-protection is induced in preclinical models by a human papillomavirus vaccine composed of L1/L2 chimeric virus-like particles. J Virol 2016; 90(14): 6314-25. [http://dx.doi.org/10.1128/JVI.00449-16] [PMID: 27147749]

[43] Peng S, Qiu J, Yang A, *et al.* Optimization of heterologous DNA-prime, protein boost regimens and site of vaccination to enhance therapeutic immunity against human papillomavirus-associated disease. Cell Biosci 2016; 6(16): 16. [http://dx.doi.org/10.1186/s13578-016-0080-z] [PMID: 26918115]

[44] Van Damme P, Bouillette-Marussig M, Hens A, *et al.* GTL001, a therapeutic vaccine for women infected with human papillomavirus 16 or 18 and normal cervical cytology: Results of a phase I clinical trial. Clin Cancer Res 2016; 22(13): 3238-48. [http://dx.doi.org/10.1158/1078-0432.CCR-16-0085] [PMID: 27252412]

[45] Ku GY, Yuan J, Page DB, *et al.* Single-institution experience with ipilimumab in advanced melanoma patients in the compassionate use setting: lymphocyte count after 2 doses correlates with survival. Cancer 2010; 116(7): 1767-75. [http://dx.doi.org/10.1002/cncr.24951] [PMID: 20143434]

[46] Lee SJ, Yang A, Wu TC, Hung CF. Immunotherapy for human papillomavirus-associated disease and cervical cancer: review of clinical and translational research. J Gynecol Oncol 2016; 27(5): e51. [http://dx.doi.org/10.3802/jgo.2016.27.e51] [PMID: 27329199]

[47] Sharma RK, Elpek KG, Yolcu ES, *et al.* Costimulation as a platform for the development of vaccines: a peptide-based vaccine containing a novel form of 4-1BB ligand eradicates established tumors. Cancer Res 2009; 69(10): 4319-26. [http://dx.doi.org/10.1158/0008-5472.CAN-08-3141] [PMID: 19435920]

[48] Vici P, Pizzuti L, Mariani L, *et al.* Targeting immune response with therapeutic vaccines in premalignant lesions and cervical cancer: hope or reality from clinical studies. Expert Rev Vaccines 2016; 15(10): 1327-36. [http://dx.doi.org/10.1080/14760584.2016.1176533] [PMID: 27063030]

[49] Yang A, Farmer E, Wu TC, Hung CF. Perspectives for therapeutic HPV vaccine development. J Biomed Sci 2016; 23(1): 75. [http://dx.doi.org/10.1186/s12929-016-0293-9] [PMID: 27809842]

[50] Kardani K, Mardani G, Bolhassani A. HPV prophylactic vaccines: Second-generation or first-

generation vaccines. J Solid Tumors 2015; 5(2): 112-9. [http://dx.doi.org/10.5430/jst.v5n2p112]

[51] Schiller JT, Nardelli-Haefliger D. Chapter 17: Second generation HPV vaccines to prevent cervical cancer. Vaccine 2006; 24S3: S3/147-53.

CHAPTER 16

Side Effects of HPV Vaccines

Afshin Khavari and **Azam Bolhassani***

Department of Hepatitis and AIDS, Pasteur Institute of Iran, Tehran, Iran

Abstract: The Human Papillomavirus (HPV) vaccines have been widely introduced in the national immunization programs of the medium and high income countries. Both bivalent and quadrivalent vaccines are generally known as safe and well-tolerated. Site injection symptoms are the most frequent adverse events reported. Among them, pain was generally the most frequently referred local symptom. It was shown that the occurrence of serious adverse events was similar in both vaccine and control groups. Regarding to the reports, no deaths from the introduction of the two vaccines have been attributed to HPV vaccination. Studies on the safety of the vaccine in some populations (men, women older than 25 years, HIV^+ girls) have given satisfactory results. However, there are some unresolved issues in the current HPV vaccines for different populations such as safety and duration of protection, cross-protection, tolerability, and side effects (*e.g.,* pain, swelling and redness, autoimmune and neurological conditions) similar to other vaccines. Briefly, we explain the possible adverse effects of common HPV vaccines in this chapter.

Keywords: HPV, Side effects, Vaccine.

INTRODUCTION

The recent human papillomavirus (HPV) vaccines are widely used to prevent HPV infections in women [1]. However, vaccine implementation in a funded immunization program for susceptible women requires consideration of both technical and social factors (*e.g.,* gender, safety, adolescent sexuality, delivery approach to the developing countries) [2]. Furthermore, it is critical to screen asymptomatic women and monitor precancerous abnormal cells. Screening methods include conventional cytology (*e.g.,* Pap smears, colposcopy), visual inspection with acetic acid (VIA), liquid-based cytology (LBC), visual inspection with lugol's iodine (VILI), and recently HPV DNA tests for triage of women with unclear cytology or for surveillance of women older than 30 years for the presence of high risk HPV DNA [3 - 5]. In high-income countries, organized

* **Corresponding author Azam Bolhassani:** Department of Hepatitis and AIDS, Pasteur Institute of Iran, Tehran, Iran; Tel: 66953311-20; E-mails: A_bolhasani@pasteur.ac.ir, azam.bolhassani@yahoo.com

Azam Bolhassani (Ed.)

programs for screening and post-screening treatment have reduced morbidity and mortality from cervical cancer; but there is the absence of effective screening programs in developing and poor countries due to some problems such as the lack of screening equipment (*e.g.*, colposcopes) and trained laboratory personnel, and inadequate knowledge about cervical cancer among healthcare workers [1]. The American congress of obstetricians and gynecologists (ACOG) recommends that screening program starts at age 21 and it is repeated once every 2 years until age 30 and then every 3 years until 65-70 [5, 6]. In general, passive surveillance systems need to be reinforced to identify any safety signal. As tested, both HPV vaccines available (Cervarix and Gardasil) are generally safe and well tolerated; Efforts should be made to increase the vaccination coverage of these vaccines as an important tool to decrease the disease burden of HPV. Regarding the reports, a second generation of HPV vaccines might be available soon. These vaccines would be cheaper and more stable, able to protect against different cancer-related strains and possess both therapeutic and prophylactic properties [5].

Unresolved Fundamental Issues

Several studies have demonstrated the safety of the bivalent (Cervarix) and quadrivalent (Gardasil) HPV vaccines. Moreover, both vaccines have shown long-term durability for protection against primary infections caused by targeted HPV viruses along with a moderate degree of cross-protection against some non-targeted HPV viruses such as HPV 31, 33, and 45 [15]. However, there are still several gaps in the current performance of HPV vaccines as described below.

Safety and Duration of Protection

The safety of the HPV vaccines has been studied in several countries such as the US and Scandinavia [7, 8]. The studies showed that the bivalent and the quadrivalent vaccines can highly protect women for at least 9 years and 8 years, respectively [9, 10]. If the protection (*i.e.,* antibody production) decreases, it can be overcome by a booster dose [11, 12].

Clinical Significance of Cross-Protection

Another important issue is the efficiency of HPV vaccines against all HPV serotypes not specifically targeted by VLPs available in the vaccine. Cross-protection against non-vaccine HPV types is an important problem, because the non-vaccine HPV types are associated with ~ 30% of cervical cancers in the world [13]. However, the cross-protection was observed for both commercial vaccines, although with a lower rate of cross-neutralizing antibody levels and an unknown duration of clinical efficiency [14 - 16]. There is also a potential theoretical risk that a vaccine will generate new viral variants that are more oncogenic but not recognized by vaccine-induced antibodies. However, as HPV uses host cell DNA polymerases and has an extremely slow mutation rate, this risk is also minimal [17 - 20].

Tolerability and Side Effects of HPV Vaccines

Many studies have evaluated safety and adverse effects of HPV vaccines (*i.e.,* Cervarix and Gardasil). The reports indicated that in the group receiving Cervarix, the most frequently reported events related to the vaccine were pain, swelling and redness. For the group receiving Gardasil, the events were pain and swelling. These effects can be due to a possible VLP-related inflammation process. Fatigue, fever, gastrointestinal symptoms, and headache were observed in some cases [21, 22]. Furthermore, HPV vaccines are not recommended for females 9 years old or individuals that are pregnant. On the other hand, Cervarix is not licensed for use in males [23].

CONCLUDING REMARKS

Regarding the commercial HPV vaccines that may not protect all vaccinated individuals, cancer screening programs should be developed irrespective to whether or not a person receives HPV vaccine. In December 2014, the FDA approved the so-called nonavalent vaccine including direct protection against HPV types 31, 33, 45, 52 and 58 as well as the HPV types 6, 11, 16 and 18 of the quadrivalent vaccine. Although, the potential of HPV vaccines to elicit side effects is relatively low, but However, it is necessary to determine and resolve the side effects of HPV vaccination in the world.

CONFLICT OF INTEREST

The author (editor) declares no conflict of interest, financial or otherwise.

ACKNOWLEDGEMENT

Declare none.

REFERENCES

[1] Graham JE, Mishra A. Global challenges of implementing human papillomavirus vaccines. International Journal for Equity in Health, The official journal of the International Society for Equity in Health 2011; 10: 27.
[http://dx.doi.org/10.1186/1475-9276-10-27]

[2] Erickson LJ, De Wals P, Farand L. An analytical framework for immunization programs in Canada. Vaccine 2005; 23(19): 2470-6.
[http://dx.doi.org/10.1016/j.vaccine.2004.10.029] [PMID: 15752833]

[3] Sankaranarayanan R, Gaffikin L, Jacob M, Sellors J, Robles S. A critical assessment of screening methods for cervical neoplasia. Int J Gynaecol Obstet 2005; 89(2) (Suppl. 2): S4-S12.

[http://dx.doi.org/10.1016/j.ijgo.2005.01.009] [PMID: 15823266]

[4] American Society for Colposcopy and Cervical Pathology. HPV Genotyping Clinical Update http://www.asccp.org/pdfs/consensus/clinical_update_20090408.pdf

[5] Stillo M, Carrillo Santisteve P, Lopalco PL. Safety of human papillomavirus vaccines: a review. Expert Opin Drug Saf 2015; 14(5): 697-712.
[http://dx.doi.org/10.1517/14740338.2015.1013532] [PMID: 25689872]

[6] Paavonen J, Jenkins D, Bosch FX, *et al.* Efficacy of a prophylactic adjuvanted bivalent L1 virus-lik--particle vaccine against infection with human papillomavirus types 16 and 18 in young women: an interim analysis of a phase III double-blind, randomised controlled trial. Lancet 2007; 369(9580): 2161-70.
[http://dx.doi.org/10.1016/S0140-6736(07)60946-5] [PMID: 17602732]

[7] Stokley S, Jeyarajah J, Yankey D, *et al.* Human papillomavirus vaccination coverage among adolescents, 2007-2013, and postlicensure vaccine safety monitoring, 2006-2014--United States. MMWR Morb Mortal Wkly Rep 2014; 63(29): 620-4.
[PMID: 25055185]

[8] Arnheim-Dahlström L, Pasternak B, Svanström H, Sparén P, Hviid A. Autoimmune, neurological, and venous thromboembolic adverse events after immunisation of adolescent girls with quadrivalent human papillomavirus vaccine in Denmark and Sweden: cohort study. BMJ 2013; 347: f5906.
[http://dx.doi.org/10.1136/bmj.f5906] [PMID: 24108159]

[9] Naud PS, Roteli-Martins CM, De Carvalho NS, *et al.* Sustained efficacy, immunogenicity, and safety of the HPV-16/18 AS04-adjuvanted vaccine: final analysis of a long-term follow-up study up to 9.4 years post-vaccination. Hum Vaccin Immunother 2014; 10(8): 2147-62.
[http://dx.doi.org/10.4161/hv.29532] [PMID: 25424918]

[10] Engels EA, Biggar RJ, Hall HI, *et al.* Cancer risk in people infected with human immunodeficiency virus in the United States. Int J Cancer 2008; 123(1): 187-94.
[http://dx.doi.org/10.1002/ijc.23487] [PMID: 18435450]

[11] Lowy DR. HPV vaccination to prevent cervical cancer and other HPV-associated disease: from basic science to effective interventions. J Clin Invest 2016; 126(1): 5-11.
[http://dx.doi.org/10.1172/JCI85446] [PMID: 26727228]

[12] Harper DM. Preliminary HPV vaccine results for women older than 25 years. Lancet 2009; 373(9679): 1921-2.
[http://dx.doi.org/10.1016/S0140-6736(09)61045-X] [PMID: 19501728]

[13] Lowy DR, Schiller JT. Reducing HPV-associated cancer globally. Cancer Prev Res (Phila) 2012; 5(1): 18-23.
[http://dx.doi.org/10.1158/1940-6207.CAPR-11-0542] [PMID: 22219162]

[14] Schiller JT, Lowy DR. Immunogenicity testing in human papillomavirus virus-like-particle vaccine trials. J Infect Dis 2009; 200(2): 166-71.
[http://dx.doi.org/10.1086/599988] [PMID: 19519255]

[15] Brown DR, Kjaer SK, Sigurdsson K, *et al.* The impact of quadrivalent human papillomavirus (HPV; types 6, 11, 16, and 18) L1 virus-like particle vaccine on infection and disease due to oncogenic nonvaccine HPV types in generally HPV-naive women aged 16-26 years. J Infect Dis 2009; 199(7): 926-35.
[http://dx.doi.org/10.1086/597307] [PMID: 19236279]

[16] Brotherton JM, Fridman M, May CL, Chappell G, Saville AM, Gertig DM. Early effect of the HPV vaccination programme on cervical abnormalities in Victoria, Australia: an ecological study. Lancet 2011; 377(9783): 2085-92.
[http://dx.doi.org/10.1016/S0140-6736(11)60551-5] [PMID: 21684381]

[17] Dillner J, Arbyn M, Unger E, Dillner L. Monitoring of human papillomavirus vaccination. Clin Exp

Immunol 2011; 163(1): 17-25.
[http://dx.doi.org/10.1111/j.1365-2249.2010.04268.x] [PMID: 21062269]

[18] Poljak M. Prophylactic human papillomavirus vaccination and primary prevention of cervical cancer: issues and challenges. Clin Microbiol Infect 2012; 18(5) (Suppl. 5): 64-9.
[http://dx.doi.org/10.1111/j.1469-0691.2012.03946.x] [PMID: 22862799]

[19] Basu P, Banerjee D, Singh P, Bhattacharya C, Biswas J. Efficacy and safety of human papillomavirus vaccine for primary prevention of cervical cancer: A review of evidence from phase III trials and national programs. South Asian J Cancer 2013; 2(4): 187-92.
[http://dx.doi.org/10.4103/2278-330X.119877] [PMID: 24455618]

[20] Bonanni P, Boccalini S, Bechini A. Efficacy, duration of immunity and cross protection after HPV vaccination: a review of the evidence. Vaccine 2009; 27 (Suppl. 1): A46-53.
[http://dx.doi.org/10.1016/j.vaccine.2008.10.085] [PMID: 19480962]

[21] Gonçalves AK, Cobucci RN, Rodrigues HM, de Melo AG, Giraldo PC. Safety, tolerability and side effects of human papillomavirus vaccines: a systematic quantitative review. Braz J Infect Dis 2014; 18(6): 651-9.
[http://dx.doi.org/10.1016/j.bjid.2014.02.005] [PMID: 24780368]

[22] Sangar VC, Ghongane BB, Mathur G, Chowdhary AS. Safety and adverse events of prophylactic HPV vaccines among healthy women: A systematic review & meta analysis. IJPSR 2015; 6(4): 1779-91.

[23] Nicol AF, Andrade CV, Russomano FB, Rodrigues LL, Oliveira NS, Provance DW Jr. HPV vaccines: a controversial issue? Braz J Med Biol Res 2016; 49(5): e5060.
[http://dx.doi.org/10.1590/1414-431X20155060] [PMID: 27074168]

CHAPTER 17

Future Prospects in HPV Prevention and Treatment

Azam Bolhassani*

Department of Hepatitis and AIDS, Pasteur Institute of Iran, Tehran, Iran

Abstract: All countries are encouraged to introduce routine HPV vaccination into their health programs. A range of screening and treatment protocols prevent cervical cancer in women already infected with HPV. The clinical trials indicated that HPV-based screening in women above the age of 30 is the most effective option. The main problems are that the licensed HPV vaccines are too expensive for universal use and they are not targeted against all HPV genotypes. Thus, the future generation of preventive vaccines must address two main issues such as lowering the cost of the vaccine for developing countries, and increasing the number of HPV types covered in order to maximize protection against HPV-associated malignancies. Moreover, several factors demonstrate the need for a therapeutic vaccine rather than preventive vaccine. The most critical of these factors is the high prevalence of existing HPV infection worldwide. In this chapter, future prospects of preventive and therapeutic vaccines will be discussed. Among these methods, combined therapy is of interest for improvement of these vaccines.

Keywords: Cancer, HPV infection, Prospects in prevention, Prospects in treatment, Vaccine.

INTRODUCTION

High-risk human papillomaviruses (HR-HPV) infect nearly the half million cervical cancer cases annually in the world. Moreover, high-risk HPVs especially HPV16 are proposed to develop some anal, oropharyngeal, vaginal, vulval, and penile cancers. Generally, all of the HR-HPVs are responsible for approximately 5% of all cancers worldwide (~ 10% in women). However, the most prevalent HR-HPV genotype varies with geographical location. The vaccines are effective approaches when inject prior to potential virus exposure (*i.e.*, before beginning of sexual activity). Recommendations for routine inoculation of the current vaccines are in females 13-26 years of age and in males 13-21 years of age [1 - 5].

* **Corresponding author Azam Bolhassani:** Department of Hepatitis and AIDS, Pasteur Institute of Iran, Tehran, Iran; Tel: 66953311-20; E-mails: A_bolhasani@pasteur.ac.ir, azam.bolhassani@yahoo.com

Azam Bolhassani (Ed.)

Countries are strongly encouraged to offer an organized vaccination and screening program against HPV infections. Several screening tests exist to identify HPV infections such as HPV testing and cytology [5]. Recently, the studies showed that an expression ratio ≥1.5 of miR-25/92a group over miR-22/29a group might be used to distinguish cervical cancers from normal cervix [6]. Although preventive HPV vaccines are available, these vaccines do not induce strong therapeutic effects against established HPV infections and lesions. Moreover, there are three key barriers to HPV preventive vaccines including sociocultural, health systems and political. Thus, it is critical for development of therapeutic strategies against the existing HPV infections [7 - 9]. The search for a cheaper, thermostable vaccine with wider coverage against all the oncogenic viruses has resulted in the development of the new generation of prophylactic vaccines [10, 11]. These include a nine-valent vaccine, an L2-based vaccine, a capsomere vaccine and a chimeric L1/L2 vaccine [11]. Gardasil 9 or nine-valent vaccine is a second generation HPV VLP vaccine that was licensed in 2015. Indeed, the researchers are seeking to overcome limitations of the VLP vaccines, *i.e.,* limited coverage of non-vaccine HPV types and lack of therapeutic efficiency [12]. A broad and long-term protection against all oncogenic types can eliminate the need for cytological screening programs in developed countries, and L2 vaccines may also prevent the morbidity and costs associated with other non-malignant HPV diseases that frequently occur in children [13].

Future Prospects of Preventive Vaccines

Future generation of preventive vaccines should solve two major problems such as lowering the cost of the vaccine, and increasing the number of HPV types covered in vaccine. An attractive approach to reduce the cost of commercial vaccines is the use of L1 capsomers. As known, the current L1 vaccines, Cervarix and Gardasil, are generated in insect cells and yeast, respectively, but however, production of the vaccine in *E. coli* may be a cheaper method. Use of the recombinant *E. coli* to produce these L1 capsomers has been successful for induction of protective antibodies in animal models. Moreover, L1 capsomer vaccines were stable at room temperature, without the need for refrigeration. On the other hand, to overcome the genotype restriction of L1 vaccines, the highly conserved and cross-reactive L2 vaccines can be used. L2-based vaccines can also be produced using *E. coli* to reduce costs and increase availability to the developing countries. However, L2 vaccines are less immunogenic than L1 vaccines that can be improved through the use of strong adjuvants including TLR-2 agonists. Another method of generating broader protection is through polyvalent L1 vaccines increasing cross-protections against various types of HPV [14 - 17]. A novel nonavalent vaccine under phase III clinical trial has about 15-30% higher anti-cancer effect by adding the new carcinogenic HPV types 31, 33, 45, 52, and

58 than Merck's existing quadrivalent vaccine (HPV type 6, 11, 16, and 18) [15, 18]. However, the value of the nonavalent vaccine as a next-generation HPV vaccine is doubtful, because there are no studies about analysis of cost effectiveness and comparative efficiency of the novel vaccine as compared to the conventional vaccines [15]. Other attempts to reduce the manufacturing costs include the generation of L1 VLPs in other vectors such as the yeast *Pichia pastoris* [19] or in plants [20]. Alternatively, improvements in the methods of storing the vaccine, or easier administration methods such as nasal spray or patch, may result in easier and cheaper accessibility of the vaccines. Among 40 countries, the United States, the UK, Canada, and Australia were the first countries to implement HPV vaccination in their national immunization programs (NIPs) [21]. HPV vaccinations are recommended for females and also for males in several countries [21, 22]. It is unlikely that Merck and GSK will be interested in the development of different second generation vaccines. Indeed, it may be difficult to attract sufficient funding when an effective HPV vaccine is commercially available [23].

Future Prospects of Therapeutic Vaccines

Current HPV vaccines are purely prophylactic and effective only in HPV naive individuals. These vaccines lack therapeutic effect because of two main reasons: a) they are based on L1 viral capsid proteins that are undetectable in HPV associated malignancies; b) they induce only humoral immunity and not cell-mediated immunity that is necessary for a therapeutic effect. A successful therapeutic vaccine requires targeting antigens expressed actively throughout lifecycle of HPV [11, 24]. The cancer immunotherapy studies showed that the presence of tumor-specific cytotoxic cells is not sufficient for therapeutic effects in a tumor-bearing host. It is equally important to overcome the immune-suppressive mechanisms acting in the tumor microenvironment [25 - 30]. Novel polymerization technologies including macroporous polymer matrices as carriers for cancer vaccines are capable of directing the trafficking and activation of DCs *in vivo* [30 - 33]. In addition, the route of vaccine injection significantly influences the magnitude of the immune response. For instance, a preclinical study showed that the growth of HPV-related head and neck tumors was inhibited when a cancer vaccine (STxB-$E7_{43-57}$, consisting of the $E7_{43-57}$ peptide coupled to the nontoxic B subunit of Shiga toxin) was delivered by the intranasal route but not the intramuscular route. The intranasally administered vaccine elicited antigen-specific CTLs. However, a recent clinical trial showed that intramuscular therapeutic HPV16 DNA vaccination (TA-HPV) induced T cell responses. The opposite findings of these two studies may be due to different nature of the vaccines used (peptide *vs.* DNA) [30, 34, 35]. Moreover, immunization in novel humanized mouse models (*e.g.,* HLA-A2.1-/HLA-DR1-transgenic H-2 class I-

/class II-knockout mouse) may represent better predictions for the outcome in humans. The data obtained from advanced mouse models should be exactly described, since beside the humanized parts, these mice still have a murine immune system that largely differs from the human one [30, 36]. On the other hand, immunomonitoring studies show relevant mechanisms of immune induction and tolerance, and assist in defining patient subpopulations with a higher potential of response to vaccination [30, 37, 38].

CONCLUDING REMARKS

Great progress has been done to improve new therapeutic HPV vaccines and treat existing HPV infections; but however, it is required to do further work. Many promising therapeutic approaches have been developed that some of them achieved to clinical trial stages. Although, prophylactic HPV vaccines would definitely reduce the incidence of HPV infections, several factors highlight the need for a therapeutic, rather than preventive vaccine. These factors include the high prevalence of existing HPV infection worldwide, genomic integration in HPV-associated malignancies lacking L1 or L2 expression as well as disadvantages of current prophylactic vaccines such as limited species coverage, absence of therapeutic role, cost and affordability, immunogenicity, duration of protection and requirement of booster doses, age of vaccination, vaccine resistance, vaccination of males, and vaccine safety. Thus, therapeutic vaccines are required to stimulate a strong cell-mediated immune response against HPV in order to control infection and kill tumor. Thus, the next generation vaccines need to have a therapeutic effect so that they can be used in HPV-infected individuals for preventing future infections and also in the treatment of HPV-associated cancers.

CONFLICT OF INTEREST

The author (editor) declares no conflict of interest, financial or otherwise.

ACKNOWLEDGEMENT

Declare none.

REFERENCES

[1] Bruni L, Barrionuevo R. 2015.http://www.hpvcentre.net/ statistics/reports/XWX.pdf

[2] Bosch FX, Lorincz A, Muñoz N, Meijer CJ, Shah KV. The causal relation between human papillomavirus and cervical cancer. J Clin Pathol 2002; 55(4): 244-65. [http://dx.doi.org/10.1136/jcp.55.4.244] [PMID: 11919208]

[3] Schiller JT, Lowy DR. Vaccines to prevent infections by oncoviruses. Annu Rev Microbiol 2010; 64: 23-41. [http://dx.doi.org/10.1146/annurev.micro.112408.134019] [PMID: 20420520]

[4] Pogoda CS, Roden RB, Garcea RL. Immunizing against anogenital cancer: HPV vaccines. PLoS Pathog 2016; 12(5): e1005587.
[http://dx.doi.org/10.1371/journal.ppat.1005587] [PMID: 27196109]

[5] Bosch FX, Broker TR, Forman D, *et al.* Comprehensive control of human papillomavirus infections and related diseases. Vaccine 2013; 31 (Suppl. 5): F1-F31.
[http://dx.doi.org/10.1016/j.vaccine.2013.10.001] [PMID: 24331745]

[6] Jin L, Xu ZX. Recent advances in the study of HPV-associated carcinogenesis. Virol Sin 2015; 30(2): 101-6.
[http://dx.doi.org/10.1007/s12250-015-3586-3] [PMID: 25910482]

[7] Yang A, Farmer E, Wu TC, Hung CF. Perspectives for therapeutic HPV vaccine development. J Biomed Sci 2016; 23(1): 75.
[http://dx.doi.org/10.1186/s12929-016-0293-9] [PMID: 27809842]

[8] Wigle J, Coast E, Watson-Jones D. Human papillomavirus (HPV) vaccine implementation in low and middle-income countries (LMICs): health system experiences and prospects. Vaccine 2013; 31(37): 3811-7.
[http://dx.doi.org/10.1016/j.vaccine.2013.06.016] [PMID: 23777956]

[9] Tsu V, Murray M, Franceschi S. Human papillomavirus vaccination in low-resource countries: lack of evidence to support vaccinating sexually active women. Br J Cancer 2012; 107(9): 1445-50.
[http://dx.doi.org/10.1038/bjc.2012.404] [PMID: 22955856]

[10] Hestbech MS, Lynge E, Kragstrup J, Siersma V, Vazquez-Prada Baillet M, Brodersen J. The impact of HPV vaccination on future cervical screening: a simulation study of two birth cohorts in Denmark. BMJ Open 2015; 5(8): e007921.
[http://dx.doi.org/10.1136/bmjopen-2015-007921] [PMID: 26275901]

[11] Kumar S, Biswas M, Jose T. HPV vaccine: Current status and future directions. Med J Armed Forces India 2015; 71(2): 171-7.
[http://dx.doi.org/10.1016/j.mjafi.2015.02.006] [PMID: 25859081]

[12] Pouyanfard S, Müller M. Human papillomavirus first and second generation vaccines-current status and future directions. Biol Chem 2017; 398(8): 871-89.
[http://dx.doi.org/10.1515/hsz-2017-0105] [PMID: 28328521]

[13] Karanam B, Jagu S, Huh WK, Roden RB. Developing vaccines against minor capsid antigen L2 to prevent papillomavirus infection. Immunol Cell Biol 2009; 87(4): 287-99.
[http://dx.doi.org/10.1038/icb.2009.13] [PMID: 19421199]

[14] Lin K, Doolan K, Hung CF, Wu TC. Perspectives for preventive and therapeutic HPV vaccines. J Formos Med Assoc 2010; 109(1): 4-24.
[http://dx.doi.org/10.1016/S0929-6646(10)60017-4] [PMID: 20123582]

[15] Kim KS, Park SA, Ko KN, Yi S, Cho YJ. Current status of human papillomavirus vaccines. Clin Exp Vaccine Res 2014; 3(2): 168-75.
[http://dx.doi.org/10.7774/cevr.2014.3.2.168] [PMID: 25003090]

[16] Rubin M. HPV update: what nurse practitioners need to know practical strategies for helping patients and parents understand the importance of HPV vaccination. Washington, DC: National Association of Nurse Practitionors in Woman Health 2011.

[17] Murray M. 2010.http://www.path. org/publications/files/RH-outlook-27-2.pdf

[18] Peres J. For cancers caused by HPV, two vaccines were just the beginning. J Natl Cancer Inst 2011; 103(5): 360-2.
[http://dx.doi.org/10.1093/jnci/djr053] [PMID: 21357595]

[19] Bazan SB, de Alencar Muniz Chaves A, Aires KA, Cianciarullo AM, Garcea RL, Ho PL. Expression and characterization of HPV-16 L1 capsid protein in Pichia pastoris. Arch Virol 2009; 154(10): 1609-

17.
[http://dx.doi.org/10.1007/s00705-009-0484-8] [PMID: 19756360]

[20] Rybicki EP, Williamson AL, Meyers A, Hitzeroth II. Vaccine farming in Cape Town. Hum Vaccin 2011; 7(3): 339-48.
[http://dx.doi.org/10.4161/hv.7.3.14263] [PMID: 21358269]

[21] Markowitz LE, Tsu V, Deeks SL, *et al.* Human papillomavirus vaccine introduction--the first five years. Vaccine 2012; 30(5) (Suppl. 5): F139-48.
[http://dx.doi.org/10.1016/j.vaccine.2012.05.039] [PMID: 23199957]

[22] Recommendations on the use of quadrivalent human papillomavirus vaccine in males--Advisory Committee on Immunization Practices (ACIP), 2011. MMWR Morb Mortal Wkly Rep 2011; 60(50): 1705-8.
[PMID: 22189893]

[23] Schiller JT, Nardelli-Haefliger D. 2006.

[24] Lin K, Doolan K, Hung CF, Wu TC. Perspectives for preventive and therapeutic HPV vaccines. J Formos Med Assoc 2010; 109(1): 4-24.
[http://dx.doi.org/10.1016/S0929-6646(10)60017-4] [PMID: 20123582]

[25] Galluzzi L, Senovilla L, Zitvogel L, Kroemer G. The secret ally: immunostimulation by anticancer drugs. Nat Rev Drug Discov 2012; 11(3): 215-33.
[http://dx.doi.org/10.1038/nrd3626] [PMID: 22301798]

[26] Emens LA, Asquith JM, Leatherman JM, *et al.* Timed sequential treatment with cyclophosphamide, doxorubicin, and an allogeneic granulocyte-macrophage colony-stimulating factor-secreting breast tumor vaccine: a chemotherapy dose-ranging factorial study of safety and immune activation. J Clin Oncol 2009; 27(35): 5911-8.
[http://dx.doi.org/10.1200/JCO.2009.23.3494] [PMID: 19805669]

[27] Hodi FS, O'Day SJ, McDermott DF, *et al.* Improved survival with ipilimumab in patients with metastatic melanoma. N Engl J Med 2010; 363(8): 711-23.
[http://dx.doi.org/10.1056/NEJMoa1003466] [PMID: 20525992]

[28] Callahan MK, Wolchok JD. At the bedside: CTLA-4- and PD-1-blocking antibodies in cancer immunotherapy. J Leukoc Biol 2013; 94(1): 41-53.
[http://dx.doi.org/10.1189/jlb.1212631] [PMID: 23667165]

[29] Perez-Gracia JL, Labiano S, Rodriguez-Ruiz ME, Sanmamed MF, Melero I. Orchestrating immune check-point blockade for cancer immunotherapy in combinations. Curr Opin Immunol 2014; 27: 89-97.
[http://dx.doi.org/10.1016/j.coi.2014.01.002] [PMID: 24485523]

[30] Khallouf H, Grabowska AK, Riemer AB. Therapeutic vaccine strategies against human papillomavirus. Vaccines (Basel) 2014; 2(2): 422-62.
[http://dx.doi.org/10.3390/vaccines2020422] [PMID: 26344626]

[31] Ali OA, Emerich D, Dranoff G, Mooney DJ. *In situ* regulation of DC subsets and T cells mediates tumor regression in mice. Sci Transl Med 2009; 1(8): 8ra19.
[http://dx.doi.org/10.1126/scitranslmed.3000359] [PMID: 20368186]

[32] Ali OA, Huebsch N, Cao L, Dranoff G, Mooney DJ. Infection-mimicking materials to program dendritic cells *in situ.* Nat Mater 2009; 8(2): 151-8.
[http://dx.doi.org/10.1038/nmat2357] [PMID: 19136947]

[33] Ali OA, Verbeke C, Johnson C, *et al.* Identification of immune factors regulating antitumor immunity using polymeric vaccines with multiple adjuvants. Cancer Res 2014; 74(6): 1670-81.
[http://dx.doi.org/10.1158/0008-5472.CAN-13-0777] [PMID: 24480625]

[34] Sandoval F, Terme M, Nizard M, *et al.* Mucosal imprinting of vaccine-induced $CD8^+$ T cells is crucial to inhibit the growth of mucosal tumors. Sci Transl Med 2013; 5(172): 172ra20.

[http://dx.doi.org/10.1126/scitranslmed.3004888] [PMID: 23408053]

[35] Maldonado L, Teague JE, Morrow MP, *et al.* Intramuscular therapeutic vaccination targeting HPV16 induces T cell responses that localize in mucosal lesions. Sci Transl Med 2014; 6(221): 221ra13. [http://dx.doi.org/10.1126/scitranslmed.3007323] [PMID: 24477000]

[36] Pajot A, Michel ML, Fazilleau N, *et al.* A mouse model of human adaptive immune functions: HLA-A2.1-/HLA-DR1-transgenic H-2 class I-/class II-knockout mice. Eur J Immunol 2004; 34(11): 3060-9. [http://dx.doi.org/10.1002/eji.200425463] [PMID: 15468058]

[37] Rappuoli R, Mandl CW, Black S, De Gregorio E. Vaccines for the twenty-first century society. Nat Rev Immunol 2011; 11(12): 865-72. [PMID: 22051890]

[38] Ogi C, Aruga A. Immunological monitoring of anticancer vaccines in clinical trials. OncoImmunology 2013; 2(8): e26012. [http://dx.doi.org/10.4161/onci.26012] [PMID: 24083085]

SUBJECT INDEX

D

E

F

G

H

I

K

Q

R

S

T

U

V

Made in United States
Orlando, FL
04 November 2026

90199928R00150